MW00677543

The Biographical Series of the Sanskrit Classics

The Journey of a Himalayan Hermit
PART 2

"The greatest adventure of man is to find the Source of the mind in the state of Tranquil Breath." - Swami Satyeswarananda

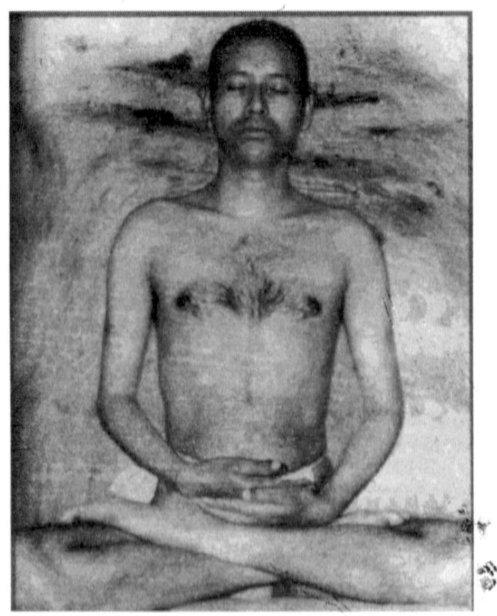

Himalayan Hermit in the Himalayan Cave
(Swami Satyeswarananda Vidyaratna Babaji Maharaj)

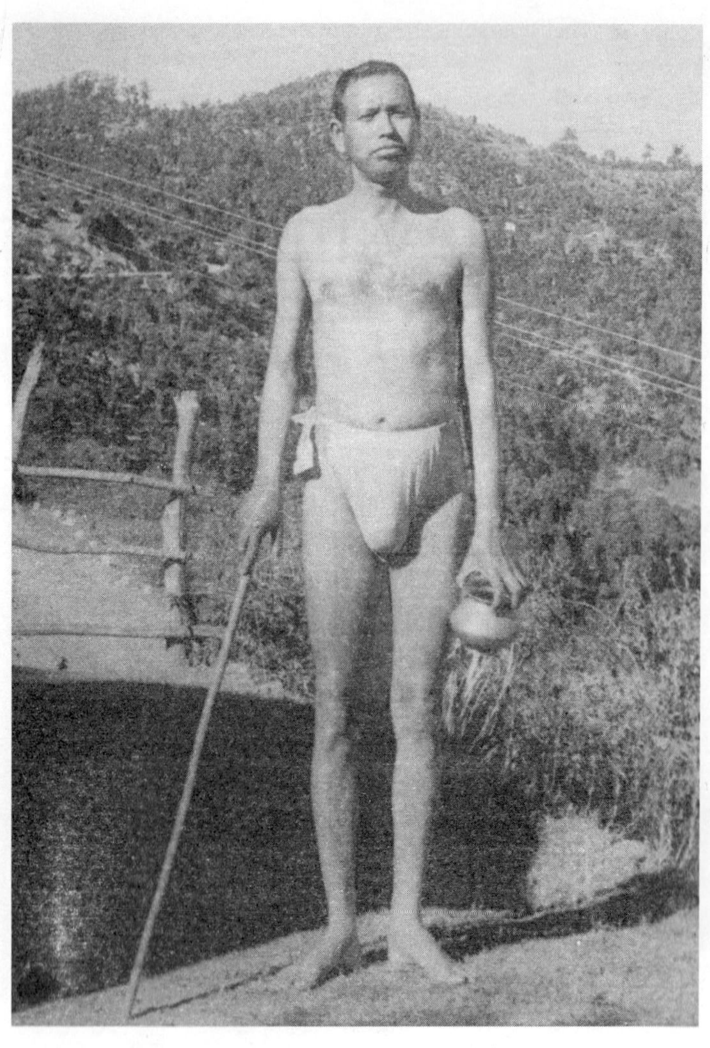

Himalayan Hermit, at Dunagiri Hill, Himalayas
Swami Satyeswarananda Vidyaratna Babaji Maharaj,
The Himalayan Yogi Vedantist.

The Biographical Series of the Sanskrit Classics

The Journey of a Himalayan Hermit

PART 2

By Swami Satyeswaranada Giri Maharaj,

(VIDYARATNA BABAJI)

The Sanskrit Classics, Publisher
P.O. Box 5368
San Diego, CA 92165, U.S.A.

www.sanskritclassics.com

Publisher: Swami Satyeswarananda Vidyaratna Babaji Maharaj, M. A. (C.U.), LL. B. (C.U.), Former Attorney (Advocate) and Law Professor, Sanskrit Scholar, Vidyaratna, Himalayan Yogi Vedantist.

First Edition 2014

ISBN 10: 1-877854-53-0
ISBN 13: 978-1-877854-53-8

Available from:

1. The Sanskrit Classics, Publisher
   P.O. Box 5368
   San Diego, CA 92165, U.S.A.
   Phone (619) 284-7779

2. Mahesh Library
   2/1 Shyamacharan De St
   Calcutta/Kolkata – 700073
   Ph: 33-2241-7479

3. Sanskrit Pustak Bhanda
   38 Bidhan Sarani.
   Calcutta/Kolkata – 700006
   Ph: 33-2241-1208

4. Sarbodaya
   Howrah Railway Station
   Howrah
   Ph: 33-2511-7767

For Availability – Contact:
B. Chakraborty, Resi: 33-2407-7477

Printed at:
Bhattacharya and Brothers
4 Harisova Lane.
Kolkata – 700060
INDIA

Printed in India

Dedication

Dedicated to:

The Ancient Sages

Swami Satyeswarananda Giri Babaji Maharaj,
(Vidyaratna Babaji, the Author).

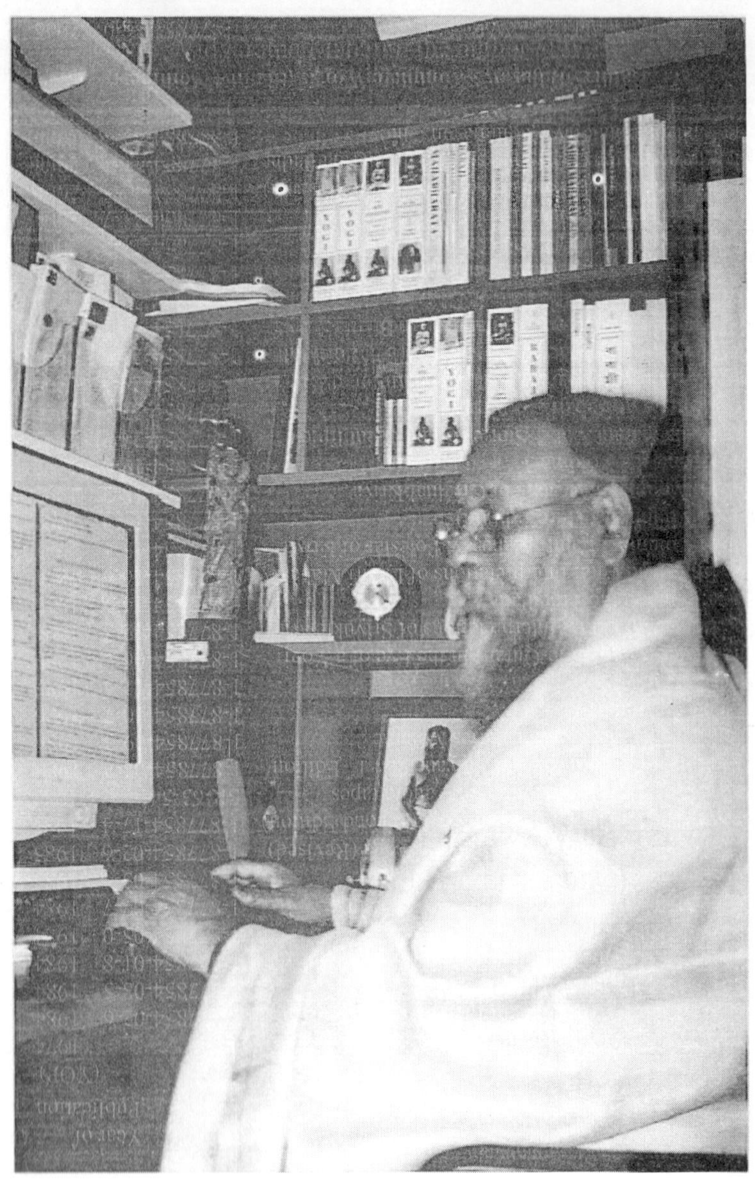

S. S. Vidyaratna Maharaj, the author at work

Published Works by Swami Satyeswarananda Maharaj

	Title	ISBN No.	Year of Publication (YOP)	Out of Print (OP)
	English			
1.	Kriya Yoga: The Science of Self Realization		1974	OP
2.	Lahiri Mahasay: The Father of Kriya Yoga	1-877854-02-6	1984	OP
3.	The Commentaries Volume 1	1-877854-08-5	1984	OP
4.	Babaji: The Divine Himalayan Yogi (First Edition)	1-877854-01-8	1984	OP
5.	The Only Bible	1-877854-05-0	1984	OP
6.	Lahiri Mahasay's Personal Letters	1-877854-07-7	1984	OP
7.	Kebalananda and Sriyukteswar	1-877854-03-4	1985	OP
8.	Lahiri Mahasay: The Father of Kriya Yoga (Revised)	1-877854-02-6	1985	OP
9.	Babaji: The Divine Himalayan Yogi (Second Edition)	1-877854-17-4	1985	OP
10.	Babaji Vol. 1, Second Edition in 4 audio tapes	SR-63-541	1985	OP
11.	Biography of a Yogi (Swami Satyananda) 1st Edition	1-877854-04-2	1985	
12.	The Mahabharata: Commentaries Volume 2	1-877854-09-3	1986	
13.	Hidden Wisdom	1-877854-10-7	1986	
14.	Inner Victory	1-877854-11-5	1987	
15.	The Bibles (Gita-Bible-Quran) In the Eye of a Yogi	1-877854-06-9	1988	
16.	The Bhagavad Gita – Interpretations of Sriyukteswar	1-877854-12-3	1991	
17.	Kriya: Finding the True Path	1-877854-14-X	1991	
18.	The Bhagavad Gita: Interpretations of Lahiri Mahasay	1-877854-16-6	1991	
19.	Babaji Volume 2 Lahiri Mahasay, Polestar of Kriya	1-877854-13-1	1991	OP
20.	Babaji Volume 1 (Third Edition)	1-877854-17-4	1992	OP
21.	Babaji: Volume 3 Masters of Original Kriya	1-877854-18-2	1992	
22.	The Upanisads Volume 3	1-877854-19-0	1992	
23.	The Mahabharata Vol. 1 Stories of the Great Epic	1-877854-24-7	1993	
24.	Kriya Sutras of Babaji	1-877854-27-1	1994	
25.	Sriyukteswar: A Biography	1-877854-28-X	1994	
26.	The Holy Bible- In the Light of Kriya (3RD Edition)	1-877854-23-9	1994	
27.	The Divine Incarnation: Sri Panchanan Bhattacharya	1-877854-30-1	1996	
28.	The Dhammapada: The Path of Dharma	1-877854-20-4	1996	
29.	Babaji and His Legacy (Revised Fourth Edition)	1-877854-31-X	2002	
30.	Biography of a Yogi (Revised Second Edition)	1-877854-26-3	2002	
31.	Essence of Kriya (Pocket Book)	1-877854-38-7	2004	
32.	The Original Kriya (Revised Second edition of Kriya)	1-877854-42-5	2005	
33.	The Eternal Silence ...Synthesis of All Dharma Paths	1-877854-41-7	2006	
34.	The Mahabharata (Two Volumes in One)	1-877854-43-3	2006	
	Lahiri Mahasay's Complete Works (Set in 4 Volumes)			
35.	The Gitas and Sanghitas – Volume 1	1-877854-36-0	2006	
36.	Chandi and the Other Scriptures – Volume 2	1-877854-39-7	2006	
37.	The Upanisads (Revised Second Edition) Volume 3	1-877854-44-1	2006	
38.	The Six Systems (Revised Second Edition) Volume 4	1-877854-45-X	2006	

Title	ISBN No.	Year of Publication (YOP)	Out of Print (OP)
39. Mahamuni Babaji & His Legacy (Revised 5th Edition)	1-877854-34-4	2008	
40. Yogacharya Sri Sri Panchanan Bhattacharya	1-877854-48-4	2010	
41. The Ultimate Book – Yoga Vasistha – Synthesis of Yoga Vedanta (Set in 2 Volumes)	978-1-877854-50-7	2011	
42. The Journey of a Himalayan Hermit	978-1-877854-49-1	2012	
43. Suddenly Silence ... Atmastha	978-1-877854-51-4	2014	
44. Siva Sanghita,Six Centers, Brahma Sanghita	978-1-877854-52-1	2014	

Bengali

45. The Bhagavad Gita of Lahiri Mahasay's Original Bengali Interpretations		1981	
46. Vedic Chantings & Kriya Masters songs, audio Tape	SR-64-698	1985	OP
47. Devotional Songs in Sanskrit, audio tape	SR-64-699	1985	OP
48. Satha Chakra (Six Centers Drawing)	VA-333-582	1989	
49. Kriya Ganga	1-877854-21-2	1998	
50. The Bhagavad Gita of Lahiri Mahasay's Original Bengali Interpretations	1-877854-25-5	2003	
51. Babaji O Tnar Parampara	1-877854-33-6	2004	
52. Kriyasar (Pocket Book)	1-877854-39-5	2004	
53. Kriya Ganga (Hard Cover)	1-877854-40-9	2008	

Hindi

54. Dunagiri Hill Himalayas (Pamphlet)		1981
55. Babaji - Himalaya Ke Dibya Yogi	978-1-877854-46-0	2013
56. Bhagavad Gita – Interpretation of Lahiri Mahasay	978-1-877854-35-4	2013

German

57. Die Kriya Sutras des Babaji 1-877854-29-8 1994

Spanish

58. Kriya Sutras de Babaji 1-877854-22-0 1994

Chinese

59. The Kriya Sutras 1-877854-47-6 2010

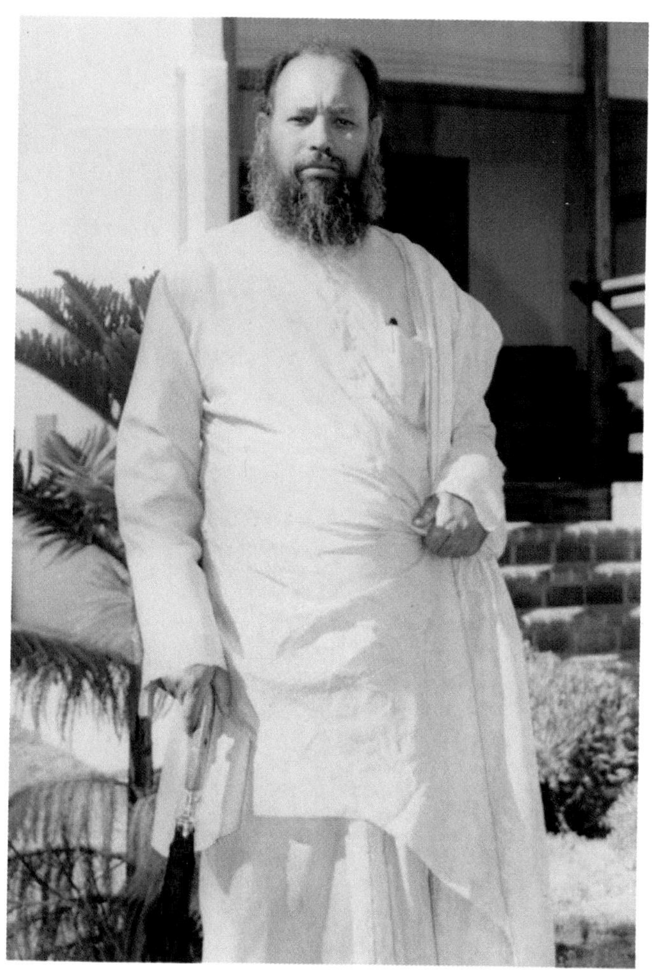

Swami Satyeswarananda Maharaj, the Author.

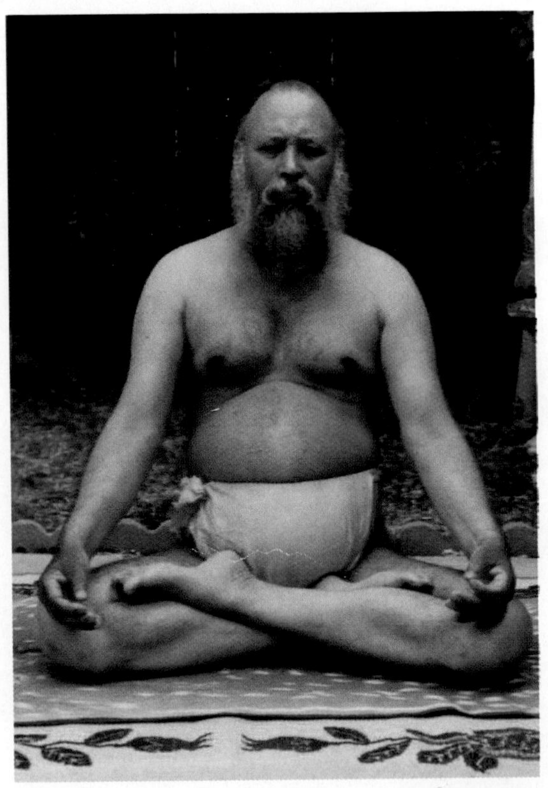

Swami Satyeswarananda Maharaj
The Himalayan Yogi Vedantist,
Former Attorney and Professor of law,
Sanskrit Scholar, Vidyaratna, and Author

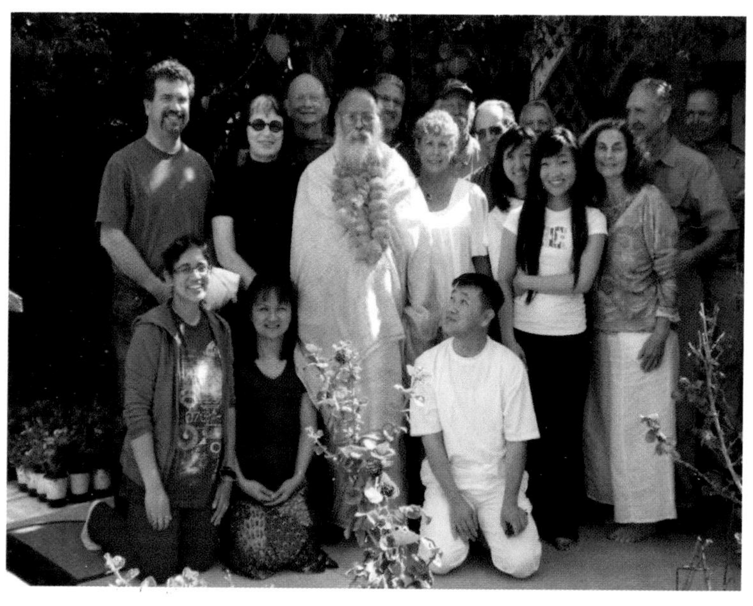

Swami Satyeswarananda Maharaj with a Group of *Kriyanwits* and *Kriyanwitas* on the *Guru* Full Moon Day, July 22, 2013

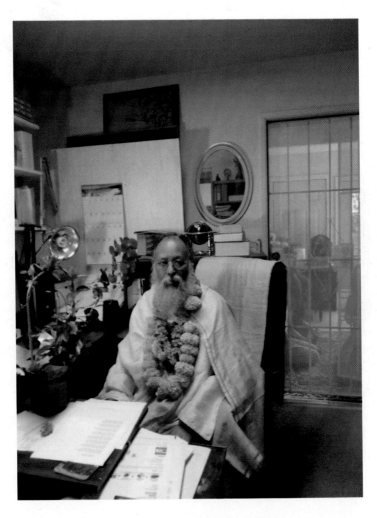

Swami Satyeswarananda Maharaj
in his home office, on the Guru Full Moon Day
July 22, 2013

Contents

The Illustrations

Cover: Swami Satyeswarananda Maharaj in Dunagiri Hill, Himalayas

SRI ANJAN KR. DAN
ESTATES & TRUST OFFICER
UNIVERSITY OF CALCUTTA

SENATE HOUSE
87/1, COLLEGE STREET
KOLKATA-700073
Phone : 2241-0071/4984
Fax : 91-033-2241-3222
Telex : 021-2752 UNIV IN.
E-Mail : eto@caluniv.ac.in

No. ET/T/53

Date 7/5/08

To
Swami Satyeswaranada Vidyaratna Maharaj,
P. O. Box No. 5368,
San Diego, CA 92165,
U. S. A.

Subject: Your donation of Rs. 5.0 lakhs for creation of two Endowment a/cs

Sir,

With reference to the above, I am sending the photocopies of the first page of the two CU A/C passbooks in the name and style "Yogiraj Sri Sri Shyamacharan Lahiri Mahasay Memorial Scholarship" and "Yogiraj Sri Sri Shyamacharan Lahiri Mahasay Memorial Lectureship" created on your kind donation.

The university will take necessary steps to hold the lecture as well as to award the scholarship on receipt of the 1st year's yield under intimation to you.

An acknowledgement in receipt is highly solicited.

With best regards,

Yours faithfully,

07.05.008
(Anjan K Dan)
Estate & Trust Officer

07.5.8
07.5.08

Introduction

Swami Satyeswarananda and The Sanskrit Classics, the Self Publishing

Swami Satyananda Giri Maharaj was the initiated disciple of Hangsa Swami Kebalananda (*Sastri* Mahasay) and chief monastic disciple of Swami Sriyukteswar who appointed him "Ashram Swami" of his Puri Asram. He also appointed him as the leader of the East and Satyananda's boyhood best friend, Swami Yogananda, was chosen by Sriyukteswar as his messenger for the West.

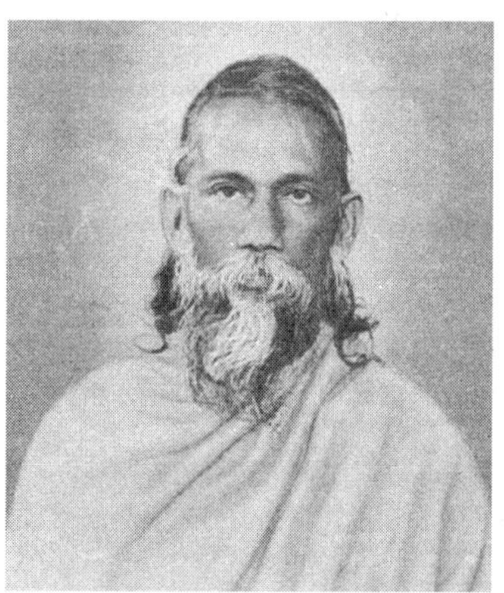

(1896-1971)
Swami Satyananda Maharaj,
Initiated by Hangsa Swami Kebalananda and
chief monastic disciple of Swami Sriyukteswar in India,
the leader of the East.

The leader of the East, Swami Satyananda, was an egoless realized Yogi. He was a harmonious person and was a peacemaker. He had good connections with all the *Kriya* groups in India as their leader.

Swami Satyeswarananda Maharaj (in short, Swamiji or Baba, also known as Vidyaratna Babaji) was very closely associated with Swami Satyananda for twenty years (1950 -1971); as a result, he knew the ins and outs of everything that was going on in all the *Kriya* groups in India.

For this reason, Swami Satyeswarananda's position was unique. He has been associated with the Original *Kriya Yoga* a long sixty five (65) years since the age of eleven. In this book, the subsequent chapters will unfold how he was harmoniously related with all.

Swami Satyeswarananda knew all the *Kriya* groups and had a good relation with them. Furthermore, Swamiji knew their systems of the *Kriya* practice including Yogananda's teaching of the Modified *Kriya,* as he was eight years, a resident student in the Vidyapith (high school).

After Satyananda's leaving the body in *Mahasamadhi* (entering into oneness attunement with the supreme Self, the final exit), Swami Satyeswarananda disassociated himself with all institutions: educational (Professor of law), professional (attorney), and the spiritual (Satyananda's hermitage Sevayatan which runs schools (boys and girls), postgraduate teacher's training college, technical school, and hospital).

Swami Satyeswarananda began to tour India on pilgrimage.

During this period there were some organizations and hermitage authorities that tried to recruit Swamiji to work for them. For example :

1) Yogoda Sat Sanga Society (YSS). They even arranged a meeting with their international visiting President, Sister Daya, at Calcutta.

2) Satya Charan Lahiri at Satyaloka wanted Swamiji to stay there at his house and conduct the evening prayer. (The story is discussed later).

3) Swami Hariharananda (not to be confused with Hariharananda of Puri) wanted to take Swamiji to Jaipur and for some reason wanted Swamiji with him. (Later, Swamiji found the reason was because Swami Satyananda had told him that Swamiji would deliver him a message in time which Swamiji himself did not even know what it was till he received it from Mahamuni Babaji, which Hariharananda

thought all along it would be from Swami Satyananda, since he had mentioned it.

4) Utarkashi Sanskrit Mahavidyalay in the Himalayas to teach Vedanta.

5) A Vaisnab Baba (Bengali Sadhu) wanted to give Baba his Asram at Nandigram, Vrajabhumi.

In brief his pilgrimage is as follows :

Leaving the Sevayatan hermitage of Satyananda, first Swamiji arrived at Calcutta. He stayed in the family of a devotee and a friend, Birendralal Choudhuri.

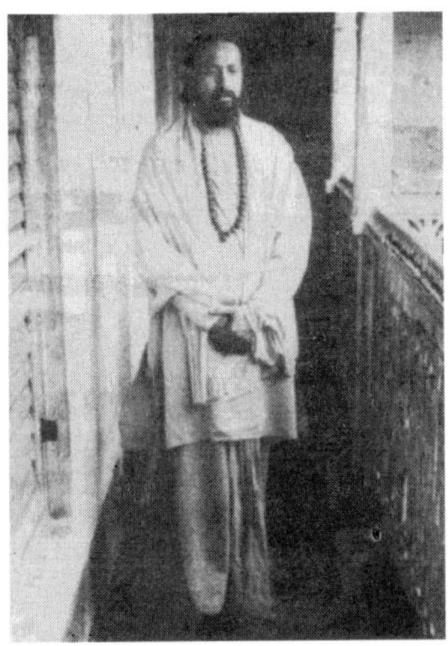

Swami Satyeswarananda at Calcutta (Kolkata)

While Swamiji was helping Swami Satyananda at Sevayatan, one founding member was not attending board meetings consecutively year after year; as a result, some members were talking about dropping his name and including some new member in it. Swami Satyananda said, "No. Sailen's name will remain there in spite of his absence in the meetings." It was a big favor to Sailen Babu. So Swamiji one day asked Satyananda about the reason for Sailen Babu's continuous absence in the meetings. Satyananda gave an answer and outlined in detail his background.

Sat Sanga with Sailendra Bejoy Dasgupta :

Sailendra Bejoy Dasgupta was a disciple of Swami Sriyukteswar, a beloved Ranchi student of Satyananda who was principal of the school for twenty years (1922 - 1941) and was founding executive general secretary of Yogoda Sat Sanga Society of India (YSS) from 1936 - 1941. As all the founding members were life members of YSS, Satyananda was a member of YSS even after leaving Ranchi till he left body.

It was a big favor to Sailendra Bejoy Dasgupta indeed because Dasgupta was a very beloved student of Satyananda. While Dasgupta was a student of ninth grade (Class IX) he wanted to take *Kriya* from Satyananda. In those days, Satyananda was permitted by Sriyukteswar to initiate others into *Kriya* but he was not acting on the permission.

The simple reason is, ideally speaking, being realized when one is in oneness with the totality of Consciousness and does not see any second existence, whom will he initiate? Having this sentiment, Satyananda was not acting on Sriyukteswar's permission. The scriptural reference to this sentiment is as follows:

Jo mang asyati sarba cha mayi pasyati.
Tasyang na pranasyami sa cha me na pranasyati. Bhagavad Gita 6:30

The verse says, "He, who sees me [the supreme Self] present in all beings [in totality of Pure Consciousness] and all beings exist in me [the supreme Self], never loses sight of [the Lord] and I never lose sight of him."

This was the position of Satyananda; being realized, he did not see the second existence; as a result, he did not like to initiate others since he did not see others except the Lord in every one.

(One day, Satyananda said to the author, "Sriyukteswarji one day said to me, 'I am old and Yogananda is not here so you have to initiate people.' "

(When he insisted, Satyananda said to the author, "I told him that I will bring your message door to door."

(With this sentiment of Satyananda, one can conclude that Satyananda never considered himself a teacher or *Guru*. Satyananda loved the author as his own son. (Mahamuni Babaji too loved the author as his son. He referred to that on a few occasions). Satyananda wrote eighty letters to the author. In some of them he mentioned the author as his son. So Satyananda maintained his original sentiment and never considered himself as *Guru*.

(Again on June 11, 1968, Satyananda pursued the subject with the author. A portion of his handwritten letter is reproduced here:

("You are my affectionate 'son.' This is true.

(Thereafter, Satyananda wrote to the author again. A portion of his handwritten letter dated March 11, 1970, is reproduced below:

(In the same handwritten letter he once again repeated his demand to the author. This portion is reproduced below:

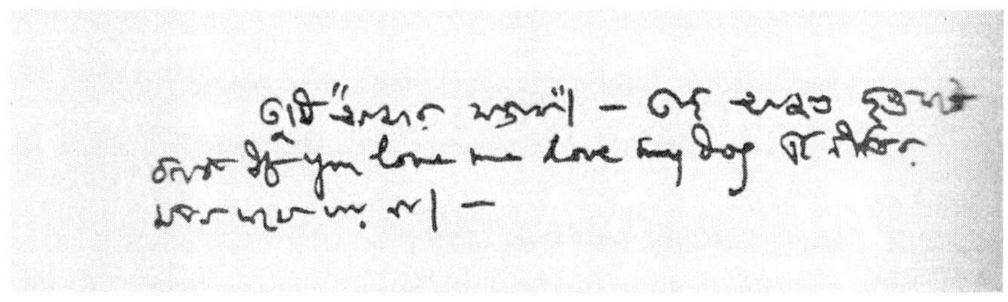

("You are 'my son', so even today I will pronounce at the top of my voice, 'if you love me, love my dog.' This maxim will not lose its value."

(Thus Satyananda was able to maintain his sentiment remaining in oneness with the pure Consciousness; he did not initiate others seeing as second existence. He had a unique way to compromise without compromising with his idealism).

Sriyukteswar usually visited Ranchi School each year at least once for a few days, as he had to preside over the annual prize distribution day and would give awards to the first boys of the different classes and the winners of the sports games. On one such occasion, Satyananda brought Dasgupta and asked him to take *Kriya* from Sriyukteswar.

At this time Dasgupta was a teen-aged boy. He remarked frankly to Satyananda, while pointing to Sriyukteswar, "I am not going to take *Kriya* from this old man; I will take *Kriya* from you and you only." Sriyukteswar was gently smiling at Dasgupta's comment. Dasgupta had such love and respect for Satyananda. Eventually, Dasgupta was initiated by Sriyukteswar.

One day, on a subsequent visit to Ranchi Sriyukteswar asked a devotee to bring Sailen. When he saw Sriyukteswar, he initiated Dasgupta the second *Kriya* of the tranquil breath, also known as *Thokkar Kriya* because Dasgupta's practice of the *Khecharimudra* or the *Talabya Kriya* was successful. Dasgupta was a lucky one.

When Dasgupta was studying in college, they were poor financially. Satyananda said that he traveled in a tram in Calcutta in the second class and saved money to give to Sailen so that he could have his breakfast in the morning.

After college, Dasgupta enrolled in the Calcutta University in the Anthropology Department where there were only fourteen students enrolled that year. In the final examination, Dusgupta stood first in the first class and became a gold medalist.

Just after that when Yogananda visited India, Satyananda was sick so he recommended Dasgupta to be Yogananda's private secretary for a year while he would stay in India. Yogananda was so impressed with Dasgupta he wanted to make him a *brahmachari*; but Dasgupta's father was an astrologer. He said that he had seen a marriage line in his son's palm so he could not be made a *brahmachari*. Yogananda made two graduate students of Ranchi, Sudhir Chandra Roy to Swami Sevananda and Panchkori Dey *Brahmachari* Shantananda, but failed to make Sailen Babu a *brahmachari*.

(It should be mentioned here that Yogananda, being liberal, his giving *sannyas* or Swami order, was liberal too. He had a tendency to violate the Vedic rules; Satyananda always cautioned him in this regard; pointing out the Vedic rules, and then left it to him, whatever he would do. When Swami Sevananda left Puri Asram, he joined his beloved Principal, Satyananda, at Sevayatan. Then at a certain point of time he felt to move close to the Himalayas. Swami Satyananda recommended his good friend, Swami Mahadevananda Giri, chief of Swami Bholananda Giri Sannyas Asram at Haridwar. As a result, he joined

Swami Bholananda Giri Asram at Haridwar, the famous place. The chief of the asram asked him, if "*Viraja Homa*" a very significant segment of the *sannyas* vow was performed during his entering into the order of Swami. Sevananda said, "No, he does not think so." Swami Mahadevananda Giri, said, "Then he has to go through it again with *sannyas* vow with *Viroja homa*, only then he could accept him. Sevananda went through it again and was accepted. Once, he became general secretary of the asram).

Dasgupta found a job teaching anthropology in Bangabasi College for only one hundred rupees a month salary, but left after a year to join a jute mill as a labor officer.

Now came Dasgupta's marriage issue. It was decided with a rich and famous man, Kiron Sankar Roy, in whose name there is an important street near the New Secretariat.

At this stage, Sailen Babu was trying to have guidance in his life from Satyananda through letter correspondence. He wrote to him on the issue. Satyananda replied to support his sentiment and wrote indirectly if he could avoid getting married, he should.

So accordingly, he said that he was not going to get married. In fact, it was too late. The invitation letters were printed and distributed by the Roy family. Having heard this message from Dasgupta, one younger daughter of Mr. Roy came to Dasgupta's office and started shouting very loudly to Dasgupta that he had to marry her elder sister. They have a social standing, The marriage cards were printed in different languages and thousands of them were distributed. It was very late. He had no chance to avoid now. Dasgupta could not stand her shouting so loudly in the office. He said well he would marry her sister. Thus it was settled. The marriage was solemnized. Mrs. Dasgupta was a high school teacher, eventually she became a principal of the school.

After the marriage, Dasgupta had a son, Mukul Dasgupta, and a daughter. He kept the file of letter correspondence with Satyananda in his office. One day, his daughter found it and gave it to her mother. Finding the letter of Swami Satyananda, she was furious. She began to think that she had a curse of a *sannyasi* in her married life. She put injunctions on Dasgupta's life that he could not have any connection with Satyananda or with any Swami for that matter. She also controlled Dasgupta's movement. It created a heavy strain on his life.

This was the reason Dasgupta could not attend board meetings year after year.

There was other trouble in Dasgupta's life. It was very serious.

During 1967 to 1970 in Bengal there was a great disturbance in the State. Politically, the Congress government ended. The congress party broke, a new party began as Bangla Congress with the leadership with Mr. Ajoy Kumar Mukherjee, student of the first chief minister, Dr. Prafullya Chandra Ghosh, D. Sc. Even he rejoined politics with his former student, Mr. Mukherjee. Panchkori Dey, principal B. Ed. College of Sevayatan, who also joined the party.

The National Congress Party failed to get an absolute majority. The United Front was made with Bangla Congress and other communist parties with Ajoy Mukherjee and then they formed the government in the state of West Bengal Ajoy Mukherjee as chief minister and Mr. Jyoti Basu, who was a hardcore communist, as deputy chief minister. Actually, the deputy chief minister Mr. Basu, held the real power. With his domination, the government did not last long. In such a chaotic situation, the law and order in the city of Calcutta, as well as in the countryside of West Bengal, increased between the poor, middle class on the one hand, and the big land lords on the other. In the next election, the left communist party gained an absolute majority and they formed the government. This time, in the countryside each day, ten to twelve people were killed and the bodies brought to the sub-divisional towns.

People of Calcutta in those days were so afraid, the wives, the sons and daughters were waiting at their doorssteps looking for their loved ones whether they would return from their offices or be kidnapped and killed. The people did not visit their relatives living in the other parts of the city because when they arrived near their relative's houses, the local communist boys standing on the intersection, seeing unfamiliar faces, captured and killed them. It was such a horrible time in Calcutta.

(Once, the dissatisfied workers of the company Dasgupta was working for, brought their agitation to the door of the office. The six feet two inches (6'2") tall British officer was afraid to face the angry and agitated workers outside the office. They looked like an unruly mob. Then they decided to send short figured S. B. Dasgupta, the labor officer, to face them. Sailen Babu calmly came out of the office and faced them and cooled them down. The British officers were watching from the upstairs. They were stunned. Dusgupta might be a short figured man but they did not know that Dasgupta was a *Khecharisiddha* (successful in *Khecharimudra*), fearless Yogi.

(After this incident, Dasgupta earned tremendous respect and also a promotion.

(Sailen Babu told the author, "When I walked sometimes with an intoxicated state of bliss, they thought I was drunk.")

The communist supported labor unions started trouble in a big way in Calcutta. They started killing officers who stood against their interests. Dasgupta, being associated with the Alliance Jute Mill Co. as a labor and personnel officer, got a threat to be killed. It was a serious matter and not a joke. He rented out his own house to a bank and rented a house for six months to live secretly; then started changing houses every six months. Mrs. Dasgupta controlled the entrance with an intercom buzzer.

On one of these days, Dasgupta invited Swamiji to visit his flat where he was living at that time with his family. In his neighborhood, lived another Ranchi ex-student of Satyananda, Paresh Chandra Bardhan, working in a high position as a sales commissioner, for the government of West Bengal. Dasgupta suggested Swamiji should first visit Paresh Babu and then let Paresh Babu inform him by the phone that Swamiji was coming soon to see him.

Paresh Chandra Bardhan was a Yogi, not a Kriya Yogi, but he was disciple of Principal Akshaya Kumar Banerjee (who was Yogi of the *Nath* sect - Gorakhanath group).

Prior to visiting Dasgupta he said to the author that when Mrs. Dasgupta would ask, "who is it?" He had to answer, "From Calcutta High Court for labor consultancy." Then he was allowed to enter. He was living on the third floor. Dasgupta personally toured the apartment to show the author. He pointed out his seat (*asana*) for practicing *Kriya*. He said that he was not allowed to sit and practice by his wife and his daughter since they feared he would renounce the world and leave them.

This second problem also handicapped Mr. Dasgupta from visiting Sevayatan for attending board meetings.

Once Satyananda said, "Sailen writes well. He should write something."

When Swamiji arrived at Calcutta after leaving Sevauatan, Dasgupta had retired. Swamiji was looking for him to tell him that Satyanada said he should write something. Through a common friend, Swamiji found out where Dasgupta was living and contacted him. He mentioned that he would be visiting a lawyer's chamber in the High Court area. We could meet there. Actually, Sailen Babu was sharing an office space with his former deputy, Mr. Asok Kumar Chattarjee, an Attorney in the High Court area. Usually we met in the office and then his driver in his small car, Standard, drove us to a big green field, *maidan*; the driver stayed in the car and we moved a little far and sat on a blanket for almost two hours for *Sat Sanga*. This continued for almost two months. We talked about alot of things. Sailen Babu began to tell his life's story which Swamiji had partly already heard from Satyananda.

In regards to his practice, his comment was that, just for the harmony in the civil life, he accepted the demand of his wife and daughter. He said that he discovered Sriyukteswar's advanced household disciple, Amulya Charan Santra Mahasay, and had occasional *Sat Sanga* in his house. Santra Mahasay was in Calcutta which was a Muslim dominated area.

(Swamiji happened to live in the same postal zone in the Hindu dominated area. Swamiji visited Santra Mahasay's house.)

Usually Santra Mahasay did not like to receive visitors. There was a system. After pressing the button one has to wait. If he responded and the green light was on, it indicated he would accept the visitor; if the red light was on then it indicated that he would not accept the visitor.

Dasgupta said that he received the third *Kriya* from Amulya Babu and commented the rest may be in the next life.

Dasgupta once started talking about his personal life. He said that Mukul, his son, after receiving M. Sc in physics, moved to the United States for higher studies. He did pretty well there and got a job. He mentioned that his only regret was that he could not manage to get his son married in his own house because of the threat to his life. He had to arrange for it somewhere else. The girl was from a Chatterjee family and her subject was Chemistry. His daughter at that time was studying History. She wanted to sit for an Administrative examination. He also mentioned that if he could buy a house for Mrs. Dasgupta at Camac Street he would be glad. Camac Street in Calcutta is a safe place where the rich people live.

Dasgupta mentioned that he had two frustrations in his life:

1) Although he was connected with Sevayatan from the very beginning, because of Swami Satyananda's unconditional love for his beloved student, as well as a brother disciple; yet, he could not remain engaged under the circumstance of his life. The author smelled a bit subtle jealousy in this regards, that he was not able to remain engaged while the

others like Swamiji were fortunate to be associated a long twenty years.

2) Regarding the second frustration of life, he mentioned that to maintain the harmonious life at home with his wife and daughter, he could not practice *Kriya* during the energetic period of life in his early middle age.

There were four founding members of Sevayatan, the hermitage of Swami Satyananda as follows:

1) Swami Premananda as Founder Trustee, since he donated the money to start with. He lived in the United States and had never seen the place.

2) Shailesh Mohan Mazumder (brother of Swami Satyananda, who later became Swami Suddhananda, in whose name the land was purchased. He donated the land to the Trust and became its secretary).

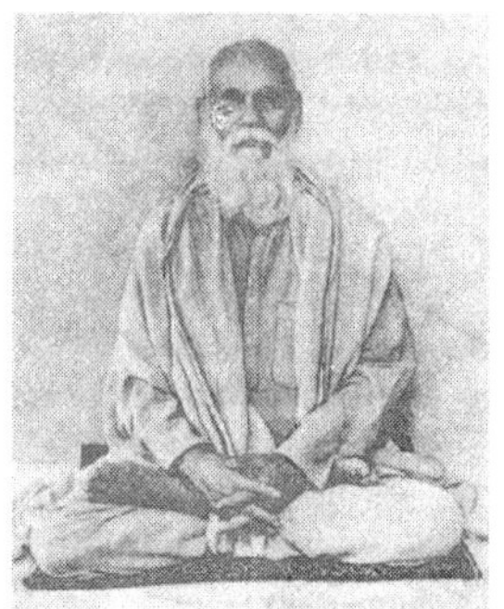

Swami Suddhananda

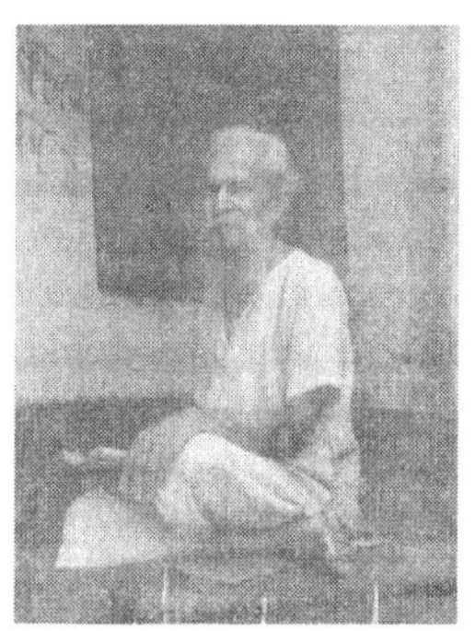

Panchkori Dey
(*Brahmachari* Shantananda)

3) Panchkori Dey, disciple of Hangsa Swami Kebalananda (Yogananda made Mr. Dey *Brahamachari* Shantananda),

4) Sailendra Bejoy Dasgupta, disciple of Sriyukteswar (Yogananda failed to make Mr. Dasgupta a *Brahmachari*).

All four members were very dear students of Swami Satyananda at Ranchi. When these students tried to bring him to Sevayatan, he mentioned that he had enough of hermitages and organizations; they would have to work on their own, he would simply be present there and if they wanted his advice he would render it.

However, it did not work that way. Although Satyananda kept himself out of the trust board and was not even an ordinary member, yet, because of the absence of the founder Trustee, Swami Premananda, they co-opted Swami Satyananda onto the board and made him President of the Sevayatan Trust board.

Once Swamiji mentioned to Dasgupta in one of our *Sat Sangas* that Satyananda had mentioned to him that Sailen writes very well and he should write something. The moment Swamiji mentioned it Sailen Babu's eyes were lifted up. He said that he was thinking to write something too. The message inspired him.

The next day, he asked Swamiji if he had any first copy of Sriyukteswar's book - The *Kaibalya Darsanam* (*the Holy Science*), which was published by King Atul Chandra Choudhuri, Sriyukteswar's disciple, founder secretary of Sadhu Sobha. King Atul Chandra Choudhuri was a publisher also, who wrote a small introduction in English. Dasgupta said that way he could avoid the copyright problem with Daya [Sister Daya, president of SRF (Self Realization Fellowship, Yogananda's organization)]. Also if Swamiji had a good copy of *Yoga Sutras* of Patanjali.

Swamiji said that he had to look in his library, with its rare collection of books.

The next day, Swamiji handed over the *Yoga Sutras* of Patanjali by Hariharananda Aranyak, published by Calcutta University, which Swami Satyananda suggested to Swamiji when he was a Philosophy M. A. student at the Calcutta University. This version contained the Buddhist version of the interpretation which impressed Satyananda.

In a few days Dasgupta wrote about fifty pages and showed them to Swamiji. We discussed it and Swamiji pointed out something he should consider to include.

At this time, Dasgupta requested Swamiji to write a book on Lahiri Mahasay with his twelve (12) disciples. Swamiji said, "It is easy for me to write on the scriptures but writing biographies needs more accurate facts and figures from history which is difficult to gather."

Dasgupta said, "You are the right person for this job in my opinion. You were associated with Swami Satyananda for twenty years and so you know many things from him which others do not know."

When the book was published in 1979, Dasgupta sent a copy in 1980 through his former deputy, Asok Kumar Chatterjee who mentioned that Mrs. Dasgupta passed away and Mr. Dasgupta became a widower. He moved to Barrakpore area to live.

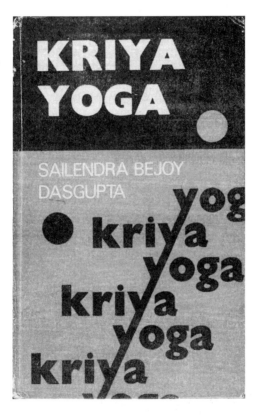

The cover page of Kriya Yoga
by Sailendra Bejoy Dasgupta, disciple of Sriyukteswar

Swami Satyeswarananda briefly at Benaras:

In the meantime two months passed, Swamiji, without telling Sailen Babu and Biren Babu, suddenly left for Benaras on his pilgrimage.

Swamiji made it a habit in his life, that whenever he had to go to the Himalayas, he used to stop at Benaras, the holy city, the citadel of Hinduism. He used to take a bath at Dasaswamedh *ghat*, visit the Lord Biswanath Temple, pay respects visiting Lahiri Mahasay's original house at Garureswar, then visit Satyalok near Chawsatti Yogini *ghat.*

This time arriving at Benaras first thing Swamiji shaved his hair and beard; took a bath in the Ganges at Dasaswamedha *Ghat*, and visited the Lord Biswanath Temple. He prayed in the temple to the Lord Biswanath that he bless Swamiji to meeti at least two realized persons in his pilgrimage.

Then Swamiji visited Lahiri Mahasay's original house at Garureswar, met Prof. Banamali Lahiri who lived there, visited Satyalok near Chawsatti Yogini *ghat* but Satya Charan Lahiri was not there on that day.

After spending a week at Benaras, Swamiji moved to Vrindavan, the heart of *Vaisnavism* in India.

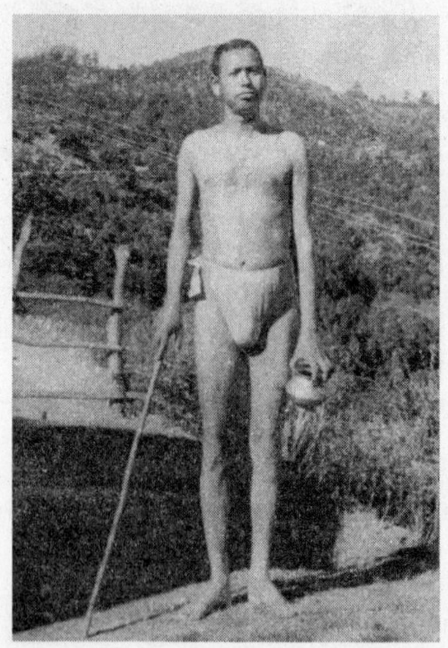

Swami Satyeswarananda, a wandering Vedantist.

Swami Satyeswarananda in Vrindavan:

Swamiji visited Vrindavan several times. When he visited Vrindavan the first time he was in his teens. He was totally surprised to see Lord Banke Bihari because he had *darsan* (meeting)with the deity in his dream exactly the way his altar was. Lord Banke Bihari was the family deity. It is the most important temple in Vrindavan.

While traveling in Vrindavan, sitting in a bus near the window, Swamiji saw at a distance the shape of two boys in the air. The boys were moving in the air towards the bus and fell on the face of Swamiji. He felt as if something happened; he did not understand what it was. Next thing he realized that he could not talk. He became silent. It continued days after days. As a result, Swamiji was forced to observe silence. He did not take a vow, but it happened in, natural way. In Vrindavan, he visited Banke Bihari Temple which drew the largest number of devotees each day.

An old college student recognizes his professor.

One day in Vrindavan an old college student of the author recognized him. He was a law student for only a month and then left the college. He graduated from *Vidya Mandir* (college) of Sri Ramakrisna Mission. Later, he was initiated in *Mantra* from Rama Krisna Mission but did not join the Mission. He left for Vrindavan and was observing silence.

It was a big surprise that several years before, after attending law classes for just one month that he could still recognize his professor in a totally different circumstance; meaning, the author was silent and was wearing a jute bag from the waist to the knee.

He found a piece of charcoal lying on the ground and wrote on a broken wall certain things, including the fact that the author used to wear Vidyasagar's *Chappals* (sandals) and then in the sand he wrote with his finger to convince him that he was not mistaken.

Now, the problem began. It was about ten o'clock in the morning. He wanted to see Raman Reti which was far away from Vrindavan. He did not know how far. The author being a *Mouni*(silent), wrote in the sand that it would be practical to start early tomorrow morning as it was far away and the sun was getting strong.

However, the student would not listen to this suggestion, he wanted to leave then and so the author's repeated requests fell on deaf ears.

Being helpless at the hands of a devoted student, the author proceeded to Mathura, then Baldeo [Balaram], then Gokul [old town] and finally to Raman Reti. It was the month of June, at high noon and after noon it was so hot that the pitch of the road started melting. Walking with bare feet on such a hot day and such a long distance was not an easy task.

When they arrived there it was afternoon. At Raman Reti there was a temple in the center of Raman Reti asram. There were many huts where many Vaisnab Sadhus (hermits) lived. They cultivated an agricultural farm and lived together in those huts around the temple and carried out their *sadhana* (meditation). It was a peaceful place. Seeing two *Mouni Babas* the manager asked a devotee to find some *prasad,* even at that late hour. The *bhoga* [food] was offered at noon in the temple and then all had their *prasad*.

The student wanted to return to Vrindavan immediately. It was a crazy idea but he insisted and started walking for the return journey. Walking in such hot weather on the hot pitch road for several hours, the author began to feel that one of his feet at the bottom was beginning to swell; the author had difficulties walking but did not let the student know. The author continued walking though gradually was falling behind.

At sundown, one private bus (the name of the bus was BABA) stopped and the driver came out and insisted the author must get in the bus. The student who was ahead did not know what was happening. He came back to know the situation; all of a sudden the driver pushed him into the bus and thus gave both a ride up to some distance. Then he put the bus in the company garage.

Now both the *Mouni* Babas (silent wandering seekers) were on the road again.

After having a short break the author's foot was giving him more pain and then he discovered that the bottom of his other foot had also begun to swell. It was almost 7:30 or 8 o'clock in the evening with still a long way to go. Somehow the author began to walk with the help of the front part of his foot.

The author struggled in his mind about whether he should let the student know the condition of his feet. He still continued with a lot of pain and decided when it would be completely impossible to walk then he would disclose the problem. Both arrived at Mathura around 8:30 or 9 P.M. Vrindavan was still far away. Eventually they arrived at Vrindavan, also stopped at an old Vana-prasthi's place. The student stayed there but the author left.

It was late evening, the author's feet were taking him to Kesi *ghat*. It suddenly struck his mind, well! what an attachment. Why does he have to go to that particular *ghat,* especially Kesi *ghat* where there were some secure places to stay. The author turned away and began to consider that he might not be able to walk for several days, so he better not go far away. Accordingly, he moved to a lonely place on the bank for the rest of the night.

As expected, the condition of his feet was very bad, so painful that the author could not walk. He intended to go off the *Parikrama Marga* (there is a traditional earmarked path to make a round of Vrindavan, many devotees make a round morning or evening, mostly morning. It takes several hours to make one round).

He laid down far away from Shyam Kuti. He thought he might be there for several days, but the Lord of Providence had a different plan. At about eleven o'clock two American devotees who lived at Shyam Kuti were also looking for a lonely place to meditate.

Seeing a renunciate Baba, they approached, and soon realized the wandering mendicant was a silent sage. They noticed his feet and their condition. The Americans would not listen to any objections of the author. They forcibly brought him to their place at Shyam Kuti where an old Homeopath doctor was a resident. They brought the Doctor Maharaj to look at his feet and give him medicine. Thus Swamiji met these two American devotees in Vrindavan.

Meeting Deoria Baba in Vrindavan.

In those days, Deoria Baba, a very old reputed Raja Yogi with a large number of followers, was camping with his devotees at Vrindavan for a few days. Deoria is a district in the state of Uttar Pradesh. He hailed from there; as a result, he was known as Deoria Baba.

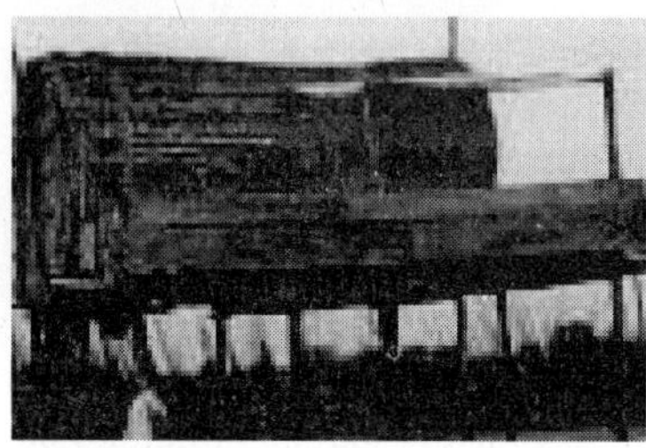

Temporary stand made by
Deoria Baba's devotees

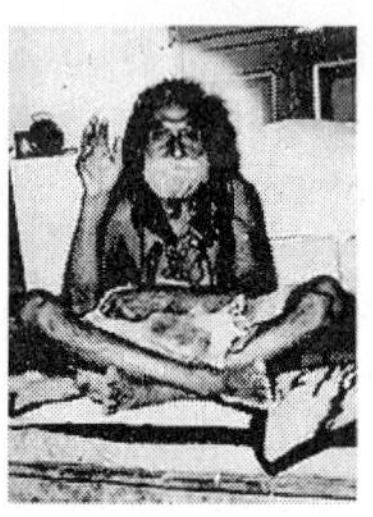

Yogi Deoria Baba

One day, the American devotees whom Swamiji met recently practically forced the author to have *darsan* of Deoria Baba. It should be mentioned here that in those days, the author was in continuous silence (*akhanda mouna*). At the camp, there was a rule that the visitors must stay at least fifty feet away from the temporary stand made by his followers where Baba was supposed to be sitting and give *darsan* (meeting).

When the author arrived there, about fifty people were sitting near the sand on the bank of the Yamuna River for his *darsan*. Deoria Baba was returning from his nature's call and after sometime he climbed on the stand and sat there. Everybody had his *darsan*.

All of a sudden, one of his devotees called for Mouni Baba. He called for Mouni Baba again. At this point no one was responding. Then one of the American devotees said to the author, "Babaji! He is calling you. No one is Mouni Baba here except you." The author was totally surprised. The American devotee repeatedly urged the author to stand up and go near the stand where Deoria Baba was sitting. The author reluctantly was about to oblige; then the devotee of Baba came forward and guided the author to the stand and asked him to go under the stand. When the author was under the stand, Deoria Baba put his one leg down through a hole. The author made *pranam* to him. Deoria Baba asked his devotee to give the author one piece of cloth to wear; since the author used to wear a piece of jute made to cover the mid section. The devotee also gave some fruits. The author returned to his seat and gave the fruits to the American devotees.

The very next day, one young devotee took away the piece of cloth from the shoulder of the author saying, "Nobody gives me a cloth when I really need one; Mouni Baba does not need cloth; he wears *tat* [jute made bag] and people give him cloth." The author smiled within.

The two American devotees who brought the author to their asram had some friends among the American devotees of Nim Karoli Baba, who had an asram at Vrindavan. The visas of these two American devotees were shortly about to expire so they were interested to get some advice on how to extend their stay in India from the American devotees of Nim Karoli Baba.

They requested the author to lead them to Kainchi, in the Himalayas, to Nim Karoli Baba's asram. The author happened to know Bhuwali, and not Kainchi, which was on the way to Dunagiri Hill, Himalayas, where the author had visited many times and practiced *Kriya*. Then the American devotees mentioned that they had heard that Kainchi was only about eight miles from Bhuwali. At this point, they insisted that the author guide them to Nim Karoli Baba's asram.

The author meets Nim Karoli Baba at Kainchi, Himalayas.

So all set out for Kainchi. From Vrindavan one has to come to Mathura by bus, then take a train to Haldwani, from there a direct bus goes to Kainchi. It takes almost a day. When the author arrived at Kainchi with the two American devotees, Nim Karoli Baba was outside. He was about to re-enter his room for lunch. Nim Karoli Baba received the author warmly; he asked his devotee, Mr. Sharma, to make all necessary arrangements for the author's stay in the asram. He also found out that the author was observing continuous silence. So he addressed the author as "Mouni Baba."

The author stayed there for twenty days. During this period, one day, Nim Karoli Baba said in Hindi, "Mouni Baba! *Mai apke liye pratiksha kar raha tha. Ek Himalay ke Yogi ne mujhe ek samachar diya ki ap job inha ayenge to batana ki ap Dunagiri Vaisnabi Mata ke mandir me jana. Apko to onha se pyar hai.*

(Meaning, "I was waiting for you. I have a message for you from a Himalayan Yogi. You must go to Dunagiri Hill, you have attraction there. Stay at the Mother's temple.")

Then Nim Karoli Baba asked Mr. Sharma to give bus fare. The author was about to leave for Dunagiri Hill, but the only bus which came from Haldwani had already left Kainchi for the day. Nim Karoli Baba called the author back and asked him to stay a few days more.

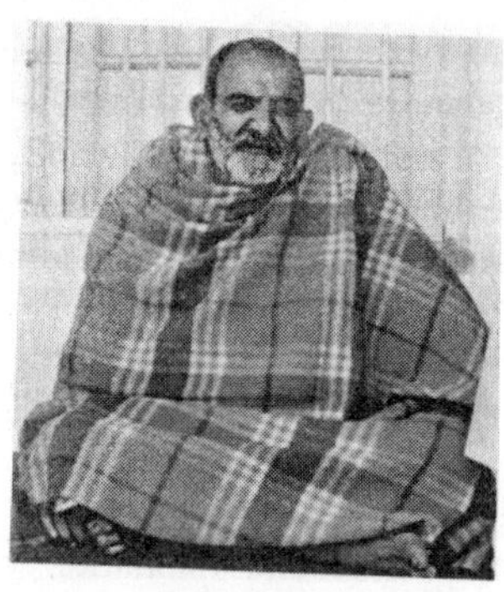

Nim Karoli Baba, Disciple of Babaji.

Another day, Nim Karoli Baba said, "*Apko maine samachar de diya. Ab mai iha sarir chhor dunga*. (Meaning, I have delivered the message to you now I will leave the body.")

(Almost six years later, near Gopeswar, one Yogi, a messenger of Mataji, told the author in Hindi, "Maharaj! *Us din ap der me aye Kainchi se. Mujhe map karenge. Apko kast diya. Mataji yad kar rahi thi. Kuchh din hi me ap unke darsan karenge*.

(It means, "On that day [one day, Mataji was camping in a cave near Nim Karoli Baba's Kainchi asram and wanting to see Swamiji and sent a message to him. Swamiji was late to arrive there. He saw Mataji and her party had left], you were late from the Kainchi asram. Kindly pardon me. I inflicted suffering on you. Actually Mataji [Sister of Babaji] was remembering you. This time you will see her within a few days."

(In return, the author apologized for being late. Also seeing Mataji at Anusuya Devi the author personally apologized to her.)

One day the American devotees asked Nim Karoli Baba for advice and he told them to return to their country.

Lord Siva fulfilled Swamiji's prayer. He met Deoria Baba and Nim Karoli Baba. Even got indication of Mahamuni Babaji from Nim Karoli Baba. In addition to meeting these two realized Yogis, during his pilgrimage Swamiji met Anandamoyee Ma at her asram near Daksha Prajapati, at Haridwar.

Swami Satyeswarananda meets Anandamoyee Ma at Haridwar.

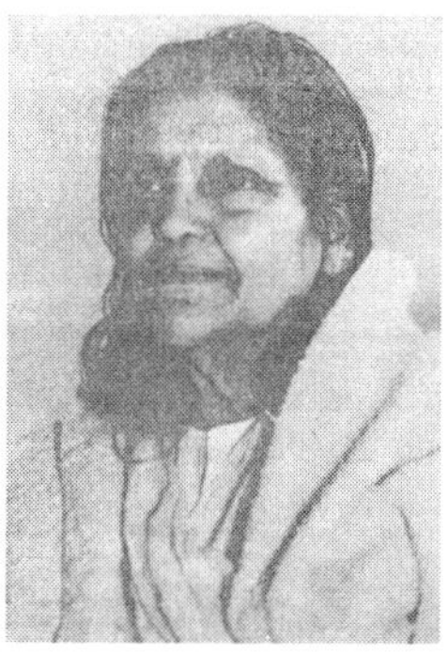

Anandamoyee Ma, a lady saint

She was sitting outside and on her left side were sitting the women devotees and on the right were the men devotees. Swamiji quietly sat down there on the right side in the men's group. One devotee was reading a scripture and the rest were listening. About forty or forty five minutes later Swamiji was thinking to leave. All of a sudden Ma looked into the eyes of Swamiji and got up and announced in Bengali, "*Keo jaben na ami na asha purjanta*," which means "nobody will leave till I return."

After a while she returned. Then she sat down like before. She brought an orange. It was in her hand. When Swamiji slowly got up to leave, he came in front her and from a distance bowed. She gestured to Swamiji to come closer. When Swamiji came closer she handed over the orange to Swamiji. It was a symbolical gesture of giving fruit (*phal*) to the journey.

Many years later when she was visiting Almora in the Himalayas at her small asram, Swami Paramananda, one of her disciples who was in charge of the trip, wrote a letter to Swamiji at Dunagiri Hill, Himalayas, at her instruction, informing Swamiji that Ma was very near, about thirty seven miles from Dunagiri Hill at the district town, Almora. She was remembering Swamiji so she asked Paramananda to inform Swamiji if he wanted to see her.

When Swamiji got the letter, there were two guests from Bengal visiting him at Dunagiri Hill. Both were *Kriyanwits*; one was a friend, a school teacher and the other was Swamiji's vice principal, Abanindra Narayan Lahiri, from the *Vidyapith* (high school). Learning the content of the letter, Principal Lahiri was highly interested to visit her. He said that long time before once he had her *darsan* (meeting) from a distance as she was always surrounded by many women devotees. It was impossible to come close. Maybe this time he would have better chance to see her close since Swamiji was invited. Two Italian devotees were also living in Dunagiri near Swamiji. They too came along. It was a good *darsan* (meeting).

Back to the pilgrimage. Finally, Swamiji Maharaj arrived at Dunagiri Hill, Himalayas, where he used to go every summer for *Kriya* practice. He retired there for his secluded meditative life. Initially, he was staying in the Rama Baba *kuti* (hut) in the temple, Bhagavati Jagadamba, Vaisnabi Mata at the top of Dunagiri Hill (height about 8, 000').

Eventually, the initiated Italian *Kriyanwits* devotees arrived to Dunagiri Hill, Himalayas. Gradually, the seekers of truth arrived to Dunagiri Hill, Himalayas from Italy, France, Germany, England, Yugoslavia, Canada, Australia and New Zealand. They rented small rooms from the hill people and began to live around Swami Satyeswarananda to learn *Kriya*, Vedic Culture, also the *Kriya* interpretation of the Holy Bible.

Swami Satyeswarananda at Dunagiri Hill, Himalayas.

Nobody knew in Bengal where Swamiji was. Dunagiri Hill of Himalayas is about 1,200 to 1,300 miles away in the state of Uttar Pradesh (Now Uttarakhanda). For the first three years, he was observing continuous silence; so people used to call him Mouni (silent) Swami or Mouni Baba.

After some years, a group of *Kriyanwits* (practitioners of *Kriya*) from West Bengal visited Dunagiri Hill temple during the worship of Goddess Durga, Bhagavati Jagadamba, Vaisnabi Mata (month of October). They were told by the official priests that Bengali Baba (Swami Satyeswarananda) lived near the bus stop. Hearing the word "Bengali Baba" they were surprised. Being curious they arrived at the holy hut (*Mouna Mandir*). Finding Swamiji they were stunned.

They were demanding that Swamiji must come down. They needed him to run the schools, college and hospital.

Swamiji said, "I am staying in this corner of the world silently without disturbing any one. You have many educated Swamis there in West Bengal. You could demand service from them. As you know, I am not a social worker; I am a seeker of truth. Hence, I am a *negta fakir* (naked renunciate). Please leave me alone."

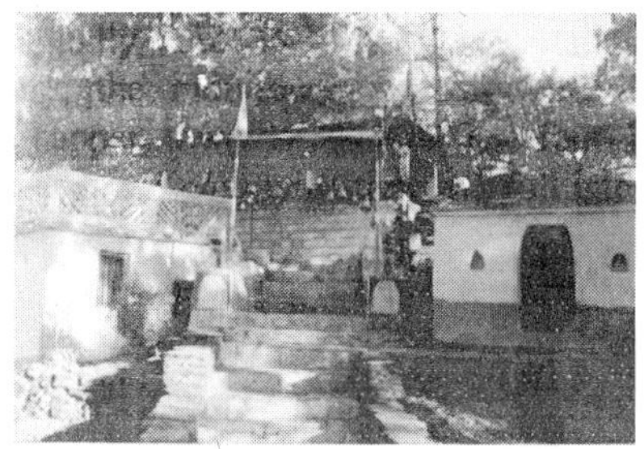

Vaisnabi Mata Temple
at Dunagiri Hill, Himalayas.

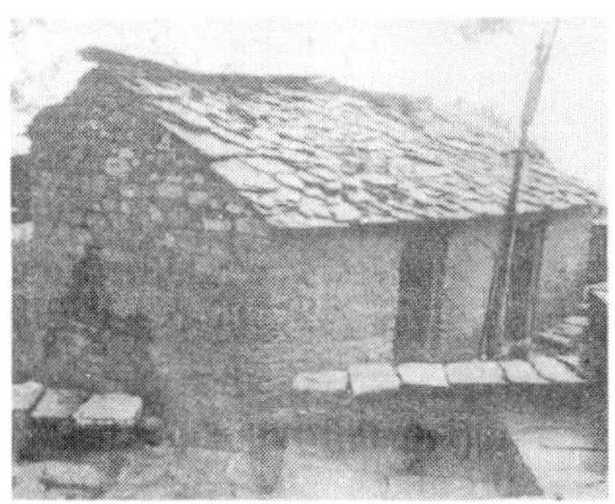

Rama Baba Kuti (hut) where initially
Swamiji lived and first saw Babaji

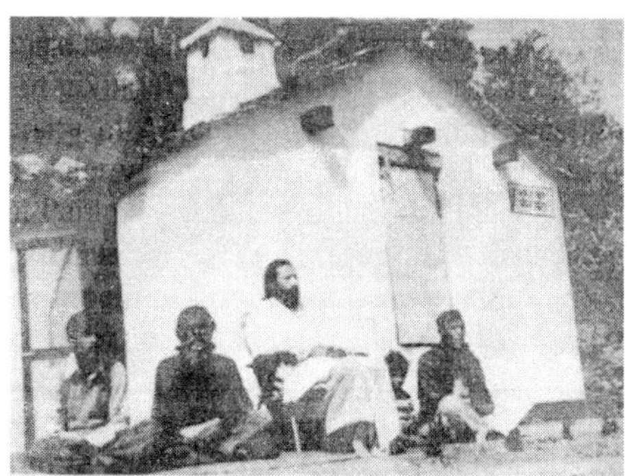

Mouna Mandir (The Holy Hut),
Built by Swamiji on private land outside the Temple complex,
(with the written Agreement with the land owner),
for solitude and lived about twelve years of his secluded meditative life.

12 Years in the Himalayas
Swami Satyeswarananda Maharaj (the author)

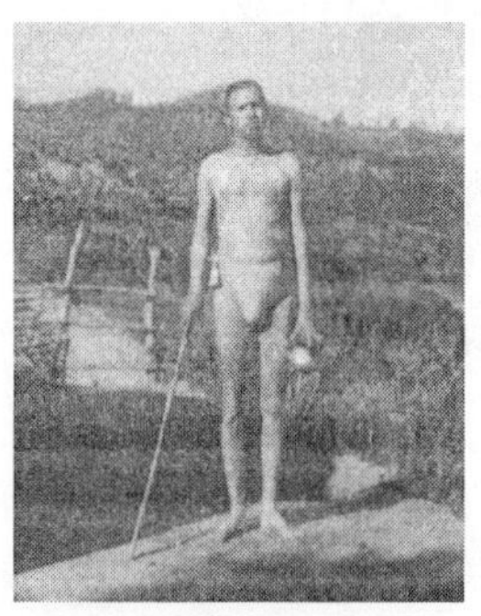

Wandering VEDANTIST

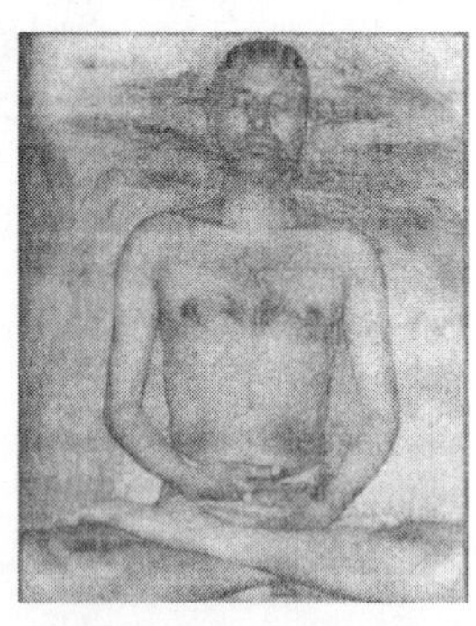

YOGI in the Himalayan Cave

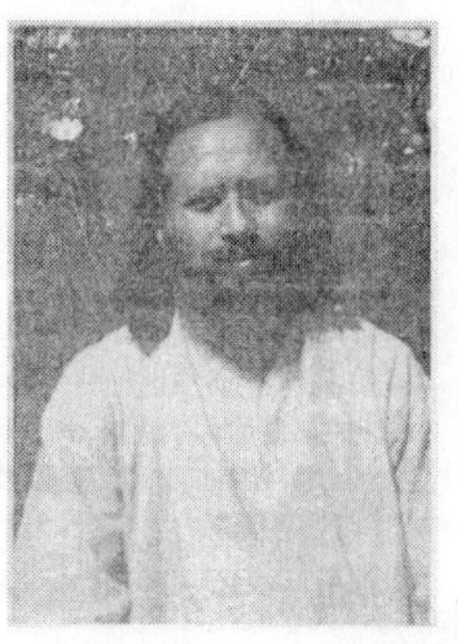

Hermit in the Himalayas

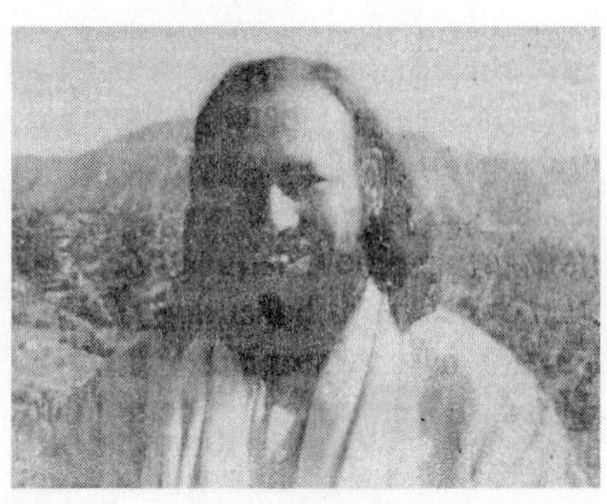

Swami in Dunagiri Hill, Himalayas

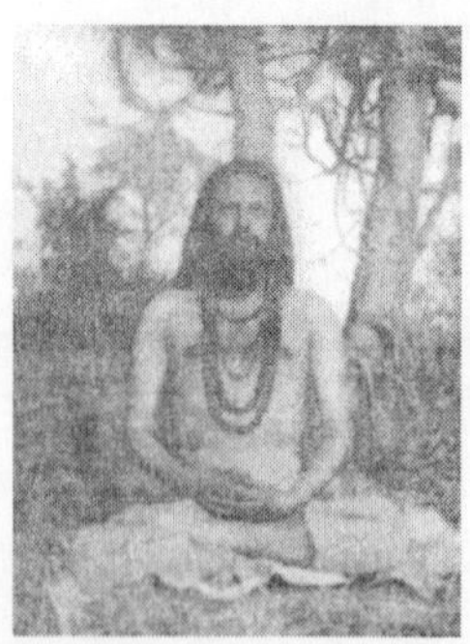

Man under the Tree

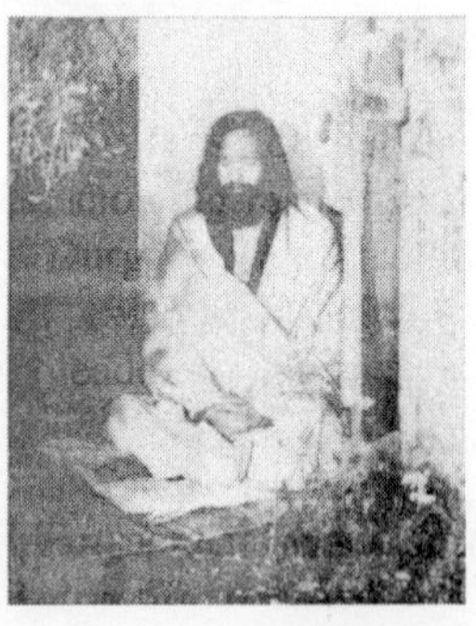

At the door of his hut
in *Dhyanmudra*

The visiting *Kriyanwits* said, "Those *brahmacharis* (celibates) and the Swamis (renunciates) were hankering after posts and positions and you have left them behind on your own voluntarily. That is the difference. Yours is the sincere selfless service. That is why we were looking for you all these months and years. We found you."

At this point, some of them said, "If you do not agree to our proposal, at least, you have to agree to our new proposal; that is, when it is snowing in the winter here, kindly Swamiji, please come down to Bengal for three months, from December to end of February each year and have your secluded life here for the rest of the year. We will be glad with that agreement.

"During your winter visit to West Bengal, the *Kriya* check up, *Kriya* review, *Kriya* advice and *Kriya* initiation, all these can be done. Kindly, you have to agree to these needs of ours. Please don't be so unkind."

They were very demanding as well as very polite. At this Swamiji said, 'I will think it over and let you know."

During this secluded meditative life time, suddenly Swami Satyeswarananda received in October 2, 1974 the message from the Divine Himalayan Yogi, Mahamuni BABAJI. He was asked to write down the message which was in Sanskrit verses.

Thereafter, one day, Paramananda Joshi (popularly known as *Sastriji*), a freedom fighter, bachelor, and an old astrologer, who used to worship in the temple of the Divine Mother (Bhagavati Jagadamba, Vaisnabi Mata) at the top of Dunagiri Hill, looking at the forehead of Swami Satyeswarananda told him, "Maharaj-ji! I am seeing on your forehead that you have to go to the foreign countries within six months. The Divine Mother has taken your hand and will bring you back within a year. At that time, if this old man still remains alive, then seriously I will try to learn from you the discipline of *Kriya Yoga*.

The Science of Self Realization
(*Kriya Yoga*: Published in 1974),
The first book of Swami Satyeswarananda

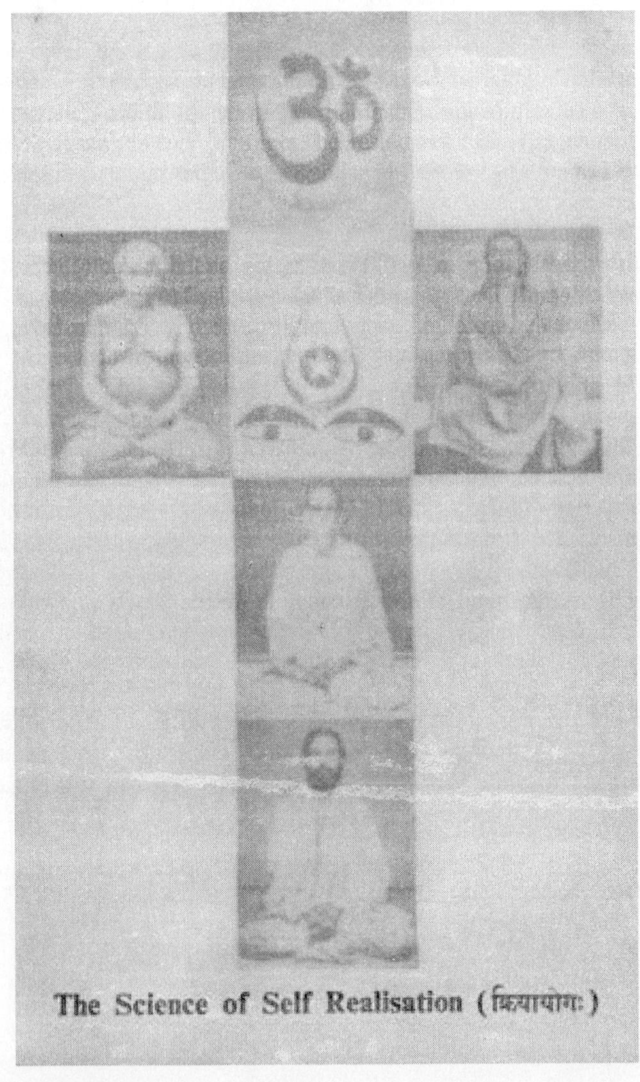

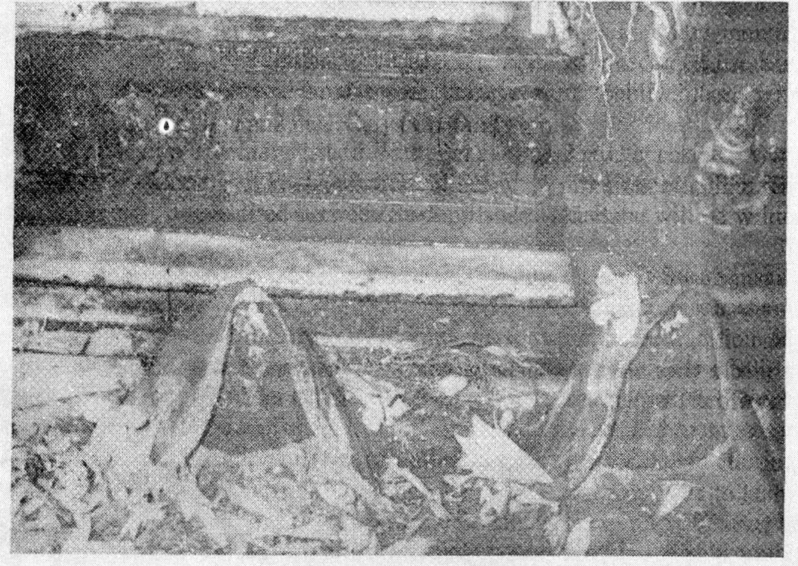

The Cover page of the small booklet with the photo of the temple of the Vaisnabi Sakti Pith, Dunagiri Hill, Himalayas (interior)

Meanwhile, one day Swami Satyananda appeared and said in Bengali, "*Musalmanra tomay nao dite pare*," which means "the Muslims may not give you." Swamiji interpreted it as that the Muslims countries may not give a Visa to visit. His statement became true when the passport officer, Mr. B. K. Dutta in Calcutta, refused to give an endorsement of Pakistan in the passport. He said, "Because of the Bangladesh war our relation with Pakistan is not good and even if I include Pakistan, they will not give you a transit Visa. So you better think to go by air to Europe."

In reply Swamiji said, "I have this Italian lady with me; if I go on the surface she would help me financially."

The Passport officer said, "Swamiji! I am sorry. You have to arrange to fly to Europe. That will be better for you."

Sastriji's observation became true as well; and as well as his anticipation, he left body just before Swamiji Maharaj returned to Dunagiri from his world lecture tour under the instruction of Mahamuni Babaji.

The message of Babaji was published in 1974 as a small booklet. The title was: *The Science of Self Realization* (*Kriya Yoga*). This was the first publication from Swami Satyeswarananda. At that time, Swamiji wrote a small booklet in Hindi about "the Vaisnabi Sakti Pith, Dunagiri Hill, Himalayas" and published it separately during the publication of the *Kriya Yoga* book. In the meantime, Swami Satyeswarananda wrote a book in English, the title was *Kriya.*

Swamiji Maharaj visited the huge "International Book Fair" at Frankfurt, Germany in 1975 during his world lecture tour. The manuscript was given to a literary agent (Edith Krispien) who said that the only publisher who would be interested was Matilal Banarasidass from New Delhi, India, but they wanted her as co-publisher donating US $ 1,000.00 which she did not have. So it did not work.

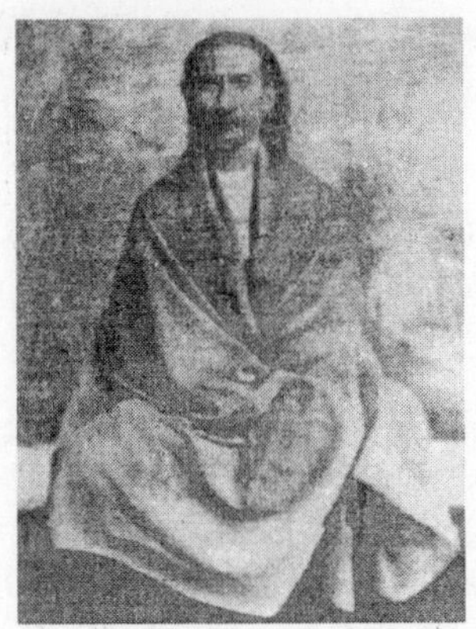

Swami Sriyukteswar Giri (in the middle age),
formerly Priyanath Karar

Later, the agent wrote Swamiji when he was back in India that Kriyananda, disciple of Yogananda, was visiting Germany and was guest of hers; so when he heard about the manuscript, he wanted to see it. At that time Kriyananda took the photo of Sriyukteswar from the manuscript and also got Swamiji's mailing address of the Himalayas.

Later, Swamiji learned from the letter of Kriyananda's correspondence secretary, Keshav, that Kriyananda took a photo from the manuscript and that it was a middle age photo of Swami Sriyukteswar. Keshav mentioned in his letter that Kriyananda never had seen that photo before in India so he took it for their altar. He hope, Swamiji would not mind.

Regarding the photo of Sriyukteswar, once, Sananda Lal Ghosh, Yogananda's brother and an accomplished artist, wrote to Swamiji at Dunagiri Hill, Himalayas (where he was living a secluded meditative life) to have a copy of this photo, mentioning that he saw it on the cover page on Swamiji's publication, "The Science of Self Realization (*Kriya Yoga*)." He mentioned that it was very urgent and important. Sananda Lal Ghosh colorizing the photo of the *Kriya* Yogis and selling them to the American devotees of Yogananda became a rich person. Swamiji thought he wanted to make a color photo out of it and add it to his product line as he had done for the *Kriya* Yogis: Lahiri Mahasay, Panchanan Bhattacharya, Sriyukteswar, Bhupendranath Sanyal, Yogananda and Satyananda. So Swamiji instructed a devotee at Calcutta, Birendra lal Choudhuri, to deliver a copy of the photo to him. Many years later in the United States, to Swamiji's utter surprise, he found it in his book *Mejda* (means the middle brother, that is Yogananda for him) in U.S.A. He never mentioned that he would require it for a book.

It brings back the memory that once Swamiji saw in Calcutta a booklet written by a group of devotees of Yogananda without mentioning their names. It became clear from the book that it was intended to create some evidence in favor of Yogananda's organization which was involved in the lawsuit about the Puri Asram of Sriyukteswar. It seems the book *Mejda* by Sananda Lal Ghosh falls in the same line.

It also brings back another memory; once Swamiji was traveling with Swami Satyananda on a bullock cart from Radhanagar to an ashram of Tripurary Har (disciple of Moti Lal Mukherjee, disciple of Sriyukteswar) in the Midnapore district of West Bengal.

(Once Sriyukteswar tried to prevent Yogananda from starting his proposed Yogoda Sat Sanga Society (YSS) in 1935-36 since he already had one (SRF) in U.S. and Sriyukteswar was giving him the Sadhu Sobha. At the insistence of Yogananda, as a last resort, Sriyukteswar forecasted that he was seeing the litigation over his hermitages. Still he was not able to prevent Yogananda. Because of Sriyukteswar's forecast of litigation, when Satyananda became the third President of Sadhu Sobha, he was extra careful about Puri Asram. Once Satyananda said to Swamiji, "It will be a failure, if during my life time the litigation takes place." That is why once he sent his disciple, Swami Ushananda also known as Swami Hariharananda who had a legal background – not to be confused with Puri's Hariharananda.

(For the same reason, because of Swamiji's legal background, Satyananda proposed once to send Swamiji there also to avoid litigation).

Being alone with Swamiji in the bullock cart (and we had to travel about eight miles), Satyananda suddenly on his own began to tell the true history of Karar Asram (Puri Asram). It was known as Karar Ashram because Sriyukteswar's family last name was Karar.

Swamiji immediately objected, "I am not at all interested to listen to the history of that ashram."

Swami Satyananda, disciple of Sriyukteswar, the Asram Swami of the Karar Asram, Puri, and the third president of Sadhu Sobha, gently said, "You have grown up. You should know the real history of the Puri Asram. It is necessary."

Satyananda's words came back to Swamiji when Mr. Banamali Das, joint general secretary of YSS, approached Swamiji at their headquarters, Dakshineswar Calcutta, to know about Puri Asram. Swamiji happened to be there by chance as the other joint general secretary, Swami Shantananda (American), arranged a meeting with Swamiji and their visiting president (Sister Daya – American) from the United States.

Mr. Das introduced himself and said, "Swamiji! I am told that you were associated with Swami Satyananda, the third president of Sadhu Sobha, a long twenty years, that is why I want a history of the Puri Asram of Sriyukteswar. We are having problems with Swami Hariharananda."

Swamiji said, "Yes, I remembered once Satyanandaji told me on his own about the Puri Asram, I had to listen reluctantly. Mr. Das! You are an eminent Barrister-at-Law, now, currently you are advocate general of the government of West Bengal. You know very well Sriyukeswar's forecast of litigation is there. The same set of people are involved in both the independently registered organizations: Sadhu Sobha and Yogoda. It does not mean Yogoda owns Sabhu Sobha. I am sorry to tell you and also you know very well your case is weak."

Later, *The Science of Self Realization* (*Kriya Yoga*) was published as the "*Kriya Sutras of Babaji*" together with three Yoga treatises: the *Yoga Sutras* by Yogi Patanjali, the *Yogopadesh* by Yogi Parasara (the father of Vyasa), and the *Yoga Rahasyam* by Yogi Dattatreya.

However, the *Kriya Sutras* part is translated into many international languages from the original Sanskrit. Such as – Bengali, Hindi, English, French, German, Italian, Spanish, Russian, Japanese and Chinese.

Under the instruction of Mahamuni Babaji, in the meantime, Swamiji Maharaj has translated the *Kriya* interpretation of the *Bhagavad Gita* by Lahiri Mahasay (*Kriya* disciple of Babaji), originally written in Bengali into English and Hindi.

After initiating Swamiji into *Purna Kriya* in 1980 and commissioning him to establish the Original *Kriya* in 1981, Mahamuni Babaji sent Swami Satyeswarananda to the United States in 1982.

Swamiji landed in the United States with a few books and manuscripts, not knowing anyone and, having no friends.

Chapter 1

Reasons For Starting The Sanskrit Classics, Self Publishing

The Sanskrit Classics is founded in 1984 by Swami Satyeswarananda Maharaj

Having arrived in the United States of America, Swami Satyeswarananda Vidyaratna Babaji Maharaj (in short Swamiji Maharaj or Baba) mentioned to a devotee that he was supposed to publish some writings of spiritual interpretations as he was instructed to by Mahamuni Babaji in the Himalayas. So the devotee asked his literary agent, a Harvard graduate, Bill Gladstone, whose father owned a publishing company to contact some publishers.

The agent suggested that since the manuscripts and the writing were on the eastern spiritual scriptures, it would be difficult to open the market. As a practical matter, there should be **first** some books on the biographies of these spiritual masters to open the market; thereafter, to consider introducing the scriptural books.

Swamiji wrote two books in two months. The titles were *Babaji, the Divine Himalayan Yogi* and *Lahiri Mahasay* and presented them to the agent. As a result, he received offers from some reputed publishers (among them was Inner Tradition from New York) who were interested in publishing them.

Commentaries Series

Kriya Sutras of Babaji

Kriya Sutras of Babaji, the Divine Himalayan Yogi
Yoga Sutras of Patanjali, the Founding Father of Yoga
Yoga Upades by Yogi Parasara, the Father of Yogi Vyasa
Yoga Rahasyam by Yogi Dattatreya, an Incarnation of Lord Siva

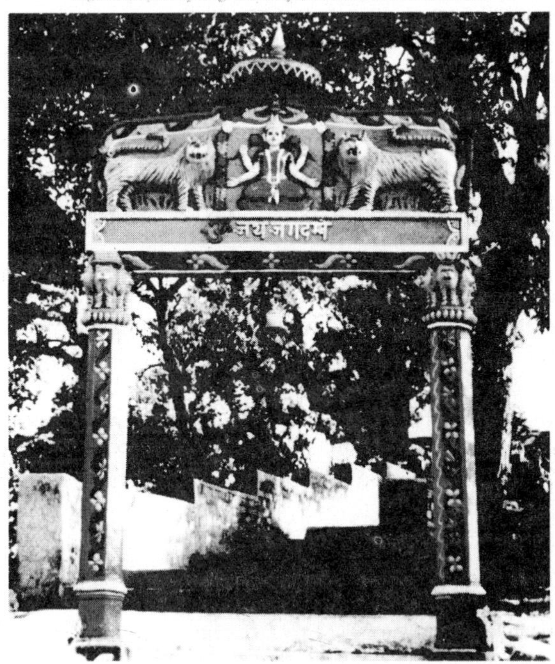

Temple Shrine of Divine Mother, Vaisnabi Mata, Bhagavati Jagadamba, Dunagiri Hill, Himalayas.

By Swami Satyeswarananda Giri Babaji, the Himalayan Yogi Vedantist.

(Once, in the young days of the present author (sixth grade – class VI) in the hermitage, under the direction of Babaji, Lahiri Mahasay possessed the right hand of the present author to communicate with him the message of Babaji. The rest of the body was in command of the author, but not the right hand. Putting a pen between the index finger and the middle finger of the right hand, by the way, which became a bit stiff, when the questions were asked, the right hand wrote the answers in brief which was the message of Babaji. Lahiri Mahasay used the same right hand of the present author again to write his predicted biography (*Biography of Lahiri Mahasay*); as well as to translate into English his complete works (*Kriya* interpretations of 26 books of Indian scriptures in four volumes) from the original Bengali.

(Thus it was the present author who was destined to write the predicted "Biography of Lahiri Mahasay," which the author wrote in 1983 and published in 1984 in the United States, as predicted by Lahiri Mahasay.)

The publishers expressed that since the writings were from an Indian gentleman they would have to edit the materials for better presentation. Mahaṛaj-ji immediately realized that he could not publish his writings with the American publishers. He did not want to compromise at all or give them the right to edit his writings. He had this strong uncompromising attitude for a valid reason; after all, these were spiritual books that needed to be presented properly.

Publishers in general have the sole interest of making a profit from their investments. Nobody can blame them in that respect; after all, it is a business for them. In that situation, the moment the author signed the contract for royalties, the publishers would own the book and do whatever they thought fit to make it publishable and profitable by their standard, and the author would lose control.

In Maharaj-ji's opinion even the highly reputed publishing companies' intellectual editors are not able to penetrate the vibrations of atoms of inner Light and atoms of inner Sound (OM) of the Letters of the Sanskrit 'words' and 'mantras' emanating and resonating mystic Energy (*Kundalini* Energy) from them.

Aksara: *A* means "No" and *ksara* means "transitory," therefore, *Aksara* literally means not-transitory. *Kutastho akara uchyate. Gita* 15:16

Aksara is called *Kutastha.* In other words, *Aksara* is "ETERNITY" or "IMMORTALITY".

The renowned editors of the publishing companies may be well equipped with their intellectual powers to understand the concepts and meanings of the words and sentences, but they lack the power and insight and have no eyes to see the inner Light of the letters and hear the inner Sound of the words. As a result, they cannot do justice to the presentation of publishing the spiritual books Maharaj-ji wrote.

For example, to an editor or an intellectual for that matter, a word is composed with combinations of letters and is defined as having a meaning, or at least, must be making a concept.

On the contrary, for a Yogi or for a spiritual person, the English word's equivalent in Sanskrit is *Sabda*, which literally means "sound" that comes from the inner Sound (*OM*).

Here the big difference between the intellectuals and the Yogis is the intellectuals tread the path of concept, word, and meanings; while the Yogis and spiritual persons follow the path of vibrations of inner Light and inner Sound from those Letters. As a result, they bypass the intellectual's limitations of concept and meaning (free of playing semantics). The intellectuals on one side and the Yogi and spiritual person on the other side, DEPART in their ways. In fact, they are in two different worlds.

Each odd letter (*Aksara*) of the alphabet contains a smaller degree and number of atoms of inner Light and atoms of inner Sound; while each even number of letters contains a greater degree and number of atoms of inner Light and atoms of inner Sound. The word, therefore, expresses the composite vibrations of inner Light and inner Sound depending on how many odd letters and even letters there are in the word.

(Similarly, a sentence carries the composite degree of vibrations of inner Light and inner Sound depending on how many words are there in a sentence.)

For example, "Sanskrit" is an English word, its equivalent is *Samaskrita*. If the word *Samaskrita* is scanned it will be two words: *Sama* means "Tranquility," and *krita* means "done." Therefore, *Samaskrita* means "the state of Tranquility;" it happens when the restless breath is made tranquil.

So the word *Samaskrita* for a Yogi and spiritual person is the "state of tranquility of the breath;" while for a linguist it is the name of an ancient language and for an intellectual it is merely a word, indicative of an ancient language. From all the words and sentences they want to make a meaningful concept which makes SENSE.

Unfortunately, Spirituality or the Self is beyond all senses including reason and thoughts. That is why the intellectuals call "Spirituality" the world of mystics. Therefore, as far as the intellectuals are concerned, they are BARRED to the spiritual world; until they get *mantras* and till they make the *mantra* conscious (*mantra chaitanya* – making the *mantra* alive by constant practice), they will remain blind and will live in the world of intellectual fools.

How then can the editors of the Western publishing companies and also of Indian Publishing companies do justice in this situation? Certainly they can't.

The internationally famous Indologist publisher - Motilal Banarasidass from New Delhi (Letter dated November 16, 1995 Ref. no. JPJ/USA/295) was interested in publishing Maharaj-ji's books, for the same reason he turned down their proposal.

Later, we will provide the lists of publishers and their correspondences in detail who were interested to publish the writings of Swamiji.

That was the main reason Swami Satyeswarananda Vidyaratna Babaji Maharaj had to start "The Sanskrit Classics," for self publishing in 1984. It becomes imperative to make it clear here that it is a publishing company and NOT a spiritual organization.

The Sanskrit Classics publishes writings on the essential classical scriptures of the Vedic culture, as interpreted in the light of Realization by various Masters of Yoga.

When the self-publications started and the books were in the hands of practitioners of *Kriya*, we received some letters, we produce some of them later.

Chapter 2

The List of Publications

Published Works by Swami Satyeswarananda Maharaj

English

Title	ISBN No.	Year of Publication (YOP)	Out of Print (OP)
1. Kriya Yoga: The Science of Self Realization		1974	OP
2. Lahiri Mahasay: The Father of Kriya Yoga	1-877854-02-6	1984	OP
3. The Commentaries Volume 1	1-877854-08-5	1984	OP
4. Babaji: The Divine Himalayan Yogi (First Edition)	1-877854-01-8	1984	OP
5. The Only Bible	1-877854-05-0	1984	OP
6. Lahiri Mahasay's Personal Letters	1-877854-07-7	1984	OP
7. Kebalananda and Sriyukteswar	1-877854-03-4	1985	OP
8. Lahiri Mahasay: The Father of Kriya Yoga (Revised)	1-877854-02-6	1985	OP
9. Babaji: The Divine Himalayan Yogi (Second Edition)	1-877854-17-4	1985	OP
10. Babaji Vol. 1, Second Edition in 4 audio tapes	SR-63-541	1985	OP
11. Biography of a Yogi (Swami Satyananda) 1st Edition	1-877854-04-2	1985	
12. The Mahabharata: Commentaries Volume 2	1-877854-09-3	1986	
13. Hidden Wisdom	1-877854-10-7	1986	
14. Inner Victory	1-877854-11-5	1987	
15. The Bibles (Gita-Bible-Quran) In the Eye of a Yogi	1-877854-06-9	1988	
16. The Bhagavad Gita – Interpretations of Sriyukteswar	1-877854-12-3	1991	
17. Kriya: Finding the True Path	1-877854-14-X	1991	
18. The Bhagavad Gita: Interpretations of Lahiri Mahasay	1-877854-16-6	1991	
19. Babaji Volume 2 Lahiri Mahasay, Polestar of Kriya	1-877854-13-1	1991	OP
20. Babaji Volume 1 (Third Edition)	1-877854-17-4	1992	OP
21. Babaji: Volume 3 Masters of Original Kriya	1-877854-18-2	1992	
22. The Upanisads Volume 3	1-877854-19-0	1992	
23. The Mahabharata Vol. 1 Stories of the Great Epic	1-877854-24-7	1993	
24. Kriya Sutras of Babaji	1-877854-27-1	1994	
25. Sriyukteswar: A Biography	1-877854-28-X	1994	
26. The Holy Bible- In the Light of Kriya (3RD Edition)	1-877854-23-9	1994	
27. The Divine Incarnation: Sri Panchanan Bhattacharya	1-877854-30-1	1996	
28. The Dhammapada: The Path of Dharma	1-877854-20-4	1996	
29. Babaji and His Legacy (Revised Fourth Edition)	1-877854-31-X	2002	
30. Biography of a Yogi (Revised Second Edition)	1-877854-26-3	2002	
31. Essence of Kriya (Pocket Book)	1-877854-38-7	2004	
32. The Original Kriya (Revised Second edition of Kriya)	1-877854-42-5	2005	
33. The Eternal Silence ...Synthesis of All Dharma Paths	1-877854-41-7	2006	
34. The Mahabharata (Two Volumes in One)	1-877854-43-3	2006	

Title	ISBN No.	Year of Publication (YOP)	Out of Print (OP)
Lahiri Mahasay's Complete Works (Set in 4 Volumes)			
35. The Gitas and Sanghitas – Volume 1	1-877854-36-0	2006	
36. Chandi and the Other Scriptures – Volume 2	1-877854-39-7	2006	
37. The Upanisads (Revised Second Edition) Volume 3	1-877854-44-1	2006	
38. The Six Systems (Revised Second Edition) Volume 4	1-877854-45-X	2006	
39. Mahamuni Babaji & His Legacy (Revised 5th Edition)	1-877854-34-4	2008	
40. Yogacharya Sri Sri Panchanan Bhattacharya	1-877854-48-4	2010	
41. The Ultimate Book – Yoga Vasistha – Synthesis of Yoga Vedanta (Set in 2 Volumes)	978-1-877854-50-7	2011	
42. The Journey of a Himalayan Hermit	978-1-877854-49-1	2012	
43. Suddenly Silence .... Atmastha	978-1-877854-51-4	2014	
44. Siva Sanghita, Six Centers, Brahma Sanghita	978-1-877854-52-1	2014	
45. The Kriya Sutras (Eleven languages)	978-1-877854-54-5	2014	

Bengali

Title	ISBN No.	YOP	OP
46. The Bhagavad Gita of Lahiri Mahasay's Original Bengali Interpretations		1981	
47. Vedic Chanting & Kriya Masters songs, audio Tape	SR-64-698	1985	OP
48. Devotional Songs in Sanskrit, audio tape	SR-64-699	1985	OP
49. Satha Chakra (Six Centers Drawing)	VA-333-582	1989	
50. Kriya Ganga	1-877854-21-2	1998	
51. The Bhagavad Gita of Lahiri Mahasay's Original Bengali Interpretations	1-877854-25-5	2003	
52. Babaji O Tnar Parampara	1-877854-33-6	2004	
53. Kriyasar (Pocket Book)	1-877854-39-5	2004	
54. Kriya Ganga (Hard Cover)	1-877854-40-9	2008	

Hindi

Title	ISBN No.	YOP	OP
55. Dunagiri Hill Himalayas (Pamphlet)		1981	
56. Babaji - Himalaya Ke Dibya Yogi	978-1-877854-46-0	2013	
57. Bhagavad Gita – Interpretation of Lahiri Mahasay	978-1-877854-35-4	2013	

German

58. Die Kriya Sutras des Babaji 1-877854-29-8 1994

Spanish

59. Kriya Sutras de Babaji 1-877854-22-0 1994

Chinese

60. The Kriya Sutraṣ 1-877854-47-6 2010

History of Publications of Swami Satyeswarananda Maharaj

	ISBN Number	Out of Print (OP)
1974		
1. Kriya Yoga: The Science of Self Realization		OP
1981		
2. The Bhagavad Gita (Lahiri Mahasay's Original Kriya Interpretation in Bengali)		OP
3. Dunagiri Hill, Himalayas (Pamphlet in Hindi)		**OP**
1984		
4. Babaji: The Divine Himalayan Yogi	1-877854-01-8	OP
5. Lahiri Mahasay: The Father of Kriya Yoga	1-877854-02-6	OP
6. Commentaries Volume 1	1-877854-08-5	OP
7. The Only Bible (in the Light of Kriya)	1-877854-05-0	OP
8. Lahiri Mahasay's (L.M.) Personal Letters (Original Bengali with English Translation)	1-877854-07-7	OP
1985		
9. Kebalananda and Sriyukteswar	1-877854-03-4	OP
10. Lahiri Mahasay (Revised Edition)	1-877854-02-6	OP
11. Babaji: The Divine Himalayan Yogi (2nd)	1-877854-17-4	OP
12. Babaji (Vol,1) Audio Tape	SR-63-541	OP
13. Vedic Chanting Audio Tape	SR-64-698	OP
14. Devotional Songs Audio Tape	SR-64-699	OP
15. Biography of a Yogi (Swami Satyananda)	1-877854-04-2	
1986		
16. The Mahabharata Commentaries Volume 2	1-877854-09-3	
17. Hidden Wisdom (with 6 books of L.M.)	1-877854-10-7	

1989

18. Satha Chakra (Six Center Drawing)	VA-333-582	

1991

19. The Bhagavad Gita - Sriyukteswar	1-877854-12-3	
20. Kriya: Finding the True Path	1-877854-14-X	
21. The Bhagavad Gita - Lahiri Mahasay	1-877854-16-6	
22. Babaji Volume 2 Lahiri Mahasay	1-877854-13-1	OP

1992

23. Babaji Volume 1 3rd Edition	1-877854-17-4	OP
24. Babaji Volume 3 Master of Original Kriya	1-877854-18-2	
25. The Upanisads Volume 3	1-877854-19-0	

1993

26. The Mahabharata Volume 1 Stories of the Great Epic	1-877854-24-7	

1994

27. Kriya Sutras of Babaji	1-877854-27-1	
28. Sriyukteswar - A Biography	1-877854-28-X	
29. The Holy Bible: In the Light of Kriya	1-877854-23-9	
30. Die Kriya Sutras des Babaji (German)	1-877854-29-8	
31. Kriya Sutras de Babaji (Spanish)	1-877854-22-0	

1996

32. The Divine Incarnation of Sri Panchanan Bhattacharya	1-877854-30-1	

1997

33. Inner Victory (with 3 Books of L.M.)	1-877854-11-5	

1998

34.The Bibles: (Gita, Bible, and Quran In the Eye of a Yogi)	1-877854-06-9
35. Kriya Ganga (Bengali)	1-877854-21-2

2002

36. Babaji and His Legacy (4th Edition)	1-877854-31-X
37. Biography of a Yogi (Revised 2nd Edition)	1-877854-26-3

2003

38. The Bhagavad Gita (Bengali of L.M.)	1-877854-25-5

2004

39. Babaji O Tnar Parampara (Bengali)	1-877854-33-6
40. Kriyasar (Bengali Pocket Book)	1-877854-39-5
41. Essence of Kriya (Pocket book)	1-877854-38-7

2005

42. The Original Kriya (Re 2nd Edn. of Kriya)	1-877854-42-5
43. Kriya Ganga (Bengali)	

2006

44. The Eternal Silence ... Synthesis of All Dharma Paths	1-877854-41-7
45. The Mahabharata (Two Volumes in One)	1-877854-43-3

Lahiri Mahasay's Complete Works (Set in 4 Volumes)

46. The Gitas and Sanghitas Volume 1	1-877854-36-0
47. Chandi and the Other Scriptures - Vol. 2	1-877854-39-7
48. The Upanisads (Revised 2nd Edn) Vol. 3	1-877854-44-1
49. The Six Systems (Revised 2nd Edn) Vol. 4	1-877854-45-X

2008

50. Babaji and His Legacy (Revised 5th Edition)	1-877854-34-4
51. Kriya Ganga (Bengali)	1-877854-40-9

2010

52. Yogacharya Sri Sri Panchanan Bhattacharya 1-877854-48-4
53. The Kriya Sutras (Chinese) 1-877854-47-6

2011

54. The Ultimate Book - Yoga Vasistha
    Synthesis of Yoga Vedanta (Set in 2 Vol.) 978-1-877854-50-7

2012

55. The Journey of a Himalayan Hermit 978-1-877854-49-1

2013

56. Babaji - Himalaya Ke Dibya Yogi (Hindi) 978-1-877854-46-0
57. The Bhagavad Gita (Lahiri Mahasay, Hindi) 9781-877854-35-4

2014

58. Suddenly Silence ... Atmastha
    (The Substance Yoga Vasistha) 978-1-877854-51-4
59. The Siva Sanghita, Brahma Sanghita 978-1-877854-52-1
60. The Kriya Sutras (Eleven Languages) 978-1-877854-54-5

Chapter 3

Letters of Encouragement

The following two letters are part of eighty-one (81) letters written by Swami Satyananda Giri to the author during his monastic training from 1950 to 1971. All of the eighty-one (81) letters are published in the title "*Biography of a Yogi*" in the second edition.

Swami Satyananda Giri was initiated by Hangsa Swami Kebalananda and he was the chief monastic disciple and spiritual successor of Swami Sriyukteswar Giri in India.

Satyananda lived in the hermitages at the Karar Asram, Puri (from 1919 to 1921), at Ranchi (from 1922 to 1941), and at Sevayatan (from 1943 to 1971). When he was not at the hermitage, he would go around the country to help spiritual seekers from these hermitages and to visit the other branches. He was a divine yogi, poet, musician, educationist and philanthropist.

Satyananda held multiple positions and responsibilities as follows: He was appointed "Asram Swami" (the monk of the hermitage) at Puri Karar Asram in 1921 by Sriyukteswar. During the years 1922 to 1941, he was the principal of Ranchi Brahma-charya Vidyalaya (school). He was the founder and Executive Secretary-General of Yogoda Sat Sanga (YSS) Society of India (1936 to 1941). He was a life member of YSS and the third president of Sadhu Sova (from 1952 to 1971), a society of Swamis, founded by his mentor, Swami Sriyukteswar. In addition, he was the first president (from 1953 to 1971) of Sat Sang Mission, Sevayatan (*Seva* means "service," *ayatan* means "house"; *Sevayatan*, then, means "Service Center"). The hermitage, Sevayatan, where Satyananda lived the last twenty-seven years of his life, offers many programs, such as a postgraduate teacher training college, junior technical school, boys' high school, basic education for boys, junior high school for girls, hospital with outdoor and indoor facilities, library, press, and a yoga temple. Some of these programs are financially sponsored by the State Government of West Bengal. The institutions mentioned are residential.

The author started his monastic training under Satyananda during his teen years, simultaneously continuing to study for eight years at Satyananda's brother disciple Paramhansa Yogananda's hermitage, YSS. Satyananda was asked specifically by Babaji, the divine Himalayan Yogi, to train young Satyeswarananda, the author, in *Kriya* and to give appropriate monastic training. Later, the author lived several years with Babaji in the Himalayas to study further intricacies of *Kriya* Science.

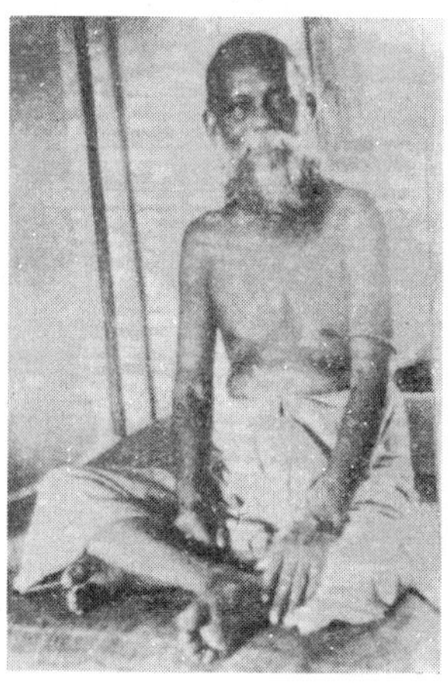

Swami Satyananda, the President of Sevayatan

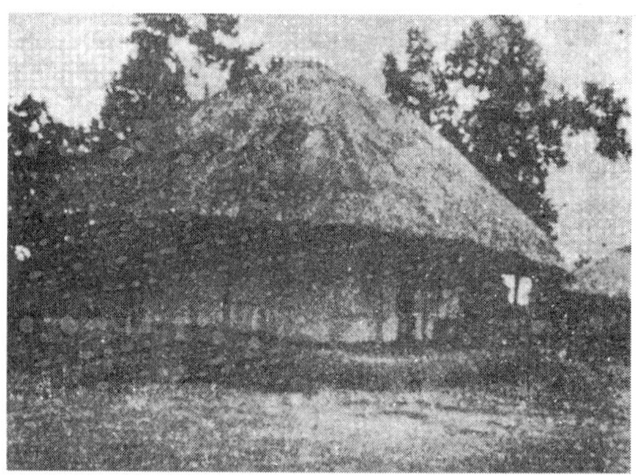

The thatched made hut of Swami Satyananda in the hermitage where Swami Satyeswarananda lived with him during the monastic training.

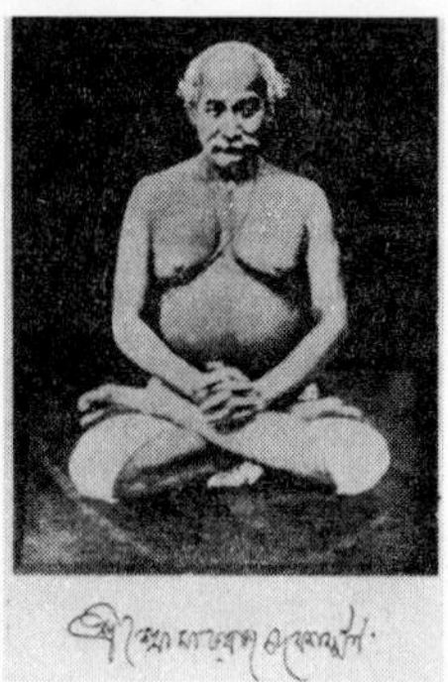

Yogiraj Sri Sri Shyama Charan Lahiri Mahasay

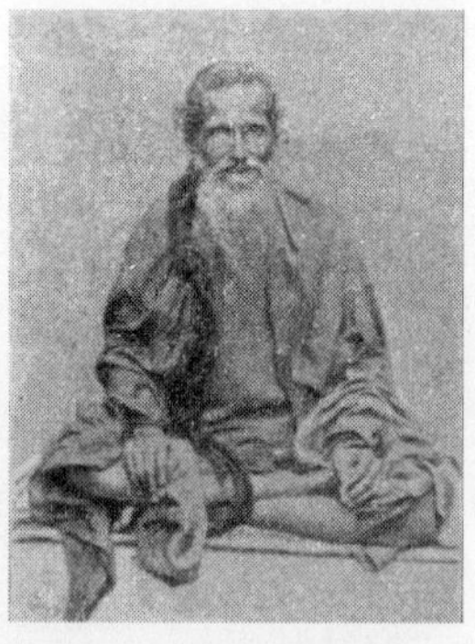

Hangsa Swami Kebalananda

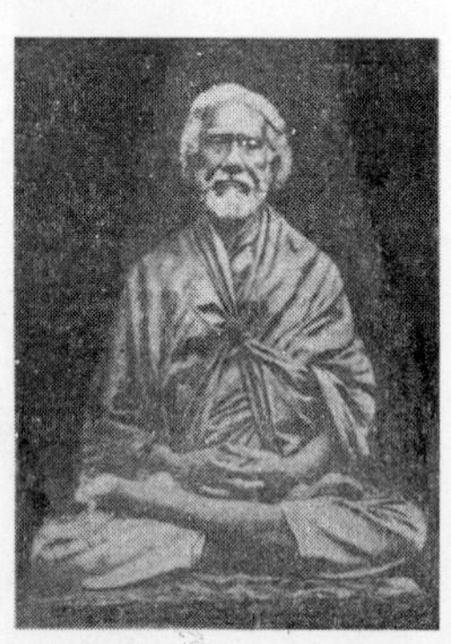

Swami Sriyukteswar

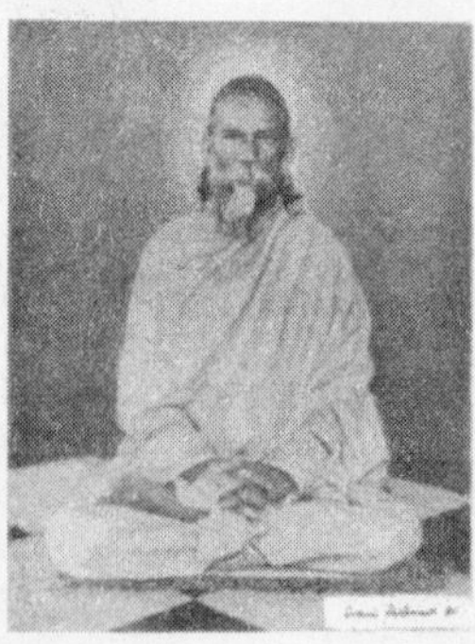

Swami Satyananda Giri Maharaj, President of Sevayatan,
Initiated by Hangsa Swami Kebalananda and
the chief monastic disciple of Swami Sriyukteswar Giri in India

The Hand Written Letter of Swami Satyananda to the Author

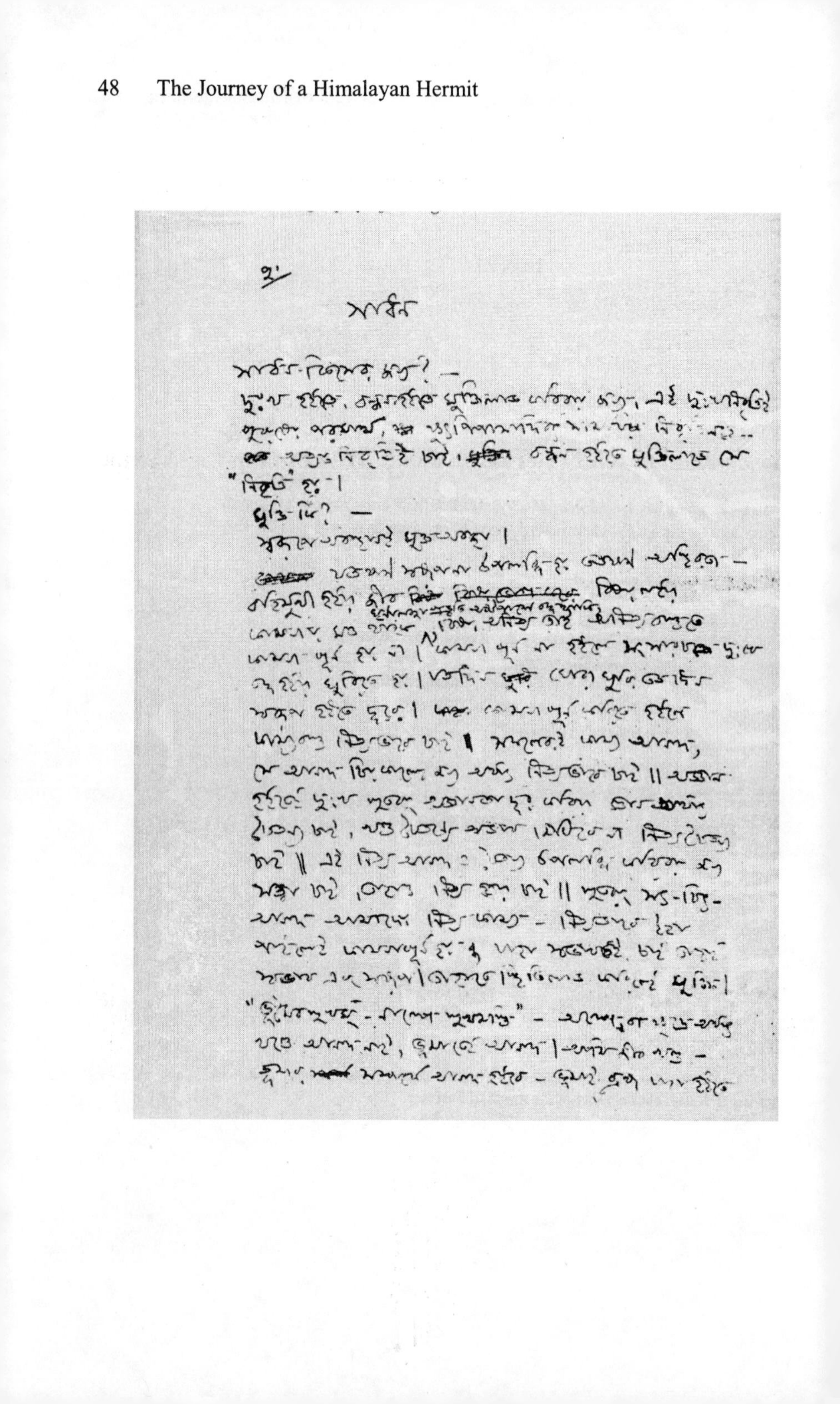

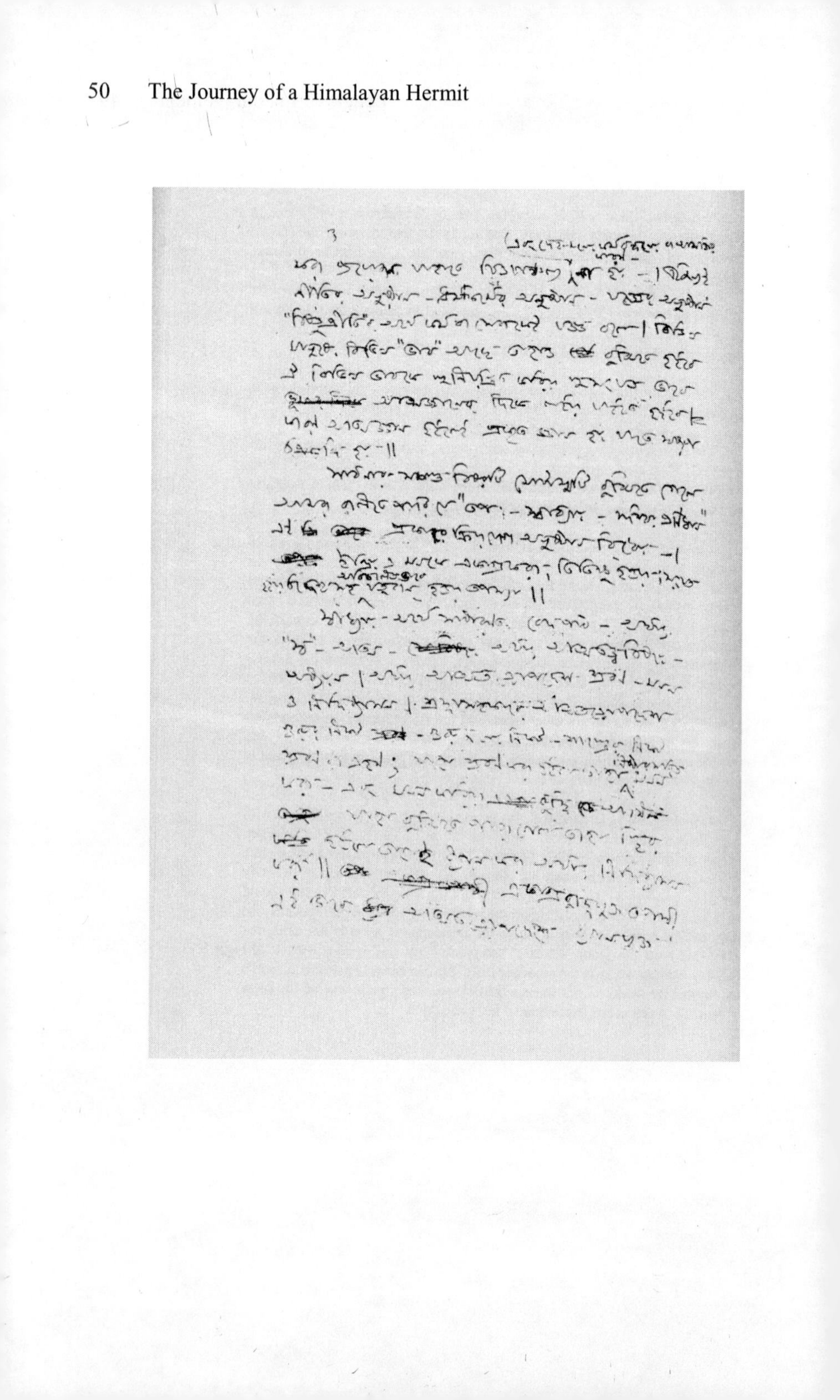

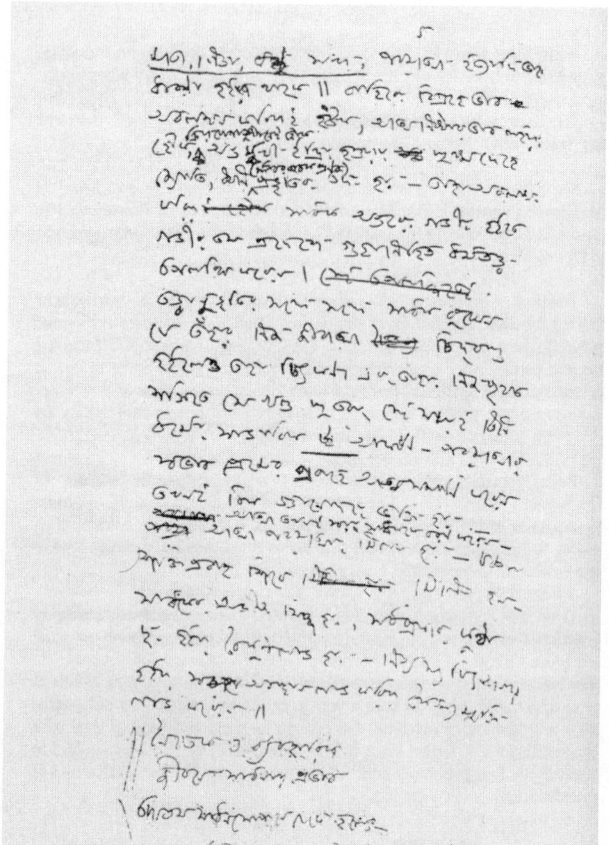

The English Version of the Handwritten Bengali Letter to the Author (*Brahmachari*) by Swami Satyananda

Om

Sevayatan
January 26, 1959

Kalyaniyesu, "Affectionate One,"
Brahmachari Bholanath,

Study attentively. Pay attention to the study of Sanskrit. You will be able to study the scriptures only if you learn Sanskrit very well.

I am going to Jabbalpore, Madhya Pradesh [Central Province]. I will return here on the Sri Panchami Day.[1] I cannot say exactly when I will be able to go to visit you.

You have to sit for the examination and do well in the test.

Let that abundance of welfare make abundant welfare for you.

Suvamastu ("All is well here.")
Satyananda Giri

---

1. *Sri Panchami* literally means the Holy Fifth Day of the lunar circle. It is not any fifth day, but only that of the month of February.

On this day, people throughout India generally worship the Divine Mother, Saraswati, the Goddess of learning, knowledge, music and tuning. It is a public holy day. All the schools, colleges, universities, libraries have a holiday, yet the students and the teachers attend the campus to worship Saraswati, the Goddess of Knowledge. The ordinary public also worship Saraswati, the Goddess of Knowledge, in their private homes.

Hangsa Swami Kebalananda was born on this day.

Enclosures:

Sadhana

[On Meditation]

Why should one practice *Sadhana*, meditation?

To be *nivrittva*, free, from sorrows and bondages. This *nivrittvi*, cessation of sorrows, is the *paramartha*, supreme attainment, for the *purusa*, or the self or man. This *nivrittvi*, cessation, is not temporary like having food and drink to prevent hunger and thirst. It must be *atyanta nivrittvi*, permanent cessation of sorrows. Becoming free from the bondages, one attains that state of "*Nivrittvi*."

What is *Mukti*, Liberation?

Swarupe abasthan, "to be established in one's true form," is the state of *Muktabastha*, the state of freedom.

As long as one does not realize one's own form, one is restless. The *jiva* [individual being] being outwards, and being attached, madly holds onto the *bisaya* [material objects]. The *jiva* puts himself into eight types of bondage like *lajja* [the sense of being ashamed], *ghrina* [hatred] etc.

Worldly objects are *anitya* [transitory]; that is why the desires are not completely fulfilled by them. Until the *kamanas* [desires] are permanently and completely satisfied, one has to wander in the whirlpool of the world being in bondage with sorrows and suffering [due to attachments to those transitory things, such as love, affection, name and fame, etc.].

As long as wandering continues, one is far away from *Swarup*, one's own true form [*Swa* means "Self" and *rup* means "form," so *Swarup* actually means "the form of the Self."

In other words, till one realizes the Self, one has to wander aimlessly in life for happiness.]

To satisfy the *kamanas* [desires] the object of desire must be *Nitya* [Permanent]. The desire of all is to have *ananda* [bliss]. That attainment of bliss or beatitude must be forever; that is, one has to receive the state of bliss permanently.

From *ajnan* [ignorance] *dukha* [sorrows] develop. Therefore, one needs *Jnana* [Knowledge], that is, one needs Consciousness. The *khanda chaitanya* [the relative consciousness], will not be able to satisfy desires. It has to be *Nitya Chaitanya* [pure, permanent, and absolute Consciousness]. To realize this *Nitya Ananda* [permanent Bliss], and Nitya Chaitanya [permanent Consciousness] one needs a *Sattva*, "the Substance," "the Truth." That too has to be *Nitya* [Permanent].

Therefore, *Sat*, *Chit*, and *Ananda* [respectively, Truth, Consciousness, and Bliss] is our desire forever. When we receive them permanently, our desires become fulfilled completely.

Swabhab [*Swa* means "Self" and *bhab* means "sentiment" or "nature."] That which is desired naturally is *Swabhab* and *Swarup* ["the true form of the Self"]. When one achieves the state of *Sthiti* ["Tranquility" of the Self], one attains the state of *Mukti* [Liberation].

Bhumaiba sukham nalpe sukhamasti, "There is no bliss in having a little or in something limited; that is, there is no bliss in *khanda*, or relative bliss. One attains bliss only in *Bhuma*, that is, the Absolute or the Infinite. [The average people think] that I am a *jiva*, a relative little one. The state of bliss will occur when one is attuned in Oneness with *Bhuma*, which is *Brahma*, the supreme Self - greater than That there is nothing.

That *Brihat*, Great Self, is called the form of *Satchidananda*, or *Iswara*, in the scriptures. To attain this state, that is, to be free to attain the eternal realization of *Brahma*, the ultimate Self, one needs to practice *Sadhana*, meditation.

No one can attain That state of Consciousness by putting the attention of the mind outwards because the objects outside in the world are *chanchal* [restless], *khanda* [relative] and *anitya* [transitory].

Till one forsakes *Chanchalata* [restlessness], *ajnanata* [ignorance] never is removed, nor are the bondages of *astapash* [the eightfold bondages].

The restlessness disappears when one focuses inside being inwards, and this is natural. Therefore, the first duty is to bring the mind from outside to inside. For this reason one has to obey and practice the *bidhi nisedh*: *bidhi* is *avyas*, or "practice," and *nisedh* is *vairagya*, "renunciation."

Yama [restraint] and *niyama* [observing and obeying the rules] should be practiced; to sit tranquilly one needs *asana* [steady posture]; to tranquilize the restless *Prana* [breath], one needs to practice *pranayam*; that by which the senses become inwards is *pratyahara*, [interiorization]; when one is inwards, then *Sthirata* ["Tranquility"] generates and one becomes *Sarbavyapi* [all-pervading]. Therefore, one receives *dharana* [a glimpse of Tranquility] that is pervading within myself too. Even the scripture says, *Iswara sarbabhutanang hritdese* [*Arjuna*] *tisthati*, "Iswara, God, the creator, lives in every heart." [*Bhagavad Gita* 18:61]. When one meditates or practices *dhyana*, on that *dharana*, then *Samadhi* generates, that is, *Yoga*.

In other words, all the restlessnesses are transcended; being free from bondages and being in One with the *Satchidananda* [Truth, Consciousness, and Bliss], one attains the *Paramatma* [the supreme Self] and is established in the *Brahmi Sthiti* [in the state of eternal Tranquility].

Generally, we understand that the *jiva* is considered to be constituted with three: *deha*, *mana* and *atma* [body, mind and the self.]

Therefore, it is necessary to have the development of all these three. Their development should take place in such a way that the bondage will be cut off. The development of the body should be in a way so that it enriches the mind; the mental development should be in such a way so that it will enrich the self, or *atma*.

Therefore, regulating the body and the mind one needs to move the development towards the *atma*, the self. One must not ignore the body and mind. For this reason, even in the ordinary worldly works in the mundane daily life, one needs to perform in such a way so that the works do not increase restlessness and do not become the cause of bondage of action and attachment of body and mind.

For this reason, the practice of *Niti* [rules], *Dharma* [righteousness] and *Karma* [action], and the practice of *Jagya* [ritual performances] are necessary. For the *Visnupriti*, "love for Lord Visnu," *Karma* [action] and *Seva* [service] are called *jagya* [performance of formal action of righteousness].

Understanding that many men have many minds or sentiments, one has to regulate those many sentiments and being restrained one has to direct those sentiments towards one's attainment of Self-Knowledge. Only by attaining Self-Knowledge does one truly receive perfect Knowledge and thereby realize one's true *Swarup*, the form or nature of one's true Self.

Generally, to understand the whole thing in brief, we can say that *tapa* [austerities], *swadhyaya* [self-study], and *Iswar pranidhan* [surrendering the self to *Iswara*, the Lord] is the prescription to practice *Kriya Yoga.*

Tapa or *tapasya* is to make the senses and the mind *ekagra* [concentrated] in one point; to become *titikshu* [steady in austerities]; to be *sangjata* [restrained], and to make oneself steady in practice.

Swadhyaya generally means reading *Vedas*, that is, *Swa*, the *atma* or self, and *adhyaya* means study regarding the subject matter of the Self. In other words, one needs to have *sravan* [hearing], *manan* [analyzing], and *nididhasan* [surrendering] on the advice regarding the Self.

One must listen to and receive the advice with reverence from the *Guru*, one who is like a *Guru*, and from the scriptures. One must make *manan*, or sincerely analyze advice from whatever source one has heard it and received it; and whatever is understood after analyzing, being *Sthira* [tranquil] one must make *dhyana* [meditate on it], in other words, practice *nididhyasan.*

The one-pointed *tapaswi* [serious seeker] would meditate on the advice regarding the Self, and he would walk on the path of self-development.

With this, there is *Iswar pranidhan* [self-surrender] or *Brahmanidhan* [surrendering to Lord *Brahma*, the ultimate Self].

We learn about Iswara from the mouth of the *Guru* and from the environment; again, by ourselves we gain indirect knowledge.

Satchidananda Bigraha [the form of Truth, Consciousness and Bliss] is vast. *Bhuma* [Vast] is Iswara [the Lord]. He is described as Paramatma [the supreme Self], Brahma [the ultimate Self], Pita [the divine Father] or Jagadamba [the Divine Mother].

The taste of Iswara takes place in me for a while. I do not have a headache [craving] for That which I have not tasted. During all these activities and wanderings here and there when just for a moment *Sthirata* [Tranquility] generates, particularly during waking in the morning and before going to bed, at least for a moment whatever state [of Consciousness] takes place or sometimes being attuned with tuning [rhythms of Tranquility], just for a while, I receive the taste of that state [of Consciousness, or Tranquility].

Being tranquil within, gradually the realization of the essence of Consciousness takes place. The knowledge of *Sat* or the essence of Truth, Consciousness and Bliss reveal and generate. At that time truly *Satchidananda Bigraha*, "true form of Truth, Consciousness and Bliss," are tasted and realized or true surrender, *Iswar pranidhan*, takes place.

[This was a rough draft of the enclosures. Observing the character of Satyananda's writing one can easily imagine that he has written his personal experiences. He was a man of reserved personality. As mentioned before, the author was associated with him for twenty years. It was very uncharacteristic of him to admit such things in such a way as he did in the last two paragraphs. That is why the author imagines that perhaps he wanted to write a final draft before mailing this letter but since he was pressured for time, he just mailed to the author the first and rough draft. However, as a result, this admission was revealed and known to the world.]

Because of many different sentiments in many *jivas*, this assimilation of surrendering to Iswara takes different shapes: *Mata* [Divine Mother], *Pita* [Divine Father], *Sakha* [Divine Friend], Paramatma [the Supreme Self], etc. Sentiment generates [and one becomes aware of Consciousness accordingly.]

Whether by adopting the external image of a deity, by sincerely holding onto the Self, or by practicing *Kriya Yoga*, when the senses become interiorized in *sukshma dehe* [in the subtle body], then *Jyoti* [inner Light], *Dhwani* [inner Sound], *Iswaravachaka Pranav* [Iswara as an embodiment of inner sound, *Om*] are revealed within. Adopting those, or holding onto those, the seeker realizes the essence of *Dharma*, Righteousness, in the deeper regions, in the cave of Consciousness [in between the eyebrows.]

During this time of understanding the essence of Truth, the seeker understands that his *jivatma* is merely an object of *chidbastu* [Divine Consciousness]; yet this *jivatma* is but a grain of sand and it is by its separate energy a relatively small one. Therefore, at that time, because of the natural attraction of *Dharma*, righteousness, the seeker surrenders at the current of natural love of *Paramatma* [the supreme Self].

At that time, with the revelation of true Knowledge, *Bhakti* [devotion] generates. Then the *atma*, [the self] itself, accepts the *sadhaka* [seeker]. The Oneness union between *atma* [the self] and the *Paramatma* [supreme Self] takes place. The flow of restless *Sakti* [energy] unites with Siva, "Tranquility." The seeker attains the *avista* [the desired goal in life]. Removing all *kuntha* [worries] he attains *Vaikuntha* [the sphere of Lord Visnu]. Being *Nitya* [Eternal], *Sat*

[Truth], *Chit* [Consciousness], *Anandamoy* [Blissful], establishing Oneself in *Swarup* [in the true form of Self], he attains the state of *Kaibalya* [the Eternal state of Tranquility, or the Natural state].

You have to realize the influence of *Sadhana* [meditation] in your moral and practical life. You have to rise to the highest State. Prepare yourself through the integrated development of body, mind and self.

[The advice of the above paragraph and the enclosures with this letter were to prepare the mind of the author to take the next serious step in life to be a young *Brahmachari*].

Suvamastu ("All is well here.")
Satyananda Giri

Swami Satyananda Giri's Handwritten Letter in Bengali Addressed to the Author

ওঁ

সেবায়তন
১৭-৬-৭১

কল্যাণীয়েষু,-

ব্রহ্মচারী জেমস, - তোমার 11.6. এবং 15.6.
২খানা পত্র পেয়েছি।

তোমার মনের দ্বিধা দূর হয়েছে জেনে একটু নিশ্চিন্ত
হয়েছি। [illegible] যাত্রা ও [illegible] গেলো।

[illegible] দেখে গেছে। [illegible]
[illegible] [illegible] [illegible] হবে। [illegible]
[illegible] পারছি না।

ইন্দুর খুব অবসাদ। - M.A. result এবং
অন্যান্য পরীক্ষা-ব্যস্ত সে উদ্বেগমনা।

=

যে দিন থেকে আমার "জেমস" সম্বন্ধে
একটা খুব মনে [illegible]। - তুমি দিন দিন আমার-
তোমার অন্যান্য জীবন সম্পর্কে- [illegible] আমার
নির্দেশ-পালনের জন্য প্রস্তুত হচ্ছ এবং কোনো vague
বা অস্পষ্ট ভাব না রেখে, মুখোমুখী- না হয়ে- সবই
খুলেই বলতে পারছ।

মনে পড়ছে তুমি ৮-৯ [illegible] আগে
সময় তুমি ব্রহ্মচারীর পথে যাবার জন্য ছুটে এসেছিলে,
আমি তোমাকে [illegible] করতে দেরি করেছি, তবু মনঃ

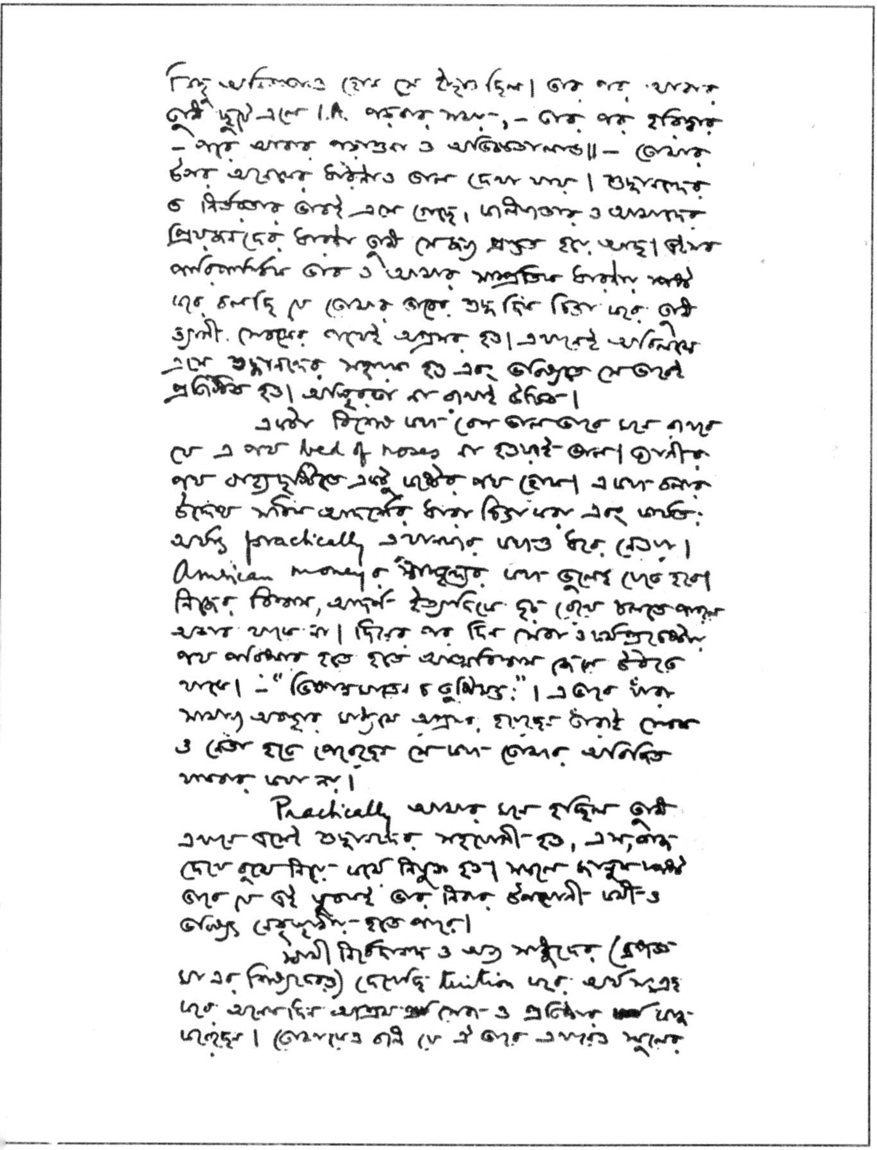

[illegible — handwritten Bengali letter, four paragraphs; legible Latin-script words include "I.A.", "bed of roses", "practically", "American money", "Practically", "tuition"]

[illegible] train-এ [illegible]
[illegible] ([illegible]) [illegible]
স্বামী [illegible]
[illegible]
[illegible] statement ছিল "[illegible]
[illegible]"। [illegible]
স্বামী [illegible]
[illegible]
[illegible]
[illegible]
[illegible] স্বামী-[illegible]
[illegible]
[illegible]।

আমি [illegible]
[illegible]
[illegible]
[illegible] "[illegible]" [illegible]। "[illegible]
[illegible]"। [illegible]
[illegible]। [illegible] qualified
[illegible] ([illegible],
[illegible]
[illegible]) [illegible]
[illegible]
[illegible]। [illegible]।
[illegible]
[illegible]
[illegible]
[illegible]। — [illegible]।

[illegible]। [illegible]
[illegible]
[illegible]।

[illegible]।
[illegible] ইতি—

[illegible]

English Translation of Satyananda's Handwritten Letter

OM

Sevayatan
June 17, 1967

Kalyaniyesu, "Affectionate One,"
Brahmachari Bhola,
I received your recent two letters dated June 11 and 15, 1967.

I am relieved to hear the news that your father is doing better. I received the information of Lakhanpur.

Subodh has gone to his village. Khokan is here. On the 21st of June Suddhananda will go to Goramahal [Subodh's village where he will attend the annual function of the asram; once the author was there with Satyananda and met Jyoti Midya, a music teacher, disciple of Yogananda]. I cannot say what Khokan [Gautam Mazumder] will do. I heard about Ivu [Iva Mazumder].[1] As if there is worry about the M.A. and other Examinations.

* * * * *

---

1. Iva Mazumder is Satyananda's niece and the sister of Khokan [Gautam Mazumder]. Iva from Y.S.S. Girl's school at Lakhanpur sat in the school examination that year, and her parents in Calcutta were worried about the results. This was another reason why Satyananda had suggested in the previous letter that the author visit Lakhanpur and find out news about the result of Iva's final examination from her school there.

Satyananda also heard news regarding the M.A. examination from the devotees who appeared as external candidates. The University of Calcutta had introduced a new system of evaluation of the answer scripts at the recommendation of the Head of the Department of philosophy from that particular year on. That was the reason why the publication of the results of the M.A. in philosophy were delayed and that created concern for some students who appeared in that year, including friends of the author and disciples of Satyananda.

In the last couple of weeks, your thoughts were thrilling, very deep in my heart, since you had asked my instructions regarding your future course of life-style, requesting me to answer you very clearly, beyond all confusion and vagueness.

I recalled in my mind you came to me from the hermitage of Paramhansa Yogananda when you were studying in the eighth grade and proposed to enter the order of *Brahmachari* and renunciate (*Tyagi*) lifestyle. I sent you back to the hermitage of P. Yogananda with the purpose in mind that you could study and gain experiences there.

Thereafter, again you came to me while you were an Intermediate Arts (I.A.) student (at the Wellesley Missionary College).

Then you went to Haridwar (in the Himalayas); thereafter, you again started your study and acquired experiences.

Many devotees have a good impression of you. Suddhananda (Swami Suddhananda Giri, the General Secretary, Sevayatan) has already decided to depend on you.

All of us here and the devotees of our Calcutta center have this understanding that you are prepared for this great responsibility.

Under these circumstances, I tell you clearly my recent considered opinion and understanding. Knowing the purity of your heart, I say you had better enter into the lifestyle of a renunciate (*Tyagi*) and a servant (*Sevaka*) of all.

Come to Sevayatan immediately, become an assistant of Suddhananda, and be established thus in your future. There should be no restlessness or confusion about this.

Please keep in mind always one important point: The path of a renunciate should not be a bed of roses. Let the path of a renunciate (*Tyagi*) apparently be a hard path. The aim of this statement is to cause you to think and to remind you of the exact nature of idealism and, practically, to understand the present situation here in the hermitage. Forget about the generous donation of American money.[1]

---

1. The hermitage used to receive generous donations from the *Kriyanwits* from the United States

If you can generate faith and idealism and be steady and determined, then there will be no problem. Day after day, through sincere service and consistent working efforts, gradually the path becomes clearer, and self reliance starts revealing from within.

"He is happy who is contented only with his alms."

[Remember the famous statement of the first Sankaracharya].

Those who started working under such circumstances became servants and spiritual leaders. This is also known to you.

Practically, I was thinking, you had better come here and be an assistant to Suddhananda. Please come, see, realize, decide and engage yourself in your works.

Let all the devotees know that this young man is qualified to take all the responsibilities and to be the future spiritual leader.

I have seen Swami Nirvedananda and other Swamis (disciples of Brahmagya Ma) teach private students to earn money to pay the bills of the hermitage. I advise you in the same way: You can teach students here and earn money to serve the hermitage (including yourself).

We (Swami Yogananda and others) earned money for a long time at Ranchi School in this way while we were renunciates. We had the statement that "We are taking money in exchange for labor for the maintenance of the hermitage." Revered Swami Sriyukteswar Giri Maharaj advised us this way. Thus we were able to keep the prestige of the hermitage by working with other teachers. About the later development of the organization, you have heard from me. Swami Bidyananda also went to teach with this attitude of service and renunciation.

After deep contemplation for a couple of weeks and knowing Suddhananda's mind clearly, today, I wish to inform you of this clear and firm decision. Generally speaking, having the blessings of the *Sri Guru* (the Lord) upon your head, jump on the path, removing "shyness, hatred, and fear."

"If you want to be great, then you must know how to be small (humble)." You also were preparing yourself in the same direction.

You are educated (qualified); therefore, your assigned works would be: working for the Mission, assisting Suddhananda, earning money for the hermitage and for yourself, including finding the ways and means to finance the Mission, etc. Nobody will admonish you; rather, you will be admired as a resident of the hermitage. This will increase our honor.

If there is self-confidence and self-respect based on sincere service and true spirit of renunciation, then the seeker can proceed on the path of idealism and be a perfect worker and a Yogi (*Tapaswi*). Reason also supports this way of service. By your enthusiasm, my enthusiasm will increase.

I told you about my heart's desire. All the members of our Calcutta center will know about it and will encourage you.

This body is in a fair way. May the Lord bless you.

Sincerely,
Signed: Satyananda Giri

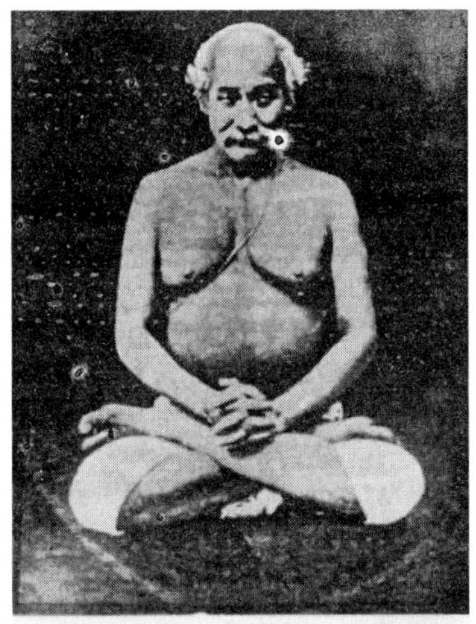

Yogiraj Sri Sri Shyama Charan
Lahiri Mahasay

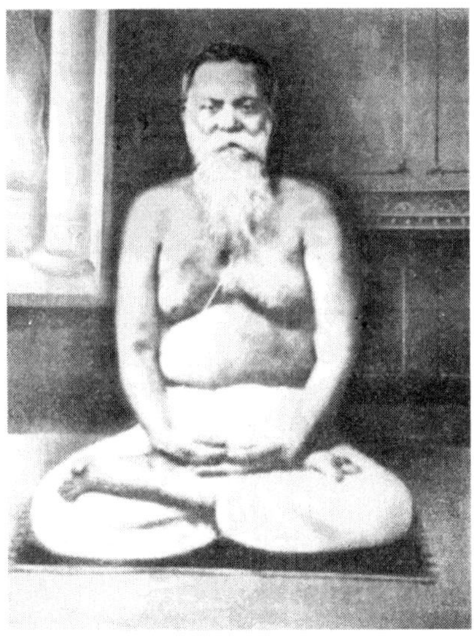

Bhupendranath Sanyal, Disciple of Lahiri Mahasay

The following three (3) letters are of twenty six (26) letters in English and in Bengali that Sunil Kumar Ghosh, attorney, wrote to Swamiji from 1982 to 1996.

Sunil Kumar Ghosh was a disciple of Bhupendranath Sanyal (Lahiri Mahasay's disciple), secretary of *Bhratri Sangha* (Fraternity of Brotherhood among the disciples of Bhupendranath Sanyal founded after Sanyal Mahasay left body in 1962).

Sunil Kumar Ghosh was a good friend of the author. Till he left body, he kept up a correspondence with Swamiji.

Swamiji was anticipating he may leave the body and may not be able to see the last publication of ours. At that time two books were in the press.

1) "The Divine Incarnation of Sri Sri Panchanan Bhattacharya", and
2) "The Dhammapada, the Path of Dharma."

So Swamiji Maharaj sent to Sunil Babu "the content pages" of the forthcoming book "The Divine Incarnation of Sri Sri Panchanan Bhattacharya." So, in case if he leaves the body, at least, he would be able to see the content of the title "The Divine Incarnation of Sri Sri Panchanan Bhattacharya." When Swamiji informed him earlier that he was writing a comprehensive biography of Sri Sri Panchanan Bhattacharya under the sudden instruction of the higher power, he expressed his interest to see it when it will be published. It was very important for him.

As a matter of fact, Sunil Babu himself wrote an article on Sri Sri Panchanan Bhattacharya at that time and published the article in their quarterly *Kriya* magazine, *Bilwadal,* of which he was the editor. Swamiji's anticipation was correct. He left the body just about three weeks before the two books arrived. His elder son, Santanu Kumar Ghosh, a Chartered Accountant (C.P.A.), informed Swamiji. Santanu's letter is reproduced here.

NOTE – **The Complete Works of Lahiri Mahasay** referred to in the following letter of Mr. Sunil Kumar Ghosh to the author, have been translated into English for the first time and published. All twenty six (26) classical books of Indian scriptures, interpreted in Bengali by Lahiri Mahasay in the light of *Kriya*, have been translated into English from the original Bengali (except for three chapters of *Vedanta Darsan*), for the **first time** and published in hard cover (set in four volumes) by Swami Satyeswarananda Maharaj for the service of the world.

Mr. S. K. Ghosh's Handwritten Letter to the Author

SUNIL KUMAR GHOSH, M.A., B.L.
ADVOCATE.: HIGH COURT & SUPREME COURT

Office:
8, OLD POST OFFICE STREET &
HIGH COURT BAR ASCN.
ROOM NO. 5.
CALCUTTA

Residence:
PHONE: 54-4047
48/2, RAMTANU BOSE LANE

Calcutta 6......30th Sept......1990.

Swami Satyeswarananda Giri.
P.O. Box 5368
San Diego. CA 92165 U.S.A.

Sraddheya Swamiji,

After a long time I have been favoured with your kind blessing on 24.9.90. Yes, I was a bit worried for not getting any news of yours for a long time though I anticipated that it may be 'Silence' on your part for some reason. Now I am glad that you are quite O.K. and are completing Sri Sri Lahiry Mahasay's remaining works by translating into English. This task is not only a huge one but very difficult and laborious and expensive too. I rarely find any other saintly or holy person so much practical and at the same time so much loving as ~~him~~ our Lahiry Mahasay. The future world will judge ~~the~~ and appreciate the great job you have done for the benefit of all mankind.

I am now running 80 and so gradually becoming unfit to shoulder heavy responsibilities.

I humbly pray to Them for your long life and success and well.

My Bijoya Pronam to you.

Yours Sincerely.

Sunil Kumar Ghosh.

Sunil Kumar Ghosh, M.A., B.L.
Advocate, High Court & Supreme Court
48/2 Ramtanu Bose Lane, Calcutta- 700006

30th September, 1990

Swami Satyeswarananda Giri
P.O. Box 5368
San Diego, CA 92165
U.S.A.

Sraddheya [Respected] Swamiji,

After a long time I have been favoured with your kind blessing on 24.9.90.

Yes, I was a bit worried for not getting any news of yours for a long time though I anticipated that it may be 'Silence' on your part for some reason.

Now I am glad that you are quite O.K. and are completing Sri Sri Lahiri Mahasay's remaining works by translating into English. This task is not only huge one but very difficult and laborious and expensive too.

I rarely find any other saintly or holy person so much practical and at the same time so much loving as our Lahiri Mahasay.

The future world will judge and appreciate the great job you have done for the benefit of all mankind. I am now running so and so gradually becoming unfit to shoulder heavy responsibilities.

I humbly pray to Him for your long life and success and well.

Yours Sincerely,
s/d Sunil Kumar Ghosh

PS: My *Bijoya Pranam* to You. S.G.

[*Bijoya Pranam* - It is a traditional salute, showing respect, at the end of Divine Mother's worship (victory of Goddess Durga over Mahisasura, the king of anti-gods, the *asuras*) in October at Bengal.

[Sunil Kumar Ghosh, disciple of Bhupendranath Sanyal Mahasay (disciple of Lahiri Mahasay) was an attorney at Calcutta High Court and Supreme Court of India, the editor of *Bilwadal Patrika*, a Bengali quarterly magazine devoted in *Kriya*, secretary of *Bhratri Sanga*, Association of Brotherhood, among the disciples of Bhupendranath Sanyal, a personal friend of the author].

Jay Paramgurudeva Yogiraj Sri Sri Shyamacharan Lahiry.
Jay Gurudeva Yogacharya Sri Sri Bhupendra Nath Sanyal.

GURUDHAM BHRATRI SANGHA

(Established 1962)

BILWADAL PATRIKA

Phone : 54-4047 Office-48/2, Ramtanu Bose Lane

Calcutta-6 20th Dec. 1982.

Respected Swamiji —

Thanks for your letter received by me on 10.12.82. I am very happy to learn that you are propagating the great messages of Sri Sri Lahiry Mahasaya, a family man becoming a Saint. He always bestowed invaluable Kriyas which are nothing but various Stages of steps to know One's Self from within, without taking anything in return of money etc. Greed has taken many a faked sadhus to foreign countries only to cheat the foreigners and to bring bad name to our Country and the Yogis. I am glad that your attempts are appreciated.

Re: Books of Sri Sri Lahiry Mahasaya, I have got only a few books viz:

1. Astavakra Samhita — which as you know is being published in Series in our Journal Bilwadal. It is still continuing. As I have got the only copy it is not possible to send it to you now. You will find

2

it already printed in last issues of Pathwaral.

2. Linga Puran — this is also being now published in our said Journal (see last two issues). Few pages are still to be published. It is in handwriting.

3. Taittiriya Upanishad — I am sending a copy now.

4. Kabir Gita — A copy of same is also being sent now. This is all for the present. A few of other books, even if they are with any person, they will not part with them as these are not now available. Even if they are available they will have to be copied.

Your task is undoubtedly a difficult one. Because the subject is too technical and literal translations of many words such as Kutastha, Linga Puran etc will bring disaster. Appropriate words shall have to be chosen to carry the proper sense.

I learn that you got a copy of "Unknown Life of Jesus Christ' by Nikolas Notovich. Perhaps you have seen my article in our Journal—"Unknown living in India for 16 years by Jesus Christ in

Jay Paramgurudeva Yogiraj Sri Sri Shyamacharan Lahiry.
Jay Gurudeva Yogacharya Sri Sri Bhupendra Nath Sanyal.

GURUDHAM BHRATRI SANGHA

(Established 1962)

BILWADAL PATRIKA

Phone : 54-4047 Office-48/2, Ramtanu Bose Lane

- 2 - Calcutta-6..................19......

search of Truth!" in Bengali. Collections from several books are given including those from Notovich's book. I shall be happy to have a copy of same if possible.

Americans are highly scientifically developed people and mostly good men. Thanks to Swami Vivekananda. They have enough of 3 W's viz - Wealth, Wine & Women but yet they are not happy. They require the Supreme Bliss 'Ananda' after which no further quest for happiness will be required. Because of their scientific achievments, matter and mind have come very closer separated only by a screen of materialism. ~~The~~ Learned people with slight effort can remove this screen and see the unseen hand working behind this screen. Churches, temples and mosques etc help only as a preliminary step in Believing. Hope I am not wrong. With Pronams & wishing you all success. Yours sincerely

Sunil Kumar Ghosh.

Gurudham Bhratri Sangha and Bilwadal Patrika

Office - 48/2 Ramatanu Bose Lane
OM Calcutta - 6
Dec 20, 1982

Respected Swamiji,

Thanks for your letter received by me on 10.12.82 [Dec 10, 1982]. I am very happy to learn that you are propagating the great messages of Sri Lahiri Mahasay, a family man becoming a saint. He always bestowed invaluable *Kriya* which are nothing but various stages of steps to know one's Self from within, without taking anything in return e,g. money etc. Greed has taken many a faked *Sadhu* [renunciate] to foreign countries only to cheat the foreigners and to bring bad name to our country and the Yogis. I am glad that your attempts are appreciated.

Re: Books of Sri Sri Lahiri Mahasay - I have got only a few books viz:

1. *Astrabakra Sanghita* - which you know is being published in series in our journal Bilwadal. It is still continuing. As I have got the only copy it is not possible to send to you now. You will find it already printed in last issues of *Bilwdal*.

2. *Linga Puran* - This is also being now published in our said journal (see last two issues). Few pages are still to be printed. It is in handwriting.

3. *Taittiriya Upanisad* - I am sending a copy now.

4. *Kabir Gita* - A copy of same is also being sent now. This is all for the present. A few of other books, even if they are with any person, they will not part with them as there are not now available. Even if they are available they will have to be copied.

Your task is undoubtedly a difficult one. Beacuse the subject is too technical and literal translation of many words such as *Kutastha*, *Linga Puran* etc., will bring disaster. Appropriate words shall have to be chosen to carry the proper sense.

I learn that you got a copy of *Unkown Life of Jesus Christ* by Nicolas Notovich. Perhaps you have seen my article in our journal - "*Unkown living in India for 16 years by Jesus Christ in Search of Truth*" in Bengali. Collection from several books are given including those from Notivich's book. I shall be happy to have a copy of same if possible.

Americans are highly scientifically developed people and mostly good ones. Thanks to Swami Vivekananda. They have enough of 3 W's viz - Wealth, Wine, & Women but yet they are not happy. They require the supreme Bliss "*Ananda*" after which no further quest for happiness will be required. Because of their scientific achievements, matter and mind have come very close separated only by a screen of materialism. Learned people with slight effort can remove this screen. Churches, Temples, and Mosques etc help only as a preliminary step in Believing. Hope I am not wrong.

With *Pronam* [bowing, traditionally] and wishing you all success.

Yours Sincerely,

Sunil Kumar Ghosh.

हवाई पत्र
Aerogramme

5.00 भारत INDIA

Srimat Swami Satyeswarananda Giri
3763 1/2 35th Street
San Diego. California 92104
U.S.A.

SECOND FOLD

In india
the festival never ends
Department of Tourism
Government of India

भेजने वाले का नाम और पता:-
Sender's Name and Address:-

Sunil Kumar Ghosh
48/2 Ramtanu Bose Lane.
Calcutta-6 India

इस पत्र के अन्दर कुछ न रखिये
No Enclosures Allowed

FIRST FOLD

48/2 Ramkanu Bose Lane.
Cal-6. 15-11-86

Param Sraddheya Swamiji —

Please accept our Subha Bejoya Pronams to your esteemed self and love and greetings to all others. May all be happy.

I have received the 2nd Copy of your English version of Mahabharata and Gita sent by Sea Mail, a few days ago. As I was indisposed for a few days, I could not write earlier.

I hope you have received Bilwadal Patrika 21st vol sent to you about 25th Aug. '86 by Air Mail. If not, please let me know it.

I am slowly reading your above book. It is needless to say that the presentation is very beautiful. It is an unique Job performed by yourself.

I have come to Cal. a few days ago after performing Sri Sri Durga Puja at my village home. A law book viz Land Acquisition Act, 7th Edn, written and edited by me, is recently published with success. Another book viz - Law of Benami Transactions in India, is in Press. As per your advice I have started writing a Life and Works of Sri Sri Bhupendra N. Sanyal Mahasay, I do not know what will happen with, because I am yet to find helpful surroundings.

— Comment on your Mahabharata will be published in 22nd vol of Bilwadal.

May God give you His blessings and a long life.

Yours sincerely.
Sunil Kumar Ghosh.

OM

48/2 Ramtanu Bose Lane
Cal - 6
15/11/86 [Nov. 15, 1986]

Param Sradheya Swamiji [supremely respectable Swamiji],

Please accept our *Bijoya Pranams* [traditional bowing or greeting at the victorious day of Goddess of Durga worship offered to each other in Bengal] to your esteemed self and love and greetings to all others. May all be happy.

I have received the 2nd copy of your English version of Mahabharata and Gita sent by sea mail a few days ago. As I was indisposed for a few days, I could not write earlier.

I hope you have received Bilwadal Patrika 21st vol. sent to you about 25th Aug'86 by Air Mail. If not, please let me know it. I am slowly reading your above book. It is needless to say that the presentation is very beautiful. It is an unique job performed by yourself.

I have come to Cal. a few days ago performing Sri Sri Durga Puja [worship of Goddess Durga] in my village home. A law book viz. Law Acquisition Act, 7th edition. written and edited by me, is recently published with success. Another book viz - Law of *Benami* Tranactions in India, is in press.

As per your advice I have started writing a Life and Works of Sri Sri Bhupendranath Sanyal Mahasay. I do not know what will happen to it, because I am yet to find helpful surroundings.

[Previously, in a letter, Sunil Babu mentioned that he wanted to write a book either on Jesus Christ or on Bhupendranath Sanyal, his *Guru*. His question to Swamiji was which of these books Swamiji would suggest him to write. Swamiji replied that on Jesus Christ many books have been written. It would be appropriate to write on Bhupendranath Sanyal since he was his disciple and in Swamiji's opinion Sunil Babu was the right person to write on Sanyal Mahasay.

[Reasons for referring to as "what will happen to it" by Sunil Babu means that since he spent money for publishing his law books, he may not have money left to print the comprehensive biography of Sanyal Mahasay written by him at the suggestion of Swamiji. Perhaps, it was a subtle hint if he could get some assistance from Swamiji in that regards. However, Sunil Babu managed to write in brief a small booklet in English on Bupendranath Sanyal from that comprehensive Bengali manuscript and published it and sent a copy to Swamiji. The cover page of the English booklet is produced here].

Comment on your *Mahabharata* will be published in 22nd vol. of *Bilwadal* [quarterly journal on *Kriya* of which Sunil Babu was the editor].

May God give you His blessings and long life.

Yours Sincerely,

Sunil Kumar Ghosh

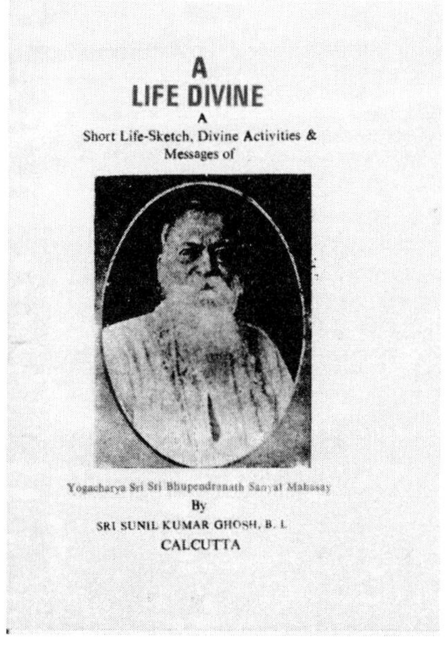

Cover page photo of the booklet
on biography of Sanyal Mahasay by Sunil Kumar Ghosh

To
Swami Satyeshwarananda Giri Babaji Maharaj
The Sanscrit Classics,
P.O Box 5368,
San Diego,
C.A. 92165
USA.

From
Santanu Ghosh,
C/O K.S AIYAR & CO
Chartered Accountants
9,Syed Amir Ali Avenue(4th floor)
Calcutta -700 017 , India
Tel/ Fax 91-33-240-3693 (Off)
Tel 91-33-334-5814 (Res)

Date - February 24,1997

Respected Swamiji Maharaj,

With profound grief and sorrow, I and my brother Shovan K Ghosh beg to inform you that our revered father **Sunil Kumar Ghosh** has left for his heavenly abode on the afternoon of 1st February,1997

While he was not keeping well for some time,particularly after the demise of our revered mother about two and half year's back,but till his last, he was absolutely active. Even on the previous evening he was making the final check up for despatch of the latest issue of Bilwadal In fact after taking his lunch around 1-30 p m he was reading the news paper and at around 3-15 p.m. he suddenly felt breath less and complained of chest pain The Cardiologist attended him within ten minutes but unfortunately nothing could be done.

The previous Sunday i.e 26th January,1997 he called a meeting of the Guru Bhratas/sisters at our ancestral house, where incidentally he requested several persons to take charge of the activities of both the Gurudham Bhratri Sangha as well as publication of Bilwadal in which he had always been taking keen interest and requested the ladies and gentlemen present there, to take appropriate action as he felt that he would not be in a position to continue any further because of his age and health. Nobody realised at that time that, he was probably advising them out of some premonition about which only HE would be knowing.

Since we are aware, that he was having a great personal respect for you and also for your valuable contribution to the international fraternity, my brother and I took the liberty of taking some of your valuable time in writting this letter to you. We apologise for not having informed to you earlier.

We also acknowledge the receipt of two very valuable publications namely 'DHAMMAPADA' and THE DEVINE INCARNATION which reached us day before yesterday

With warm regards and Pranam,

Santanu Ghosh and Shovan Kumar Ghosh

Santanu Ghosh, the eldest son of Sunil Kumar Ghosh
informed Swamiji that his father left body and they received two books

To:
Swami Satyeswarananda Giri Babaji Maharaj
The Sanskrit Classics
P.O. Box 5368
San Diego,
C.A. 92165
U.S.A.

From:
Santanu Ghosh
C\O K.S. AIYAR & CO.
Chatered Accountants
9,Syed Amir Ali Ave (4th floor)
Calcutta - 700 017; India
Tel/Fax 91-33-240-3693 (Off)
Tel. 91-33-334-5814 (Res)

Date February 24, 1997

Respected Swamiji Maharaj,

With profound grief and sorrow, I and my brother Shovan K. Ghosh beg to inform you that our revered father **Sunil Kumar Ghosh** has left his heavenly abode on the afternoon of 1st February, 1997.

While he was not keeping well for some time, particularly after the demise of our revered mother about two and half year's back, but till his last, he was absolutely active. Even on the previous evening he was making the final cheek up for despatch [dispatch] of the latest issue of *Bilwadal*. In fact after taking his lunch around 1-30 p.m. he was reading the news paper and at around 3-15 p.m. he suddenly felt breath less and complained of chest pain. The Cardiologist attended him within ten minutes but unfortunately nothing could be done.

The previous Sunday i.e. 26th January, 1997 he called a meeting of the *Guru Bhratas*/sisters at our ancestral house, where incidentally he requested several persons to take charge of the activities of both the *Gurudham Bhratri Sangha* as well as publication of *Bilwadal* in which he had always been taking keen interest and requested the ladies and gentlemen present there, to take appropriate action as he felt that he would not be in a position to continue any further because of his age and health. Nobody realised at that time that, he was probably advising them out of some premonition about which only HE would be knowing.

Since we are aware, that he was having a great personal respect for you and also for your valuable contribution to the international fraternity, my brother and I took the liberty of taking some of your valuable time in writing this letter to you. We apologise for not having informed to you earlier.

We also acknowledge the receipt of two very valuable publications namely 'DHAMMAPADA' and THE DIVINE INCARNATION which reached us day before yesterday.

With warm regards and *Pranam* [bowing traditionally].
Santanu Ghosh and Shovan Kumar Ghosh

Chapter 4

Letters of Appreciation
From the Hermitages (*Ashrams/Asrams*) and From the *Kriyanwits/Kriyanwitas*

Since Mahamuni Babaji, the Divine Himalayan Yogi, instructed Swami Satyeswarananda in the Himalayas to re-establish the Original *Kriya* by presenting the books with interpretations of Lahiri Mahasay and sent Swamiji to the United States for this purpose, the Sanskrit Classics, the self-publishing firm, was founded by Swamiji and the books were translated and released in English for the first time.

The moment some of the books were published, we sent them to some *Asrams* (hermitages), important *Kriya* persons around whom some *Kriyanwits /Kriyanwitas* gather, communicate, and seek advice from the teacher and the advanced *Kriya* persons so that the wider audience can benefit. Also some were mailed to some friends. When the word was spread in India, some people requested the books and books were sent to them.

Considering the books printed in the United States would be expensive for the Indian devotees to buy and since it was Mahamuni Babaji's instruction to re-establish the Original *Kriya*, Swamiji Maharaj gave the books to them "Free as Gifts."

We mail books to some of them on a regular basis whenever a new book is published and to some when we receive the requests from them. Some of the Asrams (hermitages) and important *Kriya* persons, and friends were regular recipients as follows:

1) Sevayatan Asram (Swami Satyananda's hermitage),
2) Satyayatan Asram, Jaipur, Rajasthan
3) Bindudham Yogasram, Barharwa, S. P. Bihar
4) Bakultola Asram, Howrah

5) Bhratri Sangha, (Sanyal Mahasay's group), Calcutta
6) Lakhanpur Asram,
7) Satyadham Asram,
8) Sevayatan B. Ed. College Library,

Among the individuals:

9) Dr. Sibaram Das,
10) Dr. Devabrata Pal,
11) Harapada Ghosh,
12) Dhiren Shee,
13) Narayan Chandra Guha Thakurata,
14) Madan Mohan Mishra,
15) Bibhuti Bhusan Mondal,
16) Sisir Kumar Chakraborty
17) Pradyot Kumar Das,
18) Dr. Amal Bikas Choudhury,
19) Mr. Sunil Kumar Ghosh, Attorney
20) Prof. Amarendranath Bhattacharya,
21) Karunamoy Bhattacharya,
22) Sibmoy Bhattachaya, and
23) Dr. Girish Chandra Joshi, Uttar Pradesh,
24) Panchan Babu,
25) Basudev Chanda,
26) Amiya Kumar Choudhuri.
27) Amiya Ranjan Sengupta, and
28) Amita Ganguly.

As mentioned in the introduction, in 1974 after receiving the message, the ***Kriya Sutras*** of *Kriya Yoga*, from Mahamuni Babaji, the Divine Himalayan Yogi, in the Himalayas, Swami Satyeswarananda wrote a book in English and the title of the manuscript was "*Kriya.*"

In that book, he wanted to publish a photo of Sri Panchanan Bhattacharya, the chief disciple of Lahiri Mahasay. Accordingly, in 1975, he wrote a letter in English to Sibmoy Bhattacharya, the youngest grandson of Panchanan Bhattacharya. Swamiji knew Panchanan Bhattacharya had two grandsons: Anandamoy Bhattacharya and Sibmoy Bhattacharya, but he did not know that he had three grandsons, the eldest of them was Karunamoy Bhattacharya. So he was totally surprised having his first letter (we are going to produce his three letters later).

Sibmoy Bhattacharya replied that he did not have a good photograph of his grandfather at Deoghar (Bihar, currently Jharkhand), but he would collect it from Calcutta (currently, Kolkata, from their parental home or from the Bakultala Asram, Sivpur, Howrah) and send it later. Since Swamiji wrote him in English (although both were Bengalis) Sibmoy Babu was very curious whether Swamiji was a Bengali or a non-Bengali from north India since the letter was written in English and from the Himalayas. He thought he could be even a non-Bengali. To make sure, he posed a question in his reply - Whether Swamiji happened to be a Bengali?

He also requested to have a copy of the book when published.

Swamiji did not answer, rather waited for the photograph. The photo came in time. Swamiji kept it in his file.

As mentioned in the introduction, an agent (Edith Krispien) tried to find possible publishers for the manuscript "*Kriya*" at the International Book Fair of 1975 in Frankfurt, Germany, but it did not work out.

In the meantime, as per Mahamuni Babaji's instruction, Swamiji arrived in America in 1982. It was also mentioned in the introduction that as per advice of literary agent, Bill Gladstone, before trying the Indian difficult Scriptural Books, the market has to open with the biographies of the wise realized Yogis and sages. Accordingly, Swamiji wrote two books: *Babaji, The Divine Himalayan Yogi* and *Lahiri Mahasay, the Polestar of Kriya* in two months.

When Lahiri Mahasay's biography was published in 1983, in which the photo of Sri Panchanan Bhattacharya was published, a copy of the newly published book was mailed to Sibmoy Bhattacharya as per his request in his letter eight years before.

Several years later in 1983 the author was able to mail from the United States a copy of the newly published title *Lahiri Mahasay* (a biography of the great yogi) to Sibmoy Babu in Deoghar. In it was the photo of Panchanan Bhattacharya he received from him. The author enclosed a note in the package asking if it would be possible to have some copies of the correspondence between Lahiri Mahasay and his grandfather, Panchanan Bhattacharya. Sibmoy Babu did not respond to this note.

Professor Bibhuti Prasanna Sinha, disciple of Nitai Charan Banerjee :

Two years later on December 22, 1985, Swamiji received a phone call out of the blue. The caller (Ashok Kumar Singha, the host of Professor Bibhuti Prasanna Sinha, a SRF student) said that a Professor Bibhuti Prasanna Sinha wanted to talk to Swami Satyeswarananda Giri Maharaj. The moment Ashok Kumar finished the sentence Swamiji heard another voice saying, "Swamiji *Pranam*, I bow to you. I'm Bibhuti Prasanna Sinha. I've a message for you from the grandson of Panchanan Bhattacharya, and I'd like to come to see you. I'm in the United States for just fifteen days, and three days have already passed."

"[Professor Bibhiti Prasanna was an internationally reputed civil engineer and close family friend of Sibmoy Bhattacharya. He visited the United States many times before. He was from Deoghar, the same town where Sibmoy Bhattacharya lived. Prof. Sinha worked for the Government of the State of Bihar. Eventually, he became the chief engineer for the Government of Bihar].

Swamiji said, "What's the message?"

Prof. Sinha said, "I must tell you in person."

Swamiji said, "Actually, it's very short notice. It's difficult to make time on such short notice since I have many appointments."

Prof. Sinha said, "I'm sorry Swamiji. You must be kind and grant my prayer. As I said, I'm only here for a few days. How about Christmas day? Aren't your American Christian devotees busy on that day celebrating?"

Swamiji said, "There is something on that day, too. Maybe an hour can be managed in the afternoon at 1 P.M.

Thus, Prof. Sinha came with his young son and his host (Ashok Kumar Singha, a Yogananda group SRF student) from Los Angeles on Christmas afternoon. After the initial courtesies, Swamiji asked, "What is the message from Bhattacharya's grandson?"

Prof. Sinha said, "Basically, he asked me to meet you and see what you're doing here. Also, I'm to say that for reasons of secrecy until now the letter correspondence between Lahiri Mahasay and Panchanan Bhattacharya has never been released to the public. This is the tradition the family has maintained. However, they are now reconsidering this. They are thinking of releasing some letters of correspondence between Lahiri Mahasay and Panchanan Bhattacharya in a selective way.

"My own father was a disciple of Panchanan Bhattacharya. I too have some letters of Panchanan Bhattacharya written to my father. However, since I don't read Bengali, I cannot read them.

"Actually, it so happened that when your package arrived from the United States with the biography of Lahiri Mahasay I happened to be there with Sibmoy Babu as I had been requested to advise him about the cost and strategies of repairing some old buildings on the Deoghar property. Thus, I watched him open the package and was amazed to see this book of my *Paramesthi Guru* (*Guru's guru's guru's guru*).

"As you can imagine since my mother language is Hindi, I feel handicapped because all the original *Kriya* literature is written in Bengali. Seeing the book title *Lahiri Mahasay* in English was a godsend for me and I understood that at long last I would be able to read about Lahiri Mahasay.

"In brief, my story is this, Swamiji. When I was a young student I was aware of *Kriya* because my father used to practice. He was a disciple of Panchanan Bhattacharya. However, I was busy with my studies. When I grew to be adult and asked my father to initiate me into *Kriya*, he refused, and advised me to take *Kriya* from his friend, Bodhisattva Bhattacharya, Panchanan Bhattacharya's only son.

"[Actually, Prof. Sinha's father got *Kriya* only four years before Panchanan Bhattacharya left body. So he was neither advanced, nor was permitted. How could he initiate Prof. Sinha?]

"So I approached Bodhisattva Bhattacharya one day. He also refused my prayerful request and said, 'Why don't you take *Kriya* from your father? '

"Then I explained to him that I had already approached my father and that it was my father who had referred him to me. But he would not budge. Then I was at a loss. I waited a long time and then approached him again with the same request and the same results. Then both my father and Bodhisattva Bhattacharya left body. I considered myself most unfortunate. *Kriya* was in my own house yet I could not get it from my own father. I did not understand why both had denied me.

"[The relation of *Guru* disciple is eternal. A father can be a well wisher for a son and would do everything for him; but the senior Sinha could not initiate his son as he was not his son's *Guru*. Both Prof. Sinha's father and Boddhisattva Bhattacharya were not permitted to initiate others into *Kriya* at that time].

"When I served our state government (Bihar) I had a responsible position with many eminent engineers working under me. Some of my colleagues advised me to take *Kriya* from Yogoda Sat Sanga where they'd received *Kriya*, but I told them I wasn't interested since I'd heard their *Kriya* was modified. They asked me again and again, but I was looking for someone from Panchanan Bhattacharya's group since my father had been his disciple. I wanted someone who could give me Original *Kriya*.

"[The ancient tradition for imparting spiritual discipline is *Guruvraktagamya* (learning directly from the mouth of a *Guru*). That is why it is called *Upanisad*. *Upa* means "near" and *nisad* means "sitting"; that is, learning sitting near the *Guru* (*padatale*). The tradition is called *Guru-param-para*)].

"In January 1962, when I was here visiting the United States for six weeks, I came to know that a direct disciple of Lahiri Mahasay, Bhupendra Nath Sanyal, was still alive at Mandar Hill, Bhagalpore, Bihar. I thought I could take *Kriya* from him since he was a direct disciple of Lahiri Mahasay and he had also learned from Panchanan Bhattacharya. Thus, I cut short my visit and flew back to India. However, when I arrived there at Mandar Hill, I was told that Sanyal Mahasay had left his body just one week before on January the 18th. It was a tremendous disappointment for me. The next five years I searched for a *Kriya* Yogi of Panchanan Bhattacharya's group. As you know, almost all *Kriya* yogis are Bengali and only a very few of them are non-Bengali. Being a non-Bengali, I felt I was at a disadvantage to seek them out.

"At last after five long years of searching, I found Nitai Charan Banerjee at Howrah in 1967. I went there and approached him for *Kriya* initiation. When he refused me, I was devastated. You can easily imagine my situation.

"However, I did not give up. I continued to look for a *Guru*, but with no result. Another ten years passed. In 1977, I decided to go back to Nitai Charan Banerjee. I approached him again. I begged him for *Kriya*. He was kind this time. He initiated me into *Kriya*, and I felt blessed.

"I said to him, 'Baba! I came to see you in 1967. I wanted *Kriya* from you then. You didn't initiate me then. Will you be kind enough to let me know the reason?'

"Baba simply looked at me and said, 'Your time was not ripe then.'

"The next year I was appointed as Chief Engineer of the entire state of Bihar, a post which is of cabinet ranking. So by virtue of the post, I became a V.I.P. and my life became very busy with heavy responsibilities. I could not find time to make *sat sanga* with my *Guru* Baba who was far away in Bengal. Then another disaster struck me. In 1979, *Guru* Baba left his body. I am still a child creeping on the ground in *Kriya* life. I don't know how I am practicing *Kriya* for there is nobody around to check my *Kriya*.

"Swamiji, are you coming back to India? When will you return? We need you there."

Swamiji said, "You see me here. I am stuck according to *prarabdha* (providence). All these books need to be finished and published."

Saying this, the author pointed to two copies of the title, *Lahiri Mahasay's Personal Letters to Kriya Disciples*, which the author had received a couple of days before from the printer for final inspection before delivery.

Prof. Sinha said, "As I mentioned, Sibmoy Babu is thinking to release some letters."

The author then interjected, "As you can see, I have already published Lahiri Mahasay's personal letters in this title from the collection of Ananda Mohan Lahiri, Lahiri Mahasay's only bachelor grandson out of eight. So at this point in time I am not in need of the letters. It's too late."

Prof. Sinha then asked, "May I have a copy of this (*Lahiri Mahasay's Letters to the Kriya Disciples*)?"

Swamiji replied, "These are the two advance copies sent by the printer for inspection. The other copies will be delivered soon. Leave your address and a copy will be mailed to you."

Prof. Sinha said, "It'll be fine if you mail it to Sibmoy Babu's address at Deoghar."

The moment Prof. Sinha ended his story, his Los Angeles host who was practicing the modified *Kriya* of Yogananda's organization and who had been present during the meeting, suddenly started defending his organization (SRF) and lesson system (Yogananda's Lesson System through mail correspondance).

Prof. Sinha then turned to his host (Ashok Kumar Singha), who happened to be from his home state, Bihar, and said, "Our ancient tradition is to learn Yoga from Master to disciple, having a personal relationship with the Master, and if possible to live with him. There are many intricacies involved here. Look at my case. My own father did not initiate me. Why? Perhaps, neither my father nor Bodhisattva Bhattacharya was my teacher. In spite of their love and affection for me, their hands were tied. They were honest. They did not like to create confusion."

Prof. Sinha's host (Ashok Kumar Singha) then turned to Swamiji and said, "Swamiji! What is your comment on this?"

Swamiji said, "Convince your guest [Prof. Sinha]."

The host said, "At least, because of Yogananda's organization I happened to know you and have your kind *darsan*."

Swamiji said to Professor Sinha, "It's interesting. In 1979 on Christmas day, your brother disciples brought this body to inaugurate the *Samadhi* Temple of your *Guru* Baba. Today you are here, talking about him."

Prof. Sinha said, "Swamiji! I do not know any advanced disciples of my *Guru* Baba. Can you please give me some names and their addresses in Calcutta?"

Swamiji gave Professor Sinha some names and addresses.

Meantime, four hours had passed. It was time to close the meeting. After making *pranam* to Swamiji, the young son of Professor Sinha and his Los Angeles host went out of the house.

Professor Sinha then closed the door and approached Swamiji to check his *Kriya*. He suspected that perhaps he was doing something wrong. Swamiji checked his *Kriya*. He was right in his guess. One *Kriya* he was doing was a bit different. It was corrected.

Thereafter, he left with his host and his son after an almost five hour meeting.

In 2009, After twenty four years (24), Swamiji received a letter from Prof. Bibhuti Prasanna Sinha. It is reproduced here. After going through the letter, Swamiji could not respond. He basically wanted Swamiji's blessing on a

Institute he proposed to start at *Bawan Bigha* (Panchanan Bhattacharya's place) at Deoghar.

He would called it "SPIRIT (Sri Sri Panchanan Institute of Research in Inner Technology)."

As mentioned before, Panchanan Bhattacharya, the chief disciple of Lahiri Mahasay, was a strict disciplinary, and anti-advertisement, a private person. Panchanan Bhattacharya started the Aryya Mission Institution at the advice of his *Guru*, Lahiri Mahasay, to publish his books and to distribute some herbal medicines. There, Bhattacharya Mahasay used to run a high school and some college classes which needed a considerably large space. The school was shifted a few times to different buildings in Calcutta. Having seen this troublesome situation the generous King Jatindra Mohan Tagore, disciple of Bhattacharya, a great philanthropist who made regular contributions to many places considering this as a service to his *Guru*, wanted to buy a building to house his *Guru's* school, the Aryya Mission Institute in a permanent building. King Jatindra Mohan knew his *Guru* very well and thought it would be very difficult to convince his *Guru*, yet, he wanted to try. Accordingly, one day he offered his proposal to Bhattacharya who flatly denied with a comment, "These things [worldly things] are temporary, should not be made permanent." Only a person like Sri Panchanan Bhattacharya could turn down such a proposal.

Swamiji could not answer Prof. Sinha's letter for an obvious reason. There is an "Injunction" of Mahamuni Babaji, also Lahiri Mahasay had prohibited his disciples to start any organization around the *Kriya* teaching. In spite of this Injunction of Babaji, there started organizations like Sriyukteswar's Sadhu Sobha, Yogananda's Self Realization Fellowship Church (SRF) and Yogoda Sat Sanga (YSS). These are started in violation with the Injunction of Babaji Maharaj. Swamiji, following the teaching of Mahamuni Babaji and Lahiri Mahasay does not support organizations and the Institutes around the teachings of *Kriya*. Thus he lives alone and eats self-prepared food (*swapak*).

After realizing the Self, the Yogis and Sages engaged themselves to serve the world in their own ways (The scriptural ref. "*Te prapnubanti mameba sarbabhutahite rata.*" *Bhagavad Gita* 12:4 which means "after realizing, they engaged themselves to serve all the beings in the world".), and from their positions they see sorrows and happiness alike, and a stone and a piece of gold as equal value. (The scriptural ref. "*Samadukhasukha swastha Samalostasama-kanchana*" - *Bhagavad Gita* 14: 24).

Therefore, why would the *Kriya* teachers need organizations and be attached to these worldly things? In Hindi, there is a proverb - *Dal me kuchh kala hai* which means that "there is something wrong in the soup of lentils."

While writing these pages, Swamiji had to look at Prof. Sinha's letter again and found a mistake as well as a comment which generated in his system as follows:

The problem of the objective scientists like Prof. Sinha is they work with the objects outside themselves in the dualistic state. As a result, they cannot reach to the absolute state. The relation of the observer and the object remains in the dualistic state. One cannot achieve absolute Knowledge which is the Self-Knowledge (*Atmajnan*). Knowing everything else except the Self is but ignorance.

On the other hand, the subjective scientist, like a Yogi who meditates on the Subject, the Self, from within and being in the state of Oneness with the formless pure Consciousness, dissolving the existence of the seeking self, the individual, gains the absolute Knowledge or the Self-Knowledge.

The objective scientist wants to objectify the object, like in the mirror he sees his own body on the dualistic plane.

Unfortunately, for the objective scientists, the Self being the formless pure Consciousness simply cannot be objectified like seeing them in the mirror.

Therefore, the objective scientists never could reach to the final state or have absolute realization no matter how they talk about "the X factor," or "The God Particle," because, from the dualistic state one can gain relative knowledge and not the absolute Knowledge; and so the Self, the eternal Truth, remains unknown and unknowable to them.

Only the Yogi, the subjective scientist, meditating on the Subject (the Self) from within, dissolving his meditative character or the character of a seer, merging in the state of Oneness with the Subject within, gains the state of absolute realization, beyond the state of comprehension by words and speech (*abangmanasagochara*) and which is inexplicable (*anirvachaniya*). Thus the Yogi becomes eternally Tranquil (*Sthira*) making himself *Atmastha* (settled within in Oneness, Peace).

The handwritten letter of Prof. Sinha to the Author.

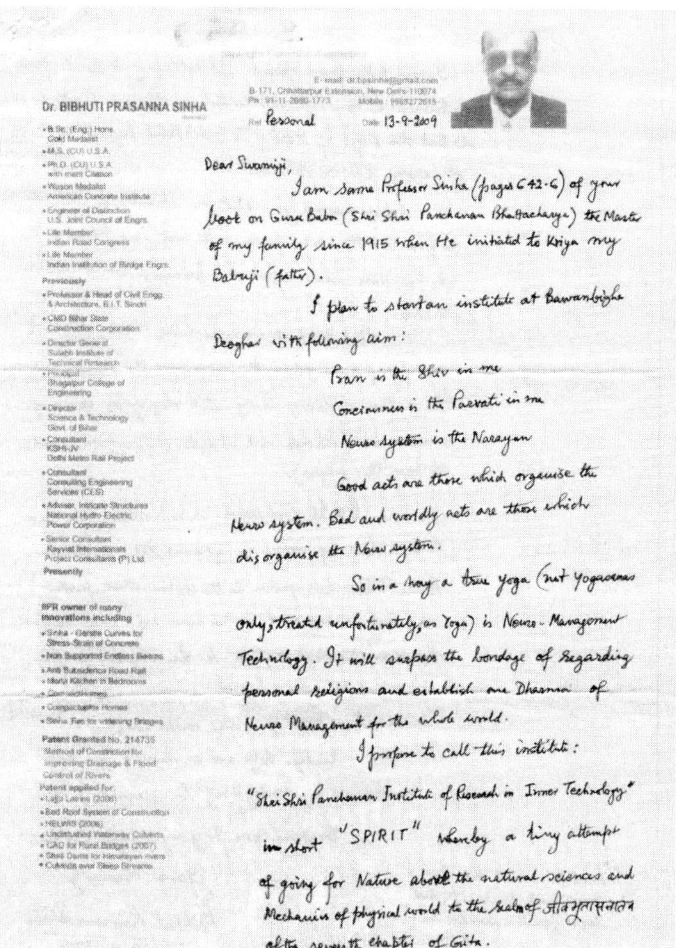

E-mail: dr.bpsinha@gmail.com
B-171, Chhattarpur Extension, New Delhi-110074
Ph: 91-11-2680-1773 Mobile: 9868272615

Dr. BIBHUTI PRASANNA SINHA

- B.Sc. (Engg.) Hons. Gold Medalist
- M.S. (CU) U.S.A.
- Ph.D. (CU) U.S.A. with merit Citation
- Wason Medalist American Concrete Institute
- Engineer of Distinction U.S. Joint Council of Engrs.
- Life Member Indian Road Congress
- Life Member Indian Institution of Bridge Engrs.

Previously

- Professor & Head of Civil Engg. & Architecture, B.I.T. Sindri
- CMD Bihar State Construction Corporation
- Director General Sulabh Institute of Technical Research
- Principal Bhagalpur College of Engineering
- Director Science & Technology Govt. of Bihar
- Consultant KSHI-JV Delhi Metro Rail Project
- Consultant Consulting Engineering Services (CES)
- Adviser, Intricate Structures National Hydro Electric Power Corporation
- Senior Consultant Kayvat Internationals Project Consultants (P) Ltd.

Presently

IPR owner of many innovations including

- Sinha - Gerstle Curves for Stress-Strain of Concrete
- Non Supported Endless Beams
- Anti Subsidence Road Rail
- Mini Kitchen in Bedrooms
- Compactcabins Homes
- Sinha Ties for widening Bridges

Patent Granted No. 214735 Method of Construction for improving Drainage & Flood Control of Rivers

Patent applied for:

- Lajja Lanes (2006)
- Bed Roof System of Construction
- HELWIS (2006)
- Undisturbed Waterway Culverts
- CAD for Rural Bridges (2007)
- Steel Dams for Himalayan rivers
- Culverts over Steep Streams

Ref: Personal Date: 13-9-2009

Dear Swamiji,

I am same Professor Sinha (pages 642-6) of your book on Guru Baba (Shri Shri Panchanan Bhattacharya) the Master of my family since 1915 when He initiated to Kriya my Babuji (father).

I plan to start an institute at Bawanbigha Deoghar with following aim:

Pran is the Shiv in me

Conciousness is the Parvati in me

Neuro system is the Narayan

Good acts are those which organise the Neuro system. Bad and worldly acts are those which disorganise the Neuro system.

So in a way a true yoga (not yogasanas only, treated unfortunately, as Yoga) is Neuro-Management Technology. It will surpass the bondage of regarding personal religions and establish one Dharma of Neuro Management for the whole world.

I propose to call this institute:

"Shri Shri Panchanan Institute of Research in Inner Technology" in short "SPIRIT" whereby a tiny attempt of going for Nature above the natural sciences and Mechanics of physical world to the realm of [illegible] of the seventh chapter of Gita.

P.T.O.

- 2 -

I need help from foreign philothropist to donate fund / instruments of very high order for tests on human's healthy brains so that the ways of Dharma is established beyond the limits of usually known religions.

Babaji, would you give your blessings to these attempts as you are the only person in the west (that I know of) who has done some effort in bringing our Guru Baba to light.

But the best service to him, I think, will be to modify present science to encompass the "Para Prakriti", the nature of living being still obeying the laws of mechanics (though with altogether different mathematics to base this subject).

If Lord says it is Prakriti, there has to be a law by which he governs this Prakrit also. Apara Prakrit has grown to the extent that further so called advancement in this line will only confuse things — the real nature is driving it to go for Para Prakriti where all the answers like the of "Expanding Universe" or "Evolution" etc. would come.

Kindly help me as much as you can by blessings, by propogation, by suggesting etc.

Thanking you for going through this letter.

Yours obediently

Bibhuti Prasanna Sinha
13.9.2009

P.S.: I am interested to know how many people purchased the book. Has it gone to a second edition?
B.P.S.

From:
Dr. Bibhuti Prasanna Sinha 13/9/2009 [September 13, 2009]

Dear Swamiji,

I am same professor Sinha (pages 642-6) of your book on *Guru Baba* (Sri Sri Panchanan Bhattacharya) the master of my family since 1915 when he initiated to *Kriya* my *Babuji* (father).

[Since Prof. Sinha is technology expert and writing about starting an Institute for Inner Technology, let us see if we can point out "technically" something here also. Panchanan Bhattacharya was his father's *Guru* and so his father could call Panchanan Bhattacharya as Guru Baba. However, "technically" speaking Panchanan Bhattacharya Mahasay was not Prof. Sinha's *Guru Baba*.

[Let us figure out the situation, Prof. Sinha's own words in 1985 when he visited Swamiji told that he received *Kriya* from Nitai Charan Banerjee, so technically, Nitai Babu was Prof. Sinha's true *Guru Baba* and not Panchanan Bhattacharya.

[How Prof. Sinha related to Panchanan Bhattacharya on his own technically would be in this order - His Guru's Guru was Bamandev Banerjee (father of Nitai Babu), so he was his *Param Guru*; now, Bamandev Banerjee's *Guru* was Panchanan Bhattacharya, so Bhattacharya Mahasay would be Prof. Sinha's *Parapar Guru*. Hence, Prof. Sinha could call Panchanan Bhattacharya, *Parapar Guru Baba*. That would be technically correct. So one must first learn the basic thing, without it the *Guru-param-para* would be lost].

I plan to start an institute at *Bawanbigha,* Deoghar with following aim:

> *Pran* [life Force] is the Shiva [Lord Siva] in me.
> Consciousness is the Parvati [Consort of Lord Siva] in me.
> Neuro System is the Narayan [Lord Narayan or Visnu].
> Good acts are those which organise the Neuro system. Bad and worldly acts are those which disorganise to Neuro system.

So in a way a true Yoga (not *yogasanas* only, treated unfortunately, as Yoga) is Neuro - Management Technology. It will surpass the bondage of regarding personal religion and establish one Dharma of Neuro Management for the whole world.

I propose to call this institute:

"Shri Shri Panchanan Bhattacharya Institute of Research in Inner Technology" in short "SPIRIT" whereby a tiny attempt of going for Nature above the natural sciences and Mechanics of Physical world to the realm of *Jivabhuta Sanatana* of the seventh chapter of *Gita*.

[Prof. Sinha has quoted one fourth of a verse in the above paragraph from the *Bhagavad Gita* and has referred to a wrong chapter. The verse actually is from the fifteenth chapter and is a part of verse number seven. The full verse is as follows:

[*Mamoubangso jivaloke* ***jivabhuta sanatana.***
[*Manasasthaniindriyani prakritisthani karsati. Bhagavad Gita* 15:7

[He quoted the second half of the first line - ***jivabhuta sanatana.*** It means "the *jiva,* the being is eternal."

[Let us see what it means in the full context of the entire verse: The front part of the first line is - *Mamaiubanhso jivaloke* which means "In the sphere of *jivaloke*, that is, in the individual sphere, the *jiva* is an eternal particle of Me (Lord Krisna)."

[So the entire first line of the verse means "The individual *jiva* is an eternal particle of Lord Krisna in the sphere of the individual (*jiva*)."

[Because of the reference of the word *Jivabhuta sanatan* ("the individual is eternal"), the devotional people love this verse.

[The actual context is the Lord said that in the sphere of individual, the individual is the eternal particle of Me. The very text still involves dualism. The Lord and the particle of Him. It is related to the part and the whole. From this relative situation only the relative knowledge accrues and not the absolute Knowledge.

[Furthermore, from the general point of view, relative knowledge is gained, but from the Vedantic point of view relative knowledge is ignorance].

I need help from foreign philanthropist to donate fund/ instruments of very high order for tests on human healthy brains so that the ways of *Dharma* are established beyond the limits of usually known religion.

Babaji [Swami Satyeswarananda], would you give your blessings to these attempts as you are the only person in the West (that I know of) who has effectively in bringing our *Guru Baba* [Panchanan Bhattacharya] to light.

But the best service to him, I think, will be to modify present scheme to encompass the "*Para Prakriti*" the nature of living being still obeying the laws of mechanics (though with altogether different mathematics to base this subject).

[Prof. Sinha wanted to modify the scheme of *Prakriti* to encompass the *Para Prakriti* (super natural). When Brahma, as per the Vedic scripture (*The Yoga Vasistha Ramayana* - Swamiji released as *The Ultimate Book in the Light of Yoga Vedanta* in two volumes over 2,100 pages putting annotations in some verses from the original Sanskrit texts), starts thinking for creation, from his warmth generates, "Niyati". The moment she was formulated, she took charge of executing the project of creation. She is extremely powerful. She is treated as Divine Mother, the mother of providence of which she is in charge. As a matter of fact, after completing the project, she went to rest in eternal Tranquility (*Sthirattva*). She did not wake up, nor will she, and that is why in the Vedic literature, there is reference to the four *Yugas*: *Satya*, *Treta*, *Dwapara*, and *Kali Yuga*. When these four *Yugas* are completed, it is called a *Kalpa*, that is a day for Brahma. Then Brahma goes to sleep for the night which makes another *Kalpa*. Thereafter, when Brahma wakes up, the creation begins for another *Kalpa*. Thus the things start repeating in this order forever. There is no change, no modification possible. Who is going to change or modify? Nobody can do anything without the permission of Niyati, the mother in charge of providence, not even Brahma. This is how she had designed it. So Brahma, Visnu, Siva and others disappear at the end of the *Kalpa*. They forget everything and at the beginning of the next *Kalpa*, they appear and repeat the same thing.

[Prof. Sinha must know the scheme of Niyati which even Brahma cannot change or modify].

If Lord says it is *Prakriti*, there has to be a law by which he governs this *Prakriti* also. *Apara Prakriti* has grown to the extent that further so called advancement in this line will only confuse things - the real nature is driving it to go for *Para Prakriti* when all the amusers [Sic] like that of "Expanding Universe" or "Evolution" etc,. would come.

[There are laws by which the *prakriti*, the nature, is governed. Prof. Sinha did not pay attention to these or perhaps is unaware. For example, when the fire burns, it goes upwards and never goes downwards; when the water flows, it goes downwards and never goes upwards; when the air moves, it can move in four directions or all directions for that matter. These are the laws of the elements. Plus, the nature is governed by the three qualities (*Gunas*): the divine or the neuter (*satta*), the positive or the active (*rajasa*), and the inactive or the lazy (*tamasa*)].

Kindly help me as much as you can by blessing, by propagation, by suggesting etc.

Thanking you for going through this letter.
Yours obediently,

Bibhuti Prasanna Sinha
13/9/2009

P.S. I am interested to know how many people purchased the book. Has it gone to a second edition?
B.P.S.

Between 1985 and 1992 several books were written and published. (see the list of publications). Accordingly, these were mailed to some hermitages (*asrams*) and *Kriya* practitioners.

Swamiji has a good relation with the Lahiri Family.

1) Starting with Sri Satya Charan Lahiri, grandson of Lahiri Mahasay (will be discussed later),

2) Banamali Lahiri, great grandson, the professor of Chemistry at Benaras Hindu University. Once Banamali Babu knowing Swamiji's legal background and from Calcutta, requested his help in buying a house in his son's name, an executive engineer who works at Calcutta. In those days, there was a disturbing trend going on between the original residents, Hindi speaking people, and the people from the other states at Benares. Banamali Babu's fear was, that even after three generations being born and living there whether they would have to leave Benares and go back to Bengal. Swamiji said that he did not have any connection with the worldly affairs but he would think what could be done.

(Initially, Banamali Babu did not like to initiate others into *Kriya*; but later, he used to initiate. An American gentleman by the name of Austin Grout wrote to Swamiji that he was a devotee of Sri Ramakrisna Mission and was interested in *Kriya Yoga*. He wrote to Yogananda's organization and was not satisfied. Later, he wrote to Swamiji for *Kriya*, but being denied *Kriya* by Swamiji went to Benares to receive *Kriya* from Shibendu Lahiri. When they instructed the rickshaw puller at Benares Railways station to take them to the Lahiri family, the rickshaw man brought them to the Original Lahiri Family house at Garureswar, instead of Shibendu Lahiri at Satyalok. So they were initiated by Banamali Lahiri. Returning to the United States, Austin Grout wrote to Swamiji and explained the whole thing. He felt gratitude to the rickshaw man. Banamali Babu mentioned to them that they should not be attracted to the organizations. He requested in his letter if he could communicate with Swamiji).

Later, it turned out that things started to normalize at Benares and tension, reduced; also another Lahiri, the wife of Prasanta Lahiri informed Swamiji that he did not have to worry about it as Banamali Lahiri's son got married in Calcutta to a rich man's only daughter and the couple moved to Bombay, currently Mumbai.

3) Prasanta Lahiri, a mining engineer who visited Swamiji at Calcutta and brought him one day to his place, at Belvedere Estate, Alipur, where several devotees of Anandamoyee Ma were attended.

During that visit Mrs. Lahiri, knowing the problem, informed what is written in the above paragraph to Swamiji. She also mentioned that her youngest uncle [she meant her husband's youngest uncle, that is, Satya Charan Lahiri] was in Calcutta in Ashok Chatterjee's house with diaries [diaries of Lahiri Mahasay] to do something.

4) Jyotirendu Lahiri (son of Tara Charan Lahiri who lived in Behala, Calcutta) came to visit Swamiji with his widowed mother at the home of Prof. Sudhin Kumar Banerjee whose father was a disciple of Tara Charan Lahiri. Swamiji was visiting Sudhin Babu's house.

5) Lastly, Shibendu Lahiri (Son of Satya Charan Lahiri). In 1992, out of the blue one day, Swamiji received a letter from Shibendu Lahiri (will be produced later). He mentioned that soon he would visit the United States and would like to see Swamiji. His father mentioned about Swamiji to him before he left body. His visit was sponsored by Roy Eugene Davis, disciple of Yogananda. He could not visit Swamiji in his first visit to the United States. It was not possible to manage.

Returning to India, he requested some books, so books were mailed to him. (Shibendu's letters will be produced later).

In his second visit with his wife, Shibendu Lahiri visited Swamiji. During the visit he mentioned that his cousin, Prasant Lahiri, asked him back in Calcutta, India, whether he had visited Swamiji in the United States. He said to him that it was not possible in the first visit but he would visit him next time. Shibendu Lahiri requested Swamiji to come to India for the celebration of the centenary of Lahiri Mahasay's leaving the body, in the forth coming year of 1995 starting in the month of October. For this reason Swamiji already had gotten many requests from India from some prominent persons and Asrams (hermitages). Swamiji did not apply his mind in this regard.

Then, one day, Swamiji received information from Lahiri Mahasay himself that his chief disciple's (Panchanan Bhattacharya's) comprehensive biography was to be presented this year. That settled the issue of Swamiji's applying the mind regarding visiting India in 1995. However, it created a big problem to Swamiji. He was instructed by Mahamuni Babaji to present Lahiri Mahasay's works and so this project was not in his mind.

It was very difficult to write about Sri Panchanan Bhattacharya who was a very strict disciplinary person and was very strict regarding advertisement. He was strict to keep everything secret. Nothing was available - all the letters with Lahiri Mahasay were kept secret. The Bhattacharya family maintained the tradition too. As mentioned, when the book *Lahiri Mahasay* was sent to Sibmoy Bhattacharya a note was included asking if some letters of Lahiri Mahasay to Sri Panchanan Bhattacharya could be shared, but Sibmoy Babu did not respond to the idea, although Swamiji has good relations with the Bhattacharya family.

So Swamiji was depending on Lahiri Mahasay on this project as it was his idea after all. In the morning, Swamiji opened a folder in his computer on the biography of Sri Sri Panchanan Bhattacharya. On the same day, in the afternoon, checking the mail from the P.O. Box, surprisingly, a letter was found from an unknown person, and it was Karunamoy Bhattacharya, the eldest grandson of Panchanan Bhattacharya who Swamiji did not know at all. His three letters we will produce here. He told Sarah Dixon that he had opened a folder in the computer that morning to write the biography of Panchanan Bhattacharya, which is a difficult job as there are no materials available since he was very strict and secret, and an anti-advertising person. Here is a letter from his eldest grandson of whom Swamiji was not aware.

Swamiji understood that it seemed Lahiri Mahasay's idea of presenting his chief disciple's, Sri Sri Panchanan Bhattachray's, comprehensive biography would be written and Lahiri Mahasay himself would do it through Swamiji's body; using his right hand like he had done before in Swamiji's young days. If on a straight string, a strike is made in the middle, the vibrations of the strike will reach to both ends. Thus, Lahiri Mahasay's strike had reached to the Bhattacharya family on the other end. Hence, this letter arrived from an unknown person but from the right person who was supposed to be helpful.

Another thing began to happen. Every night from about 3 A.M. to 6 A.M. a kind of reel appeared to Swamiji and he just had to observe and remember and then, going to the computer, just writing it all down. It was a great help. In fact, Lahiri Mahasay himself did everything on this; Swamiji was just a vehicle (*nimittamatra*). That is the reason Swamiji selected the title of the book : *The Divine Incarnation of Sri Panchanan Bhattarcharya*.

Swamiji has good relation with the Bhattacharya family too.

At least six people of the Bhattacharya family have contact with Swamiji.

1) Karunamoy Bhattacharya (eldest grandson of Panchanan Bhattacharya),
2) Sibmoy Bhattacharya (youngest grandson of Panchanan Bhattacharya),
3) Joydev Bhattacharya (great grandson of Panchanan Bhattacharya),
4) Amit Bhattacharya (great grandson of Panchanan Bhattacharya),
5) Mrs. Bhattacharya (great granddaughter of Panchanan Bhattacharya), and
6) Soumen Banerjee (great grandson of Panchanan Bhattacharya - from his mother's side).

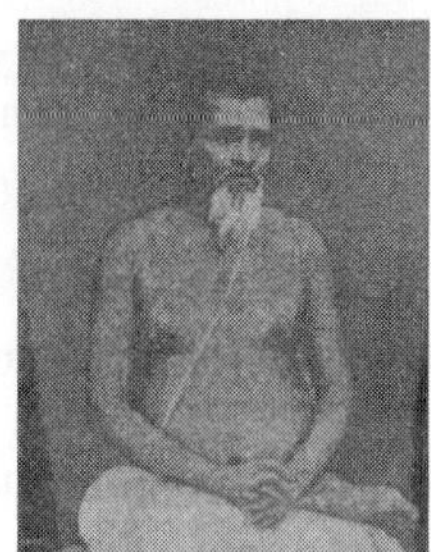

(1853-1919)
Sri Panchanan Bhattacharya,
the Chief Disciple of Lahiri Mahasay

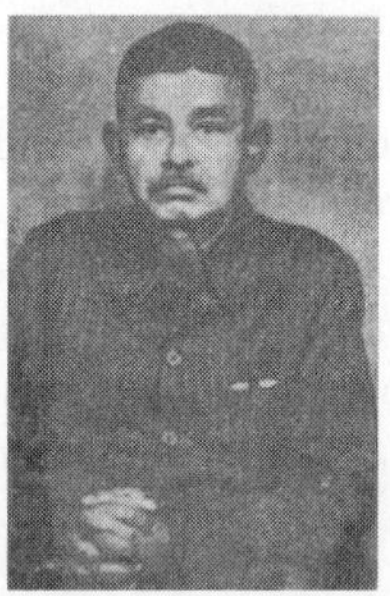

Bodhisattva Bhattacharya,
the only son of Panchanan Bhattacharya
by his second wife, Suradhani Devi

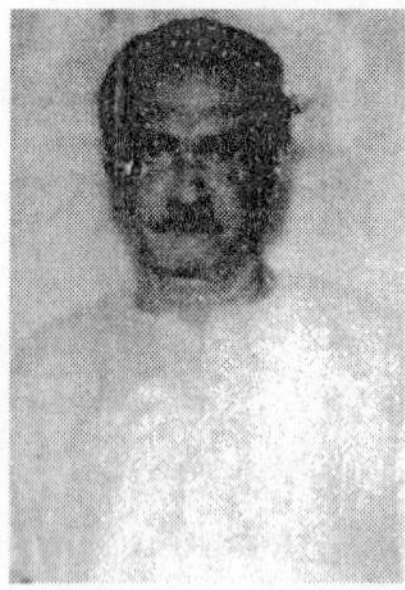

Karunamoy Bhattacharya
The eldest grandson of
Panchanan Bhattacharya

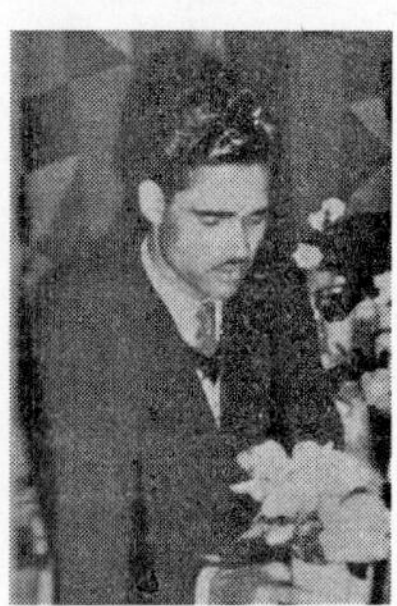

Sibmoy Bhattacharya
The youngest grandson of
Panchanan Bhattacharya

The First Handwritten Letter of Karunamoy Bhattacharya, the eldest grandson of Panchanan Bhattacharya to Swami Satyeswarananda

11, BABURAM GHOSH LANE,
CALCUTTA-700 005

'BAWANBIGHA'
B-DEOGHAR-814 112

Date 10 . 9 . 92

ওঁনমঃ

শ্রদ্ধাস্পদেষু,

গত অগাষ্টে দীর্ঘ চিঠি আপনাকে পোষ্ট করিয়াছি, আমার পত্র যদি আপনার মনে আঘাত দিয়া থাকে তবে আমি লজ্জিত এবং ক্ষমাপ্রার্থী রহিলাম।

শ্রী সুনীলকুমার ঘোষের নিকট হইতে লইয়া আমি "BIOGRAPHY OF A YOGI" পড়িয়াছি, ইহাতে মতামত এবং সংশোধন যাহা দেওয়া হইয়াছে তাহা সত্য এবং অতিরঞ্জিত নহে। কিন্তু এই বইয়ে লিখিয়াছে, যাহা আপনাকে আমি জ্ঞাপন করিতে চাই, উনি যাহা লিখিয়াছেন, সবগুলি ভুল করিয়াছেন।

(১) দুই জনের প্রতি সম্বন্ধে কিছু উল্লেখ করিলে ভাল হইত। যেমন - "কেশবী সুন্দর" এবং "দ্বিতীয় [illegible]"। এই দুইজন ভক্ত প্রতি ৺ হরিনারায়ণ বাবুর মজুমদারের নিকট দীক্ষা লইয়াছিলেন। "মহাপ্রভুর বাণী" উহারা প্রকাশ করিয়াছেন এবং ইহা সত্য ঘটনা।

(2) Rama Gopal Mazumdar (Page 77) সম্বন্ধে যাহা লিখিয়াছেন, মনে হয় উহা ঠিক নহে। অধ্যক্ষ [illegible] Principal ছিলেন ৺ রামগোপাল মজুমদার তিনি [illegible] এবং ঐ সময়ের [illegible] (বি.এ.) খুবই সুনাম ছিল। [illegible] শ্রী রামগোপাল মজুমদার "গীতা পরিচয়", original পুস্তক আমার কাছে

2

আজিপর্যন্ত ~~এখনই~~ তো, মহিমা প্রকাশন উহা ছাপ করিতে ইচ্ছুক, আমি এখনও হস্তান্তর করি নাই। Copyright করিয়াও নাই, সুতরাং উহা আমার নিকট রহিয়া গেল।
ধীরেন্দ্রনাথ মজুমদার দীক্ষা দিতেন যে প্রণাম পাইয়াছি তো তিনি কালীর ঠাকুরের শিষ্য না। আচার্য্য বসুমতীর শিষ্য তাহা আমার জানা নাই। যে কালের শিষ্য ছিলেন, ইহা লইয়া অর্থ বিতর্কেরও প্রয়োজন দেখি না। কালীর ঠাকুর বলিতেন — "গুরু কেহই নহে, সকলেই শিষ্য"

ঁ উপেন্দ্র মজুমদার, যিনি মুঙ্গেরে মিত্রাশ্রম প্রতিষ্ঠা করিয়াছিলেন ঁ বসুমতীর সঙ্গে এই কথার পর, তিনি কিন্তু প্রথমে কালীর ঠাকুরের নিকট দীক্ষা পাইয়াছিলেন; পরে মত কিছু ভবানীর আচার্য্যের নিকট হইতে। নিজে বসুমতীর ভক্তমণ্ডলী বলিতেন ইহার লইয়া আমার নিকট আছে এবং আরও কেমন হয় পাইতে পারে, তবে আর কিছু নাই।

আমার মনে কিছু সন্দেহ থাকিলে উহাদেরই সঙ্গে তাহা দূর হয়। কিছু ভুল এই থাকিলে বৈশিষ্ট্য শিষ্যমাত্রের প্রতি অবিচার করা হইবে বলিয়া আমার মনে হইল।

11, BABURAM GHOSH LANE,
CALCUTTA-700 005

'BAWANBIGHA'
B-DEOGHAR-814 112

Date

৩

সুকৃতিশীলের কবিতাগুলি আমার আছে, তবে প্রকাশক "Standard Publishers" আমার অনুমতি গ্রহণ করেন নাই। সর্বাধিকার শীলের এখন 'প্রকাশক' নাই। "ধর্ম ও সমাজ" প্রবন্ধের আমার প্রকাশিত হইল, আমাকে ঐ পুস্তকের প্রকাশের জন্য একটি পয়সা দেন নাই। copy right আমাদের নাই। 'ধর্ম ও প্রকাশক মীমাংসা' প্রবন্ধ হইতে পাওয়া যাইবেন, কাছেন দুর্লভ। উহারও copy right আমাদের নাই।

আমার জন্ম হয় ১৯৩২ সালে। ১৯৫৮ সাল হইতে ১৯৮৩ পর্যন্ত আমি এক বিহারী সংস্কৃত কলেজে অধ্যাপনা করিতেছিলাম। বিশ্ববিদ্যালয়ের কোন ছুটি না পাওয়া সত্ত্বেও ... মাসিক ২০০ টাকা বেতন পাইতাম, চাকুরী ছাড়িবার পূর্বে আমার ৩০০০ টাকা মাসিক বেতন ছিল। আমার retirement হইবার কথা ১৯৯৮ সালে, কিন্তু আমি ... premature retirement লইয়া আমি ... আমার পিতৃপুরুষের ভিটাতে। আমার পিতার ... ছিলেন এবং ... হইতে অনুমান ... বিহার প্রদেশে আসিয়া বসিয়াছিলেন। তাঁহার পিতা ... ছিলেন, তাই ... আমি ...

৪

৩২ বছর বয়সে দীক্ষা পাইয়াছিলাম। আমি দীক্ষার পর ২৫টি বছর কাটাইয়াছি এবং এখন আমার স্মৃতি অনেকখানি ক্ষীণ হইয়াছে এবং অনেক ঘটনা ভুলিয়াছি, তবুও কয়েকটি লিখিয়া রাখিতেছি (যেমন মনে আছে)।

পূর্ব সংস্কার: ১৯৪৪ খ্রীষ্টাব্দে আমার উপনয়ন হয়। বাবা গুরুদেবের সঙ্গেও দেখা হয়। সেই সময় সাধনার কথা, তাঁহার নিকট হইতে শুনিলাম। তখনই তাঁহার প্রতি শ্রদ্ধা হইল। তাঁহার সান্নিধ্য লাভ হইতেছে মনে হইল, তাঁহার সহিত নিয়মিত যোগাযোগ রাখিলাম।

"তাঁহাদের সঙ্গে এই জীবনে প্রথম দেখার সংস্কার আমার আছে। এখনও স্মৃতিতে তাহা আছে এবং আমার মনে আসে। সুতরাং আমার চিন্তাই তাঁহা। তাহার সেই ভাব, তাহা আমার স্মৃতি, অন্যের নিকটেও প্রকাশ নাই। আমার স্মৃতি তাঁহার কথা নাই, তাহাতে ইচ্ছাও নাই। তাঁহাদের নিকট আমার অনেকই চাই নাই, চাহিবও না। তাঁহার কাছে হইতে দুইটি কথা শুনিয়াছি — "সোহং ভাব, ভাব মুক্ত" আর "যোগীশ্বর ভাব আর সাধনের সংস্কার।"

স্বামী রামের এই মূর্তির কথা বলিয়া যোগী এবং সিদ্ধ পুরুষ আমার নমস্য, কিন্তু

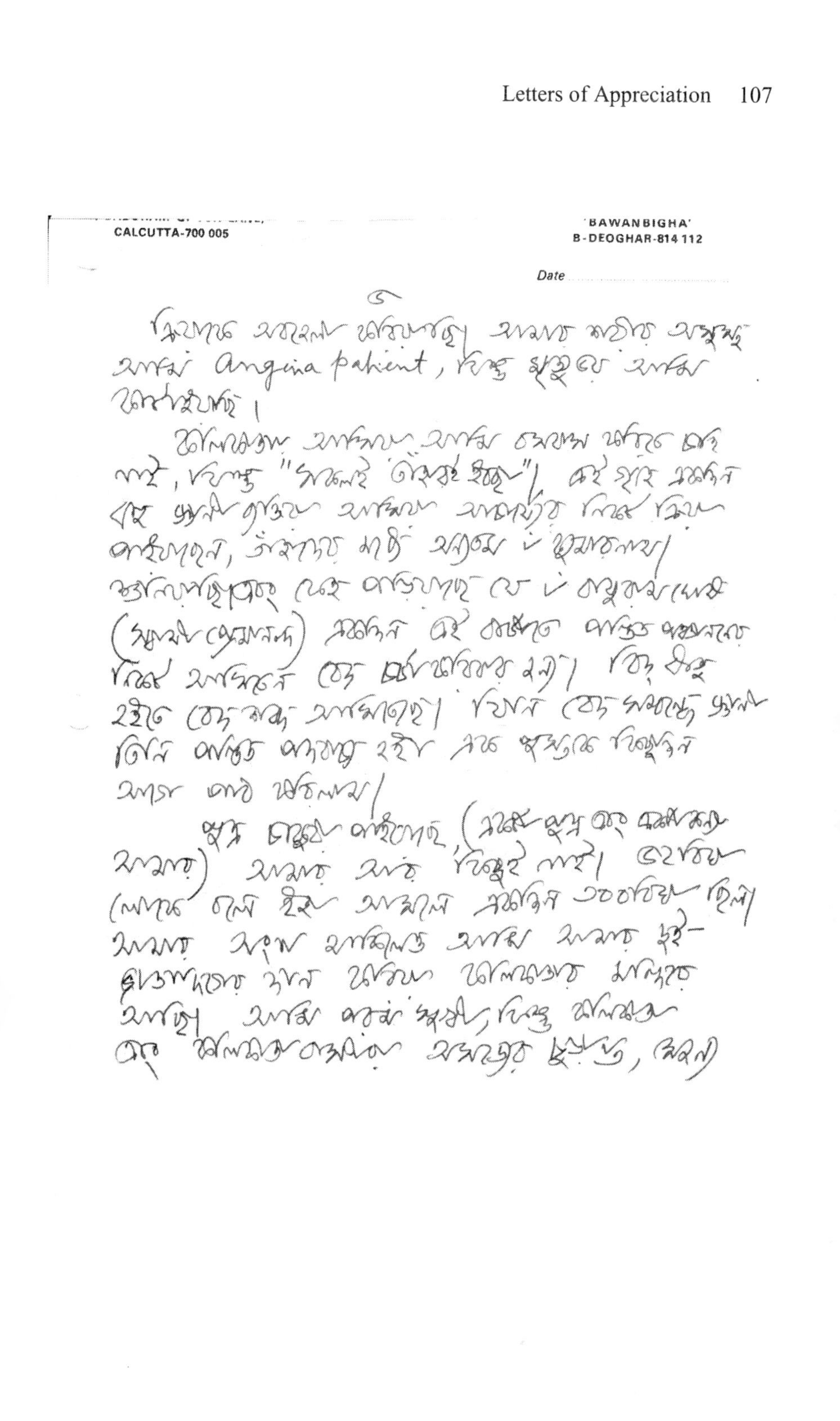

CALCUTTA-700 005

'BAWANBIGHA'
B-DEOGHAR-814 112

Date

[illegible] [illegible] কল্যাণবরেষু, আমার শরীর অসুস্থ। আমি Angina patient, কিন্তু [illegible] আমি [illegible]।

[illegible] "[illegible]" [illegible]

[illegible]

[illegible] আমার [illegible], কিন্তু [illegible] [illegible]

নির্বিঘ্নে আমাদের মধ্যে আছি।

দুইটি নিবেদন আছে।

(১) আপনাদের Publication এর যত বই কোন জায়গায় পাঠাইবেন।

(২) আমেরিকা হইতে প্রকাশিত গ্রন্থ [illegible] সামর্থ্য এবং সময় নাই।

(৩) যে কোন জায়গায় পারি [illegible] প্রকাশিত হইল।

(৪) "INNER VICTORY" - কোন লেখকের গ্রন্থ, কাহারও [illegible] হইতে কিনিতে পাঠাইবেন।

আমাদের ঠিকানা - শ্রী আচার্য্য [illegible] ব্রহ্মচারী মহারাজ [illegible], [illegible] ১১ নং [illegible] লেন [illegible] করিতেছি।

ইতি আপনাদের

শ্রী [illegible]

শ্রী [illegible] ব্রহ্মচারী

The English Version of the Handwritten First Letter of
Karunamoy Bhattacharya to Swami Satyeswarananda

Karunamoy Bhattacharya
11, Baburam Ghosh Lane
Calcutta - 700 006

Karunamoy Bhattacharya
'Bawanbigha'
B. Deoghar - 814 112
10/9/92

Respected (*Sradhaspadesu*),

One unknown poor disciple is attacking you with a letter. If this letter of mine disturbs your peace of mind, then I am ashamed and beg your pardon.

I have read the book "*Biography of a Yogi*" borrowing from Sri Sunil Kumar Ghosh [disciple of Bhupendranath Sanyal, the secretary of Bhratri Sanga, an attorney, a good friend of the author and whose letter to the author is published here]. It is extremely beautiful and what is written in brief is true and not exaggerated. Something is felt in me what I can disclose to you and that is why I am going to mention to you. Please forgive me.

1. It would have been good if two great gentlemens' names were referred to: one is late *Netaji* Subhas [Subhas Chandra Bose, a famous Bengali politician and a great patriot] and the second, Kazi Nazrul Islam [a famous revolutionary beloved Bengali poet]. These two gentlemen received *Kriya* from Baroda Mazumder of Halisahar [disciple of Panchanan Bhattacharya]. The Mahesh Library [a famous Publishing House for religious books in Calcutta] has published this information and know it for certain that it was true.

2, What you have written about Rama Gopal Mazumder (page 77) perhaps it is not correct. He was principal of Aryya Mission.

[An explanation - Actually, Karuna Babu was making a confusion between two gentlemen, both were *Kriyanwits* (practitioner of *Kriya*). One's name was Rama Gopal Mazumder and the other's name was Rama Dayal Mazumder. The middle names Gopal and Dayal made this confusion; also it was possible that Karuna Babu did not know about Rama Gopal Mazumder].

[The Aryya Mission Institution was started by Sri Panchanan Bhattacharya (the chief disciple) under the direct instruction of his Gurudev, Sri Sri Yogiraj Shyama Charan Lahiri Mahasay. Lahiri Mahasay did not advise to start organizations (rather, specifically, he prohibited it advising not to start organizations around the *Kriya*. So also did Mahamuni Babaji, the Divine

Himalayan Yogi.). However, Lahiri Mahasay made an exception and asked his chief disciple, Panchanan Bhattacharya to start an institution to publish his books (26 books, interpretation in thc Light of *Kriya* made by him) and to distribute them among the *Kriya* disciples, as well as some herbal medicines. As per his Guru's instruction Panchanan Bhattacharya named it "The Aryya Mission Institution". Later a school was added and there Rama Dayal Mazumder was appointed as Principal].

Rama Doyal Mazumder was a famous gentleman among the intellectuals. He had a good reputation. He received a degree M. A. in English. In those days, it carried a lot of good reputation. Mysteriously, the original copy of his *Gita* interpretation "*Gita Parichay*" (*Introduction to Gita*), has come to me and the Mahesh Library wants to buy it from me. I have not handed it over to them. Nobody has the copyright. Therefore, they can buy it from me. I have found proof that Sri Rama Dayal Mazumder used to give initiation to others. However, I am not sure whether he was disciple of Kashi Baba (Lahiri Mahasay) or Acharya Panchanan (his grandfather). I do not see any sense debating regarding who is whose disciple. The Lord of Kashi (*Kashir Thakur*) [That is , a reference of Lahiri Mahasay] used to say, "Nobody is *Guru*, all are disciples".

[Swamiji was fully aware of Rama Dayal Mazumder's educational background as well as his position in the *Kriya* world. He used to give *Kriya* initiation. One of his famous disciples was Sitaram das Omkarnath. Here is the hand written admission by Sitaram das Omkarnath.

[Ram Dayal Mazumder, disciple of Lahiri Mahasay and Baba Sitaramdas Omkarnath of Bengal

[Another disciple of Lahiri Mahasay was Ram Dayal Mazumder. He was permitted to initiate others. In those days, he was an M. A. in English and was a prominent educationist. He wrote interpretations of *Bhagavad Gita* in three volumes.

[One prominent Bhakta yogi of Bengal, the follower of Ramanuj *vaisnab* group was Sitaramdas Omkarnath. He was born at Dumurdaha village near Triveni, on the west side of the Ganges. His name was Prabodh Chandra Chattopadhyaya. He was educated at the toll of Yogeswar Dasarathi Smritiratna Mahasay and was initiated by him in 1922. In right time, Smritiratna Mahasay advised him to take initiation from Yogi Gaurentraji. Then he went to see him.

[Gaurentraji asked him, "Are you married?"

[Prabodh Chandra, replied, "Yes Sir (*ajnge hna*)."

["Then it will not work," commented Yogiji and continued to say, "If I advise you, your household life will be dropped off and you will enter in *Samadhi*."

[However, he advised him saying, "Fix your mind on water. *Nada* (Inner Sound, *Om*) reveals first on water."

[In 1926, Prabodh Chandra Chattopadhyaya received *Kriya* initiation from Ram Dayal Mazumder (disciple of Lahiri Mahasay).

[In 1947, being a *siddha* in *Pranab* (*Omkar*), he received the name of Sitaramdas Omkarnath. He has a large number of followers in Bengal.

[We produced a handwritten note of Baba Sitaramdas Omkarnath admitting to the effect that he received *Kriya* initiation from Dayal Maharaj (Ram Dayal Mazumder), disciple of Lahiri Mahasay.

(বাবা সীতারামদাস ওঁকারনাথ
ঠাকুরের স্বহস্ত লিখিত পত্র)

ওঁ ২৪।২।৬৯

[illegible]

[The English version of the above-mentioned handwritten letter of Baba Sitaramdas Omakarnath in Bengali.

Om

February 24. 1969

[I received *Navi Kriya*, and other *Mudras*: *Yonimudra*, *Talabya Mudra* [*Khecharimudra*] etc. Some days after practicing *Pranayam* [*Kriya*] with touching [mentally] the six centers. I could not bring down the breath and the mind. So I reported it to Dayal Maharaj [Ram Dayal Mazumder, disciple of Lahiri Mahasay].

[He said, "By the practice of *japam* (chanting *mantras*) you have finished the work. Go, you do not have to practice yoga. *Hathayogi* got vacation."

[Later, the infinite *Nada* (inner Sound of *Om*) continued infinitely.

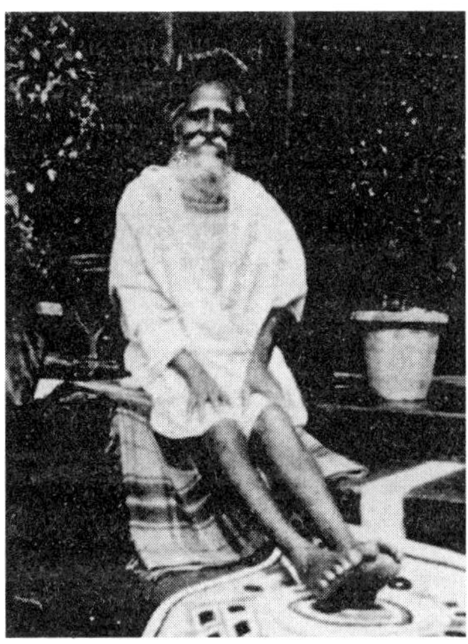

[Baba Sitaramdas Omkarnath
A *Bhakta* Yogi of Bengal with a large following of devotees.

[Back to Karuna Babu's letter].

Late Bhupal [Chandra] Mazumder who founded the *Siddhasram* at Munger (Bihar) was originally initiated by Kashir Thakur [Lahiri Mahasay]; later, all he received from the Acharya [teacher] of Bawan Bigha [means Sri Panchanan Bhattacharya]. So he used to address Panchanan Baba as "Guru Baba." Regarding this matter I have all the records, and also many can be collected, however, there is no benefit [doing so].

By their grace, any doubt arises in me, usually becomes solved. If there is any fault, then I personally think it will be an injustice to the future generations.

I have no copyrights of the *Suradhani Gita* [It refers to the *Bhagavad Gita* interpretation of Panchanan Bhattacharya, the big one and not the small (pocket) *Aryya Mission Gita*. The *Bhagavad Gita,* the interpretation by Panchanan Bhattacharya *first* published as the Suradhani Gita because his second wile's name was Suradhani Bhattacharya]. However, the "Standard Publisher" is betraying me. The *Aryya Mission Gita* is now with the Mahesh Library. *Jagat O Ami* [a Bengali book written by Panchanan Bhattacharya] just published again. I have made afford to advertize for this book. We do not have the copyright. The *Dharma O Pujadi Mimangsa* [another Bengali title written by

Panchanan Bhattacharya] is not available for a long time. I do not know the reason. We do not have copyright.

I was born in 1932. I have worked in a British Company from 1956 to 1986. Not having any degree from the University, yet, by the grace of the Guru and the great Gurus, starting from the 200.00 rupees a month, at the retirement, my salary was rupees 5,000.00 a month. My retirement was supposed to be in 1988; but I took pre-retirement and came to the paternal house at Calcutta. My father was very strict disciplinary person and so I had to learn discipline well. At that time he did not have the permission to initiate others; so in the young days, I received *Kriya* from Sri Ananda Mohan Lahiri [the only bachelor grandson out of eight of Lahiri Mahasay and B. A. classmate and good friend of Swami Satyananda at the City College, Calcutta] in our Siva Temple at Bawan Bigha, Deoghar.

By their grace, I had come in contact with many great persons. Even today, miraculously, many people come to my house. It is good to follow the dictum of the age (*Yuga Dharma*). I kept secret even from my wife, son and daughter, what happens every day. My wife did not receive *Kriya*, nor she is interested to receive. I do not expect anything from them, nor will I ask. I heard two things from the very young days - "From the greedy develops sin and from the sin brings death"; and "there is no greater sin than anger in the world."

By the great and good reputation of the past life, I was fortunate to be born to a family of Yogi and the dynasty of the *Siddhas* [realized ones]. I have neglected Kriya. My body is sick with, I am angina patient, however, I have overcome the fear of death.

I did not want to come back to Calcutta and live here. "All is His Will". Many great people had come to this house and received *Kriya* from the Acharya [Panchanan Bhattacharya]. Among them Kumarnath [Mukherjee, disciple of Panchanan Bhattacharya], Baburam Ghosh (Swami Premananda) [Sri Ramakrisna Mission and Math], one day came to this house to discuss *Vedas*. The word *Veda* is from the root verb *'bid'*. He, who is knowledgeable in the *Vedas* is called *Pandit*; I just read in a book a few days before.

My son has got a job. (I have one son and a daughter). I have nothing anymore. the people say *Bawan* (52) *Bigha*; it was actually one three hundred (300) *bighas* [100 acres]. [Karuna Babu is referring to the property his grandfather, Panchanan Bhattacharya, bought in Deoghar]. Even though I have a share, I donated my share to my two younger brothers and came here at the Calcutta Temple [Panchanan Bhattacharya's original parental house] to live. I am very happy, however, Calcutta's residents are very uncivilized, and so I am living here like a gypsy (*jajabar*).

There are two requests: [The list increases]

1) Kindly inform me how can I get your publications [published books].

2) I have no ability to purchase books from America.

3) How can I get them - Please let me know.

4) I have seen the "Inner Victory" [Published by Swami Satyeswarananda]. I do not know whether I have the fortune to read it.

I am the eldest grandson of Sri Panchanan Bhattacharya, live in 11, Baburam Ghosh Lane.

Yours
Affectionate

Sri Karunamoy Bhattacharya.

The Second Handwritten Letter of Karunamoy Bhattacharya in Bengali to Swami Satyeswarananda

11, BABURAM GHOSH LANE,
CALCUTTA-700 005

'BAWANBIGHA'
B-DEOGHAR-814 112

Date 23/10/92

[illegible]

[illegible]

২

চিন্তাধারা যাইতে যদি সত্য হয়, তবে বিশেষ কিছু ফল হইবে না। আধুনিক [illegible] সমান ভাবে সর্বদা [illegible] ও যাহা কিছু করিবে তাহা [illegible] করিবার চেষ্টা করিও। [illegible] করিতে পারিলে [illegible] যে সব কার্য্য করে তাহা ভাল ভাবেই করিতে পারিবে।"

কবিরাজের [illegible] ৪০ বছর পরে ক্রিয়া প্রভৃতি [illegible] হইতে উক্ত কবিরাজের [illegible] জানা যায়।

যেন লোকে ক্রিয়া লোপ শাস্ত্রলোপ ভবিষ্যতি।
কলিকালে শাস্ত্রাণি ভবিষ্যন্তি [illegible]॥

এই শ্লোকের ব্যাখ্যায় কবিরাজজী লিখিয়াছেন— "শাস্ত্র ও ক্রিয়া লোপ হইবে, কেবল মাত্র কলিতে সমস্ত শাস্ত্র হইবে, এইরূপ সমস্ত কলিকালে হইবে কিন্তু এই সময়েই হইয়াছে দেখা যায়।" তিনি আরও লিখিয়াছেন— "কলিকালে ক্রিয়ার লোপ জানিলে ভয় নাই, এইরূপ বিজ্ঞান একেবারে লোপ হইয়াছে সুতরাং অবিজ্ঞান, এই অবিজ্ঞান বশত সমস্ত কার্য্য, সকলেই নিজ কর্তা হইল, উহাতে বড় বড় লোক হইয়া পড়িয়াছে, বড় বড় লোকেরা মানিতে না পারিয়া, কেহও দেখেনা, শুনেও শুনেনা, যাহা হইল তাহাই প্রমাণ হয়।"

আমি কলিকাতা মহানগরীতে এত বড় পুস্তক ছাপা করিয়া [illegible] পাই নাই, অথচ তাঁহার নাম [illegible] Institute আমার [illegible], [illegible] নাই।

11, BABURAM GHOSH LANE,
CALCUTTA-700 005

Date ....

[illegible]

৪

ঈপ্সিত সুখ যখন বর্তমান যুগে কোনো বিবাহীতে নাই, তখন সৎসঙ্গ সাধনের করিলে সার্থক হইবেন।

এই প্রশ্নের উত্তর দিবেন। কেমন আছেন-বলেন। আপনাদের বহুমূল্য সময় আমি নষ্ট করিতে চাহিনা, কেননা আপনাদের চিত্ত বিনোদনে ব্যস্ত আছে।

আমি ৫০ বৎসর হইতে কণ্ঠসঙ্গীত শিক্ষা করিতে শুরু করিয়াছি। প্রায় ২০ বৎসর কাল আমি শাস্ত্রীয় সঙ্গীত শিক্ষা করিয়াছিলাম, তাহার পর নানা কারণ বশত: প্রায় ২০ বৎসর বন্ধ ছিল, কিন্তু কণ্ঠে এখনও সুর আছে।

আমার বেশী বয়স তাই ডাক্তারমতে নিষেধ, কারণ Angina আছে। আমি সকল সময় আপনাদের পাশেই আছি।

হৃদয়ে রেখো দুই চরণে,
হৃদয়ে ভেবো সাধনা।

ইতি আপনাদের স্নেহের বন্ধু
শ্রীকমলাময় ভট্টাচার্য

পু: - আপনারা সকলে আমার ৺বিজয়া ও দীপাবলীর আন্তরিক প্রীতি গ্রহণ করিবেন।

The English Version of the Handwritten Second Letter of Karunamoy Bhattacharya to Swami Satyeswarananda

Karunamoy Bhattacharya
11, Baburam Ghosh Lane,
Calcutta 700 006

Date 23/10/92

Respected (*Sradhaspadesu*),

Your address to me as "Very dear Soul" such a high esteem will remain as a means to be happy in my life. My soul is satisfied.

In the World Parliament of Religion in Chicago [1893], Swami Vivekananda had addressed the Americans as "Brothers and Sisters" ["Sisters and Brothers of America"]. Your address to me "Very Dear Soul" made an ideal example in the world.

Shyama Charan [Yogiraj Shyama Charan Lahiri Mahasay] had shelter at the feet of Shyama [Goddess Kali (Shyama), the Divine Mother], Panchanan *jiva* [the individual] became Siva [Lord Siva], I have experienced that . If I have to think beyond this, then I have to renounce the world and become a renunciate [Swami]. I do not think Babaji Maharaj was an Avatar. Who is he, I do not know, nor do I want to know. Lord Krisna was an Avatar. After Him, in the age of *Kali Yuga*, nobody was born. Those who came, they were great Persons. A few days before, one *Kriyaban* said Babaji was Aswathama [the only son of Droncahrya, the military teacher of Kaurava and Pandava]. I did not reply.

Some devotees tried to excite my grandfather [Panchanan Bhattacharya] asking a question - the question was: Who is greater Ramakrisna or Kashir Thakur [Lahiri Mahasay]? Nobody was pleased when the answer was given. He replied , "One is a [devotee] and the other is a *Sadhaka* [seeker]." In the *Gita* explanation, he had clearly mentioned what is the difference between the path of *Bhakti* (devotion) and the path of *Sadhana* (meditation). Actually, nobody study the Gita with full concentration.

I like one advice of Lord Buddha."The mind is first and then the Religion."

There is a statement in the *Jagat O Ami* [The Bengali title of the book written by Panchanan Bhattacharya the English translation of the title will be "The World and I".] "*Bhag* and *ban* are the *Purusa* [Lord] and *Prakriti* [nature]; hearing this, whosoever hears this will have knowledge." Making the English translation of it and writing something about it, can be given to the restless present generation. We are deliberately abusing the nature and causing anger to the Lord.

Panchanan Baba used to say,"You should remain engaged in thoughtful way. Only for a while you sit in Yoga practice and at that time if you allow your mind to go to think worldly objects, then you will get no results.

"Focusing the Self [the *Atmaram*] in the *Kutastha* [in between the eyebrows] whatever you try to do, make effort to do it focusing on the breath. If you are able to do this way, you will be do it better."

It is heard that Kashi Baba's [Lahiri Mahasay's] himself had made prediction that after about forty years of leaving the body] there will be *Kriya* publicity in the foreign countries.

Tena loke Kriya lop sastralop bhabisyati.
Kalpitani sastrani bhabisyati tatobhubi.

In the explanation of this verse Kashi Baba [Lahiri Mahasay] wrote, "The scriptures and *Kriya* [the Original *Kriya*] will be disappeared. Only the imagined thoughts of the mind will be the scriptures. All these will be in the age of Kali [*Kalikal*]. But these are happening now."

He [Lahiri Mahasay] has written more: "In the age of *Kali*, people are afraid hearing the *Kriya*. So the science is destroyed. Therefore, nowadays all are out of science. Therefore, all the words and conversation are unscientific. Some people have developed big ego and so their feet are not on the ground; they see yet they do not see; they hear yet they do not hear; such is the situation."

Last four years in Calcutta I tried to find one photo of Sadhak Rama Prasad Sen; yet there is an Institute after his name near my house. His photo is not there either.

In the room of Acharya [Panchanan Bhattacharya] and Kashi Baba [Lahiri Mahasay] there was never a photo of Babaji Maharaj [Because there is no real photo available of Babaji Maharaj]. In the house of Acharya Panchanan [Bhattacharya], he kept two photos : Guru Nanak and Guru Kabir. I believe for some reason that Kashi Baba [Lahiri Mahasay] is the Guru Kabir.

Once remembering Babaji Maharaj, *Thakur* of *Kashi* [Lahiri Mahasay] was in trouble. You all know this.

He used to take bath in Ganges very early morning at Chausatti Yogini *ghat*. He, who was sitting by the garbage truck, uttered three times: Shyama Charan! Shyama Charan! Shyama Charan!, It was still dark. By the strange sound of the truck, he understood that somebody has gone by giving him *darsan* (meeting). Even it is a story, yet, know it is true. Because Thakur of Kashi [Lahiri Mahasay] he used to tell his heart's story to Panchanan [Bhattacharya]. I heard this from my parents.

I have not seen you. I become free from lots of troubles simply remembering white clothes wearing the Thakur of Kashi [Lahiri Mahasay] or my grandfather, Panchanan [Bhattacharya]. In which difficult path you are progressing, you need blessings of Kashi Baba [Lahiri Mahasay]. I never see any difference between the three : Babaji Maharaj, Kashi Baba [Lahiri Mahasay] and Panchanan [Bhattacharya]. They appear to me as Union of *Tribeni* [three]. If in this life, I can get caught up with the thought of a tiny [*anu*], then I can hope in the next life, I will be able to search for an atom [*paramanu*]. *Sakali toamri ichha* - [It means "All are your desires." Actually, it is a line of a famous music composed and sung by a famous seeker, Rama Prasad Sen in Bengal. Karuna Babu quoted].

When I want to satisfy the taste of milk simply by buttermilk [*ghol*] in this age, then if the rice pudding is served, then it will not be digested.

Please do not answer this letter. If kept secret will be good. I do not want to destroy your valuable time. Also writing letter to you have a big expense.

From the last week I have started learning music on Yoga. Almost twenty years (20) I have learned the scriptural music. There after ten (10) years was stopped for many reasons. However, there is still tuning [*sura*] at the throat.

I cannot talk a lot. It is doctor's advice; as I have angina. I am always by your side.

"Where you are searching me dear. I am at your side."

[Again, Karuna Babu quoted a famous music line of (perhaps) Kabir].

Yours courtesy enchanted
Sri Karunamoy Bhattacharya

P.S. You all please accept my sincere greeting of *Bijoya* [after the worship of Goddess Durga] and *Dipavali* [after the worship of Goddess Kali, the festival of Light].

The Third Handwritten Letter of Karunamoy Bhattacharya
in Bengali to Swami Satyeswarananda

ওঁ নমঃ

১১ অক্রুর দত্ত লেন।
ওয়েলিংটন।
কলি: ৭০০০০৫ ২১/১/৯৩

শ্রদ্ধাভাজনেষু

আশা করি ভাল আছেন। আপনার ২রা অক্টোবর ১৯৯২
সালের পত্র পাইয়া উত্তর দিয়াছিলাম, আশা করি পাইয়াছেন।
আপনার পাঠানো যে পুস্তকগুলি উপহার স্বরূপ
পাঠাইয়া দিয়াছিলেন, তাহা যথা সময়ে পাইয়া প্রায় সব পড়িয়াছি।
সময়াভাবে [illegible] পারি নাই, ক্ষমা করিবেন,

ডঃ চন্দ্রশেখর রায় ([illegible]) উঁহার "যোগজীবন"
পুস্তকে যাহা লিপিবদ্ধ করিয়াছেন, তাহা সম্পূর্ণ-
সত্য ঘটনা। আরও একটি পুস্তক, যাহা সম্প্রতি-
প্রকাশ করা হইয়াছে— "ধর্মালোচনা ও সাহিত্যমালা" সুন্দর-
নির্ভর যোগ্য। এইটি পুস্তক আপনাদের নিকট-
আশা করি শীঘ্রই পাইবেন।

পত্র লিখিতে এবং পুস্তক পাঠাইতে এখন
আমার খুব অসুবিধা, তবে প্রত্যেক আপনাদের কল্যাণ
সময় নষ্ট [illegible] আমার নাই।

শ্রীভগবানের নিকট প্রার্থনা করি যেন আপনাদের
প্রচেষ্টা সফল হয়।

ইতি-
আপনাদের শুভার্থী
শ্রীকরুণাময় ভট্টাচার্য্য

The English Version of the Handwritten Letter
of Karunamoy Bhattacharya to Swami Satyeswarananda

Om Namah: Bowing to *Om* (inner Sound)

11, Baburam Ghosh Lane
Ahiritola
Calcutta- 700005
January 21, 1995

Respected One,

I hope everything is well there. I answered your letter dated October 2, 1992 in response [to my letter September 10, 1992]. I hope you have received it.

I have read all the books which you have sent to me as a present. There are some minor oversights here and there. I will let you know if you would like. [Karuna Babu is referring to some names or events the way he happens to know.]

Know it that all of what Baba of Balagar (Sris Babu) has written in his book *Yoga Jivan* ["Yoga Life" - An Autobiography of Dr. Sris Chandra Mukherjee. Dr. Mukherjee was the chief disciple of Panchanan Bhattacharya, about whom we have written in Chapter 16 in this book] are true.

Dharmalochana o Śangitmalya ["Discussion of *Dharma* or Righteousness and the Garland of Music"] is another book published recently. It is also very dependable. I will send you a book very soon.

[The title *Dharmalochana o Sangit malya* which Karuna Babu refers to was actually published by his brother, Bhattacharya. The *Iswaratattv-alochana* (Discussion of *Iswara*) part in this title was published before by their father, Bodhisattva Bhattacharya (the only son of Panchanan Bhattacharya). The author saw a copy of this book in 1971].

Nowadays it is expensive to write a letter and send books [through mail]. Anyway, I have no right to waste your valuable time.

I pray to the Lord that your efforts [in writing the biography of Panchanan Bhattacharya] be successful.

Yours Affectionately,
Sri Karunamoy Bhattacharji

The Handwritten Letter of Sibmoy Bhattacharya, the youngest grandson of Panchanan Bhattacharya in Bengali to Swami Satyeswarananda

ওঁ শ্রী গুরবে নমঃ

"Bawan Bigha"
P.O. B. Deoghar
814 112
India
7.8.1995

নমস্কারান্তর নিবেদন,

মহাশয়ের ৯/৫/৯৫ তারিখের পত্র যে সময়েই পেয়েছিলাম কিন্তু পত্রের উত্তর দিতে বিলম্ব বিশেষত: এই জন্যে যে আপনার লেখা, ইংরাজী পত্র, আমার অগ্রজের কলিকাতার ঠিকানায়, সম্ভবত: এপ্রিল মাসের শেষে এসেছিল এবং আমি তখন কলিকাতায়। বলা বাহুল্য যে সে সময়েও আমার অগ্রজ hypertension-এ খুব ভুগছিলেন কিন্তু আমি দেওঘর ফিরবার সময় তিনি বলেন যে আপনার চাহিদা মত ছবি ইত্যাদি উনি পাঠাবার ব্যবস্থা করবেন, পরে পুনরায় কলকাতা যাই (2nd July) এবং অগ্রজকে দেখে আর পর নাই বিস্মিত ও বিচলিত হই যে তিনি total nervous breakdown-এ ভুগছেন এবং চিকিৎসাদি যেমত হচ্ছিল তাতে complete rest-এ এবং sedation-এতে রাখা হচ্ছিল (দেখেছিলাম)

আপনার পত্রের উত্তর এবং যা চেয়েছেন তা শারীরিক ও মানসিক কারণে পাঠাতে পারেননি, নিজে আমায় বলেন। আমি কলকাতা থেকেই আপনার চাহিদা মত ছবি ইত্যাদি সংগ্রহ করতে চেষ্টা করে অনেক কিছু পাইনি এমতাবস্থায় দেওঘর ফিরে আসি গত দশদিন আগে। কলিকাতায় যা সংগ্রহ হয়েছিল তা নিয়ে ফিরেছি এবং এখানেও অনেক কিছু পুরাতন ছবি ও Catalogue, P. Bhattacharji & Son, Bawan Bigha, Deoghar এবং বহু পুরাতন প্রকাশিত কিছু পুস্তক যা আমার ৺দাদুর, পণ্ডিত পঞ্চানন ভট্টাচার্য মহাশয় যোগীরাজ ৺লাহিড়ী বাবার নির্দেশ অনুযায়ী প্রকাশিত করতেন, আদি সংগ্রহ করে আপনাকে এখনো Registered Parcel যোগে পাঠাতে পারিনি কারণ এরই সঙ্গেই কিছু Photostat copies of very old letters (৺তিনকড়ি বাবুর প্রতি যোগীরাজ লাহিড়ী মহাশয়ের) সংগৃহীত হয়নি যা কোনো

কারণে বর্তমানে আমার কোনো আত্মীয়ের কাছে ছিল। তিনি tour-এ আছেন, শীঘ্রই ফিরবেন এবং আমি ওগুলি নিয়ে আপনাকে যথাশীঘ্র পাঠাবার প্রবন্ধ করছি।

বিলম্বের জন্য খুবই দুঃখিত কিন্তু অবস্থা যেন could not help the situation.

ওঁকে অর্থ বাবদ সাহায্য কিছু করা বর্তমানে প্রয়োজন নেই কারণ তাঁকে মারাও যাচ্ছে। আপনার প্রকাশন ভূমিকাটি হয়ত প্রেস অভিমুখে এ আশঙ্কাও করছি। যদি সম্ভব হয় একটু বিলম্ব করবেন। বর্তমানে আপনাকে যা পাঠাবার এ সকল পাঠাতে 15th August এর আর বেশী দেরী হবে না।

আপনি কি আগামী মহাষ্টমীর পূর্বে ভারতে কাকদ্বীপে এ নূতন আশ্রম প্রতিষ্ঠা দিবসে আসছেন? আসলে দেখা ও অনেক কথা হবে।

বর্তমানে আমার অগ্রজ শ্রী কমলাক্ষ ভট্টাচার্য্যের ঠিকানায়, কলকাতায় কিছু না পাঠালেই ভাল। আপনার last package in Cambi's bag খোলাও হয়নি — দেখে এসেছি।

বিনীত

প্রীতিপূর্ণ শুভেচ্ছা সহ। শ্রী [illegible] ভট্টাচার্য্য

The English Version of the Preceding letter of Sibmoy Bhattacharya, the youngest grandson of Panchanan Bhattacharya to Swami Satyeswarananda.

Om Sri Gurube Namah

"Bawan Bigha"
P.O. Deoghar - 814112
India
August 7, 1995

After bowing,
Dear Sir!
I received your letter of May 1, 1995 in the month of May but I could not answer.

The reason is: Your letter written in English to my eldest brother [Karunamoy Bhattacharya] arrived in the last week of April. I was there in Calcutta at that time. Needless to say, during this time, my eldest brother was suffering from hypertension yet he said to me (when I was about to return to Deoghar) that he would send you the materials according to your needs.

Then on July 2nd, I visited him and I was stunned and nervous seeing his condition. He was under total nervous breakdown [neurological problems]. He was under treatment and was advised to have complete rest and I saw that he was kept under sedation.

Due to his physical and mental condition he was not able to send what you asked for. Personally he told me that.

Then in Calcutta I began to collect the photos and other things which you asked for, but I was not able to get many things. Then I returned to Deoghar just ten days ago. I have brought to Deoghar whatever I found in Calcutta. At Deoghar, I am looking for some old photos, a catalogue, "P. Bhattacharya & Sons, Bawan Bigha, Deoghar" and many old published books which my grandfather, *Pandit* Panchanan Bhattacharya Mahasay published under the directions of Yogiraj Lahiri Baba.

After collecting these, I did not send them to you by registered parcel because I am trying to collect some Photostat copies of very old letters of Tinkori Babu [eldest son of Lahiri Mahasay who was put under the supervision of Panchanan Bhattacharya], and Yogiraj Lahiri Mahasay. They have not been collected as yet as for some reason they are with one of my relatives who is currently on vacation. Very soon, he will return. Then after collecting those, I will arrange to send them to you.

I am very sorry for this delay, but under the circumstances I could not help the situation. It is not necessary for you to arrange to send anything through the mail. Many things are lost in the mail nowadays.

I suspect perhaps that your publication is on the way to the printer. If possible, please delay it a bit. At present, whatever I have collected to send will not be posted later than August 15th.

Are you coming to India for the foundation day of the new *asram* at Kakadwip? [Asok Kumar Chatterjee, disciple of Satya Charan Lahiri, was going to found an Asram there]. If you do come, we will meet and discuss many things.

It is advisable that you should not send anything to my eldest brother, Karunamoy Bhattacharya, at his Calcutta address since I have seen that your last package in a canvas bag has not been opened yet.

With love and good wishes,

Sincerely Yours,
Sri Sibmoy Bhattacharji

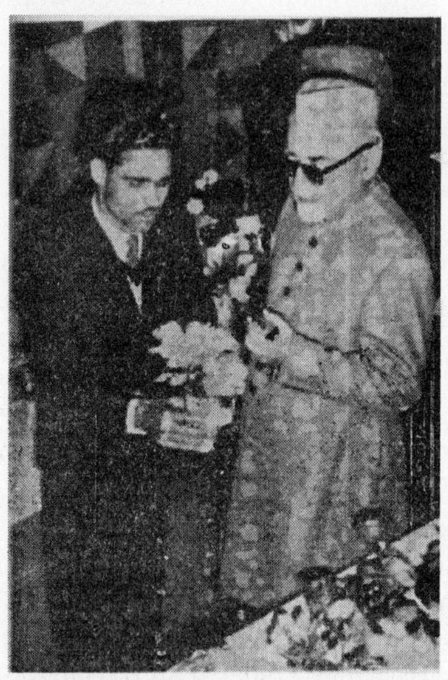

Sibmoy Bhattacharya, Youngest grandson of Panchanan Bhattacharya, Showing 'President Radhakrisna brand' to Dr. Zakir Hossain, President of India, in Delhi Flower Expo

Handwritten Letter of Joydev Bhattacharia, great grandson of Panchanan Bhattacharya in Bengali to Swami Satyeswarananda.

[illegible]

From :-
JOYDEV BHATTACHARJEE
"BANAN - BIGHA"
P.O. B - DEOGHAR
DISTT - DEOGHAR
BIHAR : 814 112

[illegible],—

[illegible] "Divine Incarnation of Panchanan Bhattacharya" [illegible] "Lahiri Mahasay's personal letters to Kriya disciples" [illegible]

P.T.O.

[illegible]

[illegible]

6/3/1999.

The English Version of the Handwritten Letter
of Joydev Bhattacharya to Swami Satyeswarananda

Om Namah

From:
Joydev Bhattacharjee
"Bawan Bigha"
P.O. B - Deoghar
Dist. Deoghar
Bihar 814 112

Worshipable Swamiji (*Pujaniya* Swamiji),

I am starting this letter with respectful *pronam* [traditional bowing] to you. If there is any fault, kindly, pardon me.

I am the eldest son of Anandamoy Bhattacharya (who is the middle grandson of Sri Panchanan Bhattacharya).

I am a *Kriyaban* [Practitioner of *Kriya*] and practice every day sincerely as far as possible. I have seen two books of yours recently with my uncle, Sibmoy Bhattacharya.

1) *Divine Incarnation of Panchanan Bhattacharya*, and
2) *Lahiri Mahasay's Personal Letters to Kriya Disciples.*

Although I did not have the opportunity to read the books well, I cannot express my feeling in languages about these two books and to collect them.

Kindly supply information to my address about these two books as well as your other books - where these can be available and what price.

My fellow *Kriyabans*, many of them are eager for these books and, I believe they will continue their interest in future.

So, in this regards, for distribution, what arrangement have you done in India, please let me know.

Again, with *Pronam* [bowing].

Joydev Bhattacharya
6/3/1999

The Handwritten Letter of Soumen Banerjee, great grandson of Panchanan Bhattacharya from his granddaughter's side. to Swami Satyeswarananda

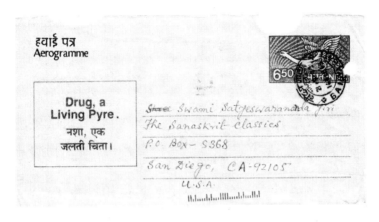

हवाई पत्र
Aerogramme

Drug, a Living Pyre.
नशा, एक जलती चिता।

6.50

Swami Satyeswarananda Giri
The Sanaskrit Classics
P.O. Box - 5368
San Diego, CA-92105
U.S.A.

Respected Sir,

I have gone through the book "Biography of A Yogi" written by you, The said book have very much impressed me. I have now learnt from my maternal uncle "Shivamoy Bhattacharya" that you have written another book Inner Victory Commentaries-IV the life and teaching of great Saint Acharya Panchanan Bhattacharya. I will be grateful if you kindly donate a copy of the said book for my own use and reading.

Incidently I beg to mention that Acharya Panchanan Bhattacharya was my great Grand father from my mother side.

Thanking you.

Yours faithfully.

Soumen Banerjee.

My address:-

SOUMEN BANERJEE
C/o. Amal Krishna Banerjee
G.T. Road, Badamtala,
P.O. Baidyabati.
Dist - Hooghly (W.B)
Pin - 712222
INDIA.

Hand written Letter of Soumen Banerjee to Swami Satyeswarananda

My Address:
Soumen Banerjee
C/O Amal Krisna Banerjee
G.T. Road, Badamtola,
P.O. Baidyabati,
Dist. Hooghly (W.B.)
Pin 712222
INDIA

Respected Sir,

I have gone through the book "Biography of a Yogi" written by you. The said book have very much impressed me.

I have now learnt from my maternal uncle "Shivamoy Bhattacharya" that you have written another book Inner Victory Commentaries -IV The Life and Teaching of great saint Acharya Panchanan Bhattacharya.

I will be grateful if you kindly donate a copy of the said book for my own use and reading.

Incidentally, I beg to mention that Acharya Panchanan Bhattacharya was my great grandfather from my mother's side.

Thanking you.

Yours Faithfully,

Soumen Banerjee

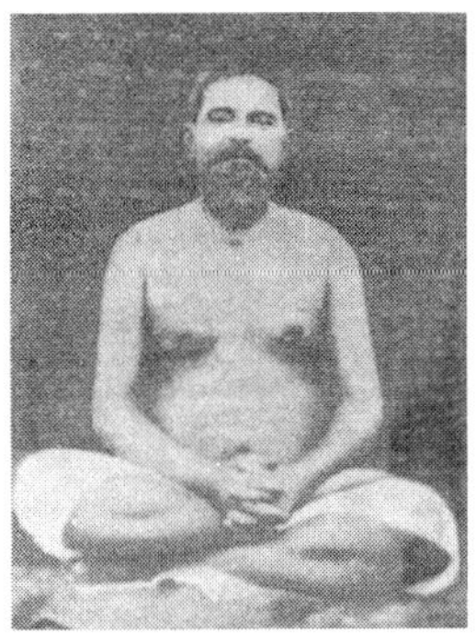

Sri Panchanan Bhattacharya,
the Chief Disciple of Lahiri Mahasay

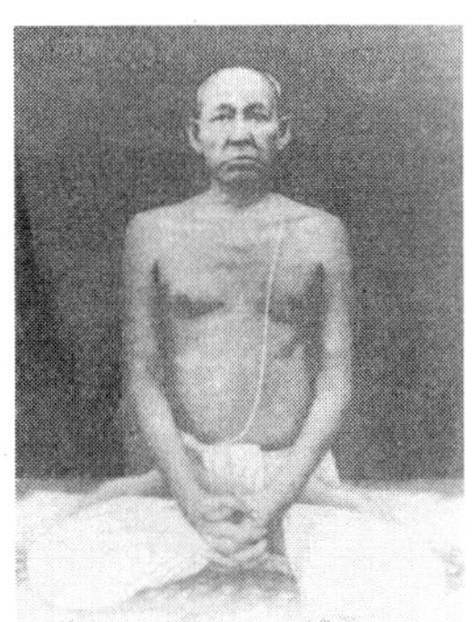

Bamandev Banerjee,
Disciple of Panchanan Bhattarcharya

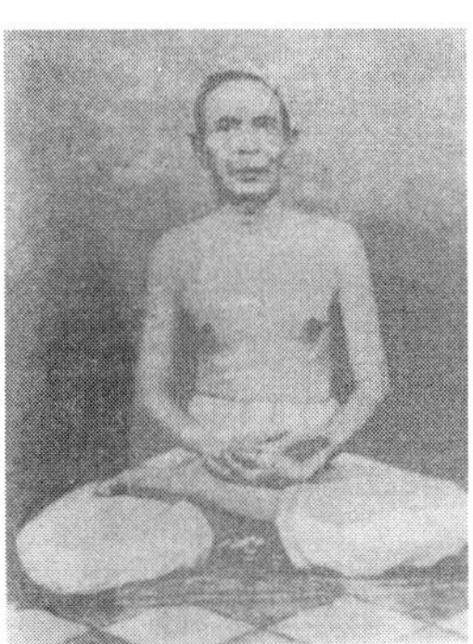

Nitai Charan Banerjee,
Disciple and son of Bamandev Banerjee

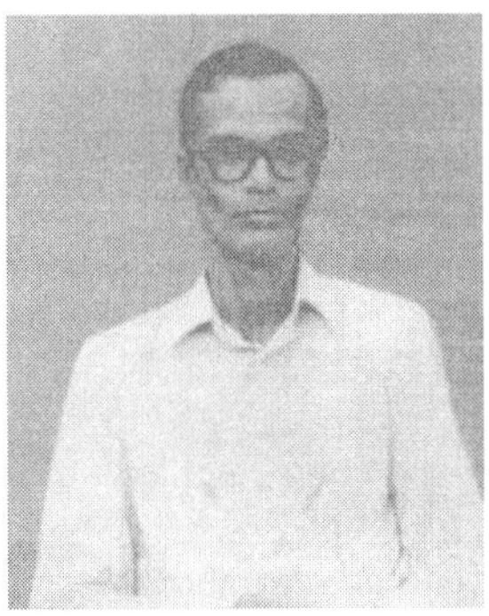

Dr Amal Bikas Choudhury,
Disciple of Nitai Ch. Banerjee

The following are the two letters of seventeen (17) letters written by Dr. Amal Bikas Choudhury to the author between 1992 - 1997.

Swami Satyeswarananda and Dr. Amal Bikas Choudhury, disciple of Nitai Charan Banerjee

Although the Swamiji did not meet Nitai Charan Banerjee personally, Nitai Babu was aware of Swami Satyeswaranada.

One day, a lady disciple, Dipti Mukherjee, asked Nitai Babu, "Baba! My husband and I received *Kriya* two years ago, and you are so old. If you should leave the body where should we go to receive further advice?"

Nitai Babu said, "You will meet a Swamiji."

Dr. Amal Bikas Choudhury was present in the room when this was said and he overheard it. Then within a few months his beloved *Gurudev* actually did leave his body. In fact, Dipti Mukherjee and her husband along with Dr. Choudhury himself would meet a Swamiji, just as their *Guru* had foretold, and this Swamiji would turn out to be the author. Here is the story of how this came about.

The author used to stay in the house of a devotee, Mr. Birendra Lal Choudhuri in Calcutta which happened to be in the same neighborhood as Dr. Amal Bikas Choudhury's chamber for practicing homeopathic medicine.

In the winter of 1979, perhaps on the 16th or 17th of February during the author's winter visit to Calcutta, Biren Babu's wife, Mrs. Asha Choudhuri, visited Dr. Amal Bikas Choudhury's chamber for medicine. There she found a photo of a *Kriya* Yogi hung on the wall.

Asha Choudhuri asked Dr. Amal Bikas Choudhury. "Isn't it a photo of a *Kriya* Yogi?"

The doctor said, "Yes. You're right. How did you know?"

Asha said, "Our Swamiji is from that discipline."

Surprised, the doctor asked, "Swamiji? Who is he?"

Asha said, "He is a Himalayan Yogi. He comes to our house every year in the winter."

Remembering his *Guru* Baba's recent comment to his lady disciple about meeting a Swamiji, the Doctor asked, "When will he come this year?"

Asha said, "He is in our house now."

The doctor said, "I'd like to go with you and visit him. Please wait for me to treat these patients, and I'll give you your medicine last so I can accompany you home."

Thereafter, the doctor examined the patients who were there, closed up his chamber and accompanied Asha to her home four or five minutes's walk away.

Meanwhile, on the eastern balcony of the second floor of the Choudhuri home, the author was looking at *Jugantar*, one of two major Bengali daily newspapers (the other being *Ananda Bazar Patrika*). It was almost eleven or eleven thirty in the morning. The obituary page had caught his attention for there was a passport-sized photo with a small note written about Nitai Charan Banerjee, the *Kriya* Yogi.

Just then Dr. Amal Bikas Choudhury was led by Mrs. Asha Choudhuri to the balcony. The moment Dr. Choudhury entered there he made *pranam* to Swamiji and looking at the page said, "Swamiji! That's my *Guru Baba*. Last week, he left us. My heart is breaking. I have become an orphan."

The doctor stayed for thirty minutes or so. When he left to have lunch, he contacted as many fellow disciples as possible with the news of meeting a Swamiji from the Himalayas of *Kriya* discipline. He gave them the address of where the Swamiji was staying. Word spread rapidly because some seventy-two families of the locale had received *Kriya* from Nitai Charan Banerjee. For the bereaved devotees who had lost their beloved *Gurudev* only a week before, this was sensational news. Within a few hours almost twenty brother and sister disciples of his had showed up to have Swamiji's *Darsan*. Dr. Choudhury who had to see patients from three to five joined them when he was free in the late afternoon.

The following year Swamiji made his annual trip to Bengal, and as usual he had a busy itinerary. An attorney devotee practicing in the Calcutta High Court had invited Swamiji to his home town at Krisna Nagar, the birth place of Lahiri Mahasay, and so Swamiji had been escorted by him there where he had stayed for three days. At one in the afternoon on Christmas day Swamiji had returned to Calcutta to the residence of the Choudhuri family where he often stayed. He found two devotees waiting for him.

One was Dulal Mukherjee who wanted to take some snap shots of Swamiji for his personal use and who had brought a photographer.

The second was Ranganath Tewari, an advanced disciple of Nitai Babu who wanted to bring Swamiji to Bakultola Asram to inaugurate the *Samadhi* temple of his Gurudev. Nitai Babu had gone to stay at Bakultola Asram on Christmas Day. It proved to be his last visit, for it was there he left his body on February ninth. Afterwards his devotees had built the *Samadhi* temple. Though the temple was not completely finished (the final cement of the verandahs around the temple was not yet poured), they felt Christmas Day would be an auspicious day to inaugurate it, and they wanted Swamiji to preside over the inaugural ceremony.

Ranganath Tewari said, "Swamiji, I have been awaiting your arrival. My brother and sister disciples have all requested me to take you to our Bakultola Asram to inaugurate our *Guru Baba's Samadhi* Temple.

"You must be kind and agree to come with me. Everyone's waiting for you there. They sent me saying if anyone could bring you it would be me. It was unanimous. I told them this: 'You all know how busy Swamiji is. His winter itinerary in Bengal is usually prearranged for six months in advance before he even arrives in Bengal from the Himalayas, so don't expect him to be able to make changes of this kind on short notice.' Still they're hopeful, and that's why they entrusted me with this difficult task. So kindly grant all of our prayers to come with me now. If not it will be a devastating disappointment for all of us."

When Mrs. Asha Choudhuri heard this request of Ranganath Tewari's addressed to Swamiji, she complained to her husband saying, "Just a few days before, Swamiji returned here at one o'clock in the morning after visiting the *Kriyanwitas* of Midnapore. Then he left for Krisna Nagar after a two-hours' rest and a bath. Now, that he has returned from there within thirty minutes he has to go to Bakultola. Incredible! Where does all this energy come from? What about his spending some time in our house? According to his original itinerary which was agreed on by all the devotees, he is scheduled to stay at our house.

"If he decides to go with Ranganath Tewari, you must go with him and bring him back in the evening. Otherwise, they'll keep him there."

Meantime, Tewariji was concerned over traffic in Howrah at Sibpur where Bakultola was. It was an eleven-day holiday in the schools and colleges, a time of picnicking for Bengalis at the famous Sibpur Botanical Garden near the Ganges with its ancient banyan tree with thousands of props, its beautiful groves of various kinds of trees and its grassy open spaces. Hundreds of buses and cars full of picnickers would be arriving and then leaving. Any sort of delay would make it impossible to reach the asram in time.

Tiwariji extended the invitation to Birendra Lal Choudhuri, but asked him to hurry. Biren Babu said, "I need to shave."

Finally, all set off for Bakultola and arrived there in time despite the crowds of picnickers. Bakultola was situated on grassy gentle slopes dotted by shady trees. The slopes converged in what seemed to have once been a streambed. Here at this quiet, idyllic spot where bodies were cremated, a visitor would be struck with the momentariness of life and turn, if only for a time, introspective and philosophic.

Swamiji found the vibrations at Bakultola to be even more peaceful than other cremation spots. This was where Brahmachari Nirad Baran had meditated for several years awaiting information of the whereabouts of his *Guru*, Nitai Charan Banerjee, the name given him by the voice while he was in the Himalayas. It was truly an ideal place for meditation.

That evening Swamiji presided over the inauguration ceremony and gave a speech which was taped. (This happened in 1979. On May 29, 1995, Dr. Amal Bikas Choudhury wrote Swamiji in San Diego that the devotees at Bakultola had printed his speech in newsletter form and distributed it for personal use. He requested Swamiji to send them some more tapes in Bengali.)

The devotees of Bakultola fed Swamiji in the evening after the meeting. It was his first meal of the day since he had left Krisna Nagar by train for Calcutta early in the morning and once arriving had rested in Calcutta for only thirty minutes before taking off again, this time for Bakultola. Dr. Dandapani Banerjee, the only son of Nitai Charan Banerjee, greeted Swamiji warmly saying, "Swamiji! It's a pleasure to meet you." It was he who personally supervised the serving of the meal. Later Dr. Amal Bikas Choudhury requested Swamiji to come to Bakultola every year on that day.

That evening Biren Babu brought Swamiji back to Calcutta.

After this, every year during his winter visit in Calcutta, Swamiji would visit Dr. Amal Bikas Choudhury's house at Santoshpur usually on a Sunday.

Swamiji was touched by the love and affection shown to him by the devotees of Santoshpur. Reciprocally each and every one is felt in Swamiji's heart.

Once, Dr. Amal Bikas Choudhury told the author the following: "Swamiji! My parents were *Kriyanwitas*. As a young man, I came by myself to this great city of Calcutta from East Bengal. I didn't know anyone here who practiced *Kriya*, and I wondered where I could get the connection to *Kriya* discipline. It wasn't easy to find that connection because, as you know, according to the tradition real *Kriya* people maintain secrecy.

"One day in my office during lunch break, a colleague of mine was discussing topics of a spiritual nature with some other colleagues. I listened with interest, and later I took him aside to another room and confronted him. I told him that he should admit that the information he had mentioned was from the book *Dharma O Pujadi Mimangsa* by Panchanan Bhattacharya. My parents had had that book and I had read it. He then admitted that it was so. I suspected that he must know some *Kriya* Yogi here in town, and I requested him to help me by providing me with the address of a *Kriya* Yogi. He then wrote the address of my *Guru* Baba on a sheet of paper and handed it to me. The same week I went to see him and received *Kriya*. This colleague was our beloved Pravat Kumar Das, an advanced disciple of *Guru* Baba."

(Pravat Babu had come to visit Swamiji a few times and had once brought a gentleman with him who had later received *Kriya* from Swamiji.)

Dr. A. B. Choudhury also told the following to Swamiji, "The American secretary of Yogoda approached my Baba [Nitai Charan Banerjee] with the proposal that he join them so that he could give *Kriya* guidance and advice to their followers. My Baba said, 'You would have to surrender unconditionally. Only then could I consider this.'

"Yogoda's secretary was surprised to hear this and said he would not be able to do so.

"Then my Baba told him that he was sorry but that he could not accept his proposal. He also told the secretary of Yogoda: 'You will remain stagnant.' "

The three advanced disciples of Nitai Charan Banerjee that Swamiji met were Pravat Kumar Das, Dr. Amal Bikas Choudhury, and Ranganath Tiwari, a school teacher.

The Handwritten Letter of Dr. Amal Bikas Choudhury, disciple of Nitai Charan Banerjee to Swami Satyeswarananda

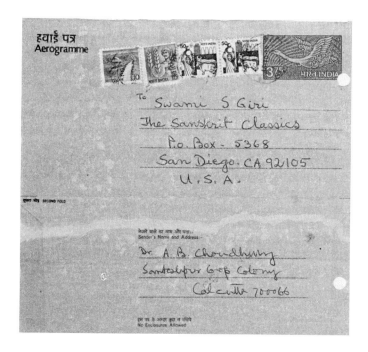

हवाई पत्र
Aerogramme

भारत INDIA

To
Swami S Giri
The Sanskrit Classics
P.O. Box - 5368
San Diego. CA 92105
U.S.A.

SECOND FOLD

Sender's Name and Address:-

Dr. A.B. Choudhury
Santoshpur Co-op Colony
Calcutta 700066

No Enclosures Allowed

ॐ

A.B. Chowdhury.
Santoshpur Co-op Colony
12.10.88

Revered Swamiji.

Thousands Pranams to you. I received your The Bibles 2nd Edition in my sick bed and felt your blessings poured down on my head. This made me forget my sickness. I feel fortunate that you have not forgotten us. We all the Kriyabans in Santoshpur pray your presence among us within a shor period. We know that you are busy with mission under direction of Maha Muni Babaji.

For the last 30 days I am very sick. Kindly write a few lines.

With kind regards

A.B.Chowdhury

OM

A. B. Choudhury
Santoshpur Co-op Colony
12/10/88

Revered Swamiji,

Thousand *Pranams* [bowing head in traditional manner] to you. I received yours the Bibles 2nd edition in my sick bed and felt your blessing poured down on my head. This made me forget my sickness.

I feel fortunate that you have not forgotten us. We all the *Kriyabans* [practitioners of *Kriya*] in Santoshpur pray your presence among us within a short period.

We know that you are busy with mission under direction of Maha Muni Babaji.

For the last 30 days I am very sick.

Kindly write a few lines.

With Kind regards.

A. B. Choudhury.

The Handwritten Letter of Dr. Amal Bikas Choudhury, disciple of Nitai Charan Banerjee, in Bengali to Swami Satyeswarananda

ॐ

Dr. A. B. Choudhury
Calcutta-66
Dt 6.4.94

[illegible] Kriya Sutras of Babaji [illegible]
2nd April 94 [illegible]

[illegible]

[illegible] Secretary. Nityananda
Yogashram. Nityananda nagar
Thana Makua Howrah.

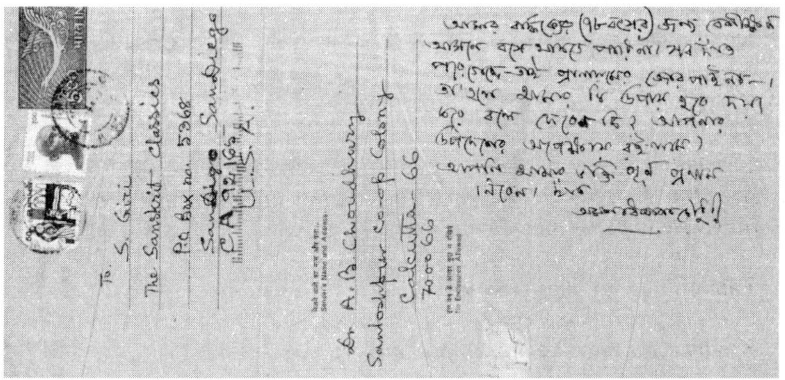

The English version of the previous letter

OM

Dr. A. B. Choudhury
Calcutta – 66
6/4/94

Param Sradheya Swamiji (Supremely Respectable Swamiji),

Kindly accept my devotional *pranam*. Kindly give your sheltered devotees my heartfelt love.

I received the book – *Kriya Sutras of Babaji* written by you. As if the scripture brought blessing to us.

You have discussed the mysteries of Yoga in this scripture. The educated *Kriyanwits* (practitioners of *Kriya*) of the western hemisphere will be benefited; there is no doubt about it.

Will you come to India on the centenary birth celebration of Lahiri Mahasay in 1995? We are all hoping you will come.

Whatever you had said in our Bakultala Ashram, as far as possible, we printed them and distributed among us. All are eagar to receive from you this type of advice and good words. If you kindly send (to the following address) some advice to this hermitage it will be very beneficial to all. It will be better in Bengali than in English (as many people do not know English).

Secretary
Nityananda Yogashram,
Nityananda Nagar,
Thana Makua, Howrah.

I cannot sit longer on the *asana* (seat) because of my old age (78 years old). I have lost all teeth. So I cannot find energy on practicing *Pranayam*. Kindly will you tell (advise) me on this matter?

I am waiting for your kind advice.

Kindly accept my devotional *pranam*.

Yours,

Amal Bikas Choudhury

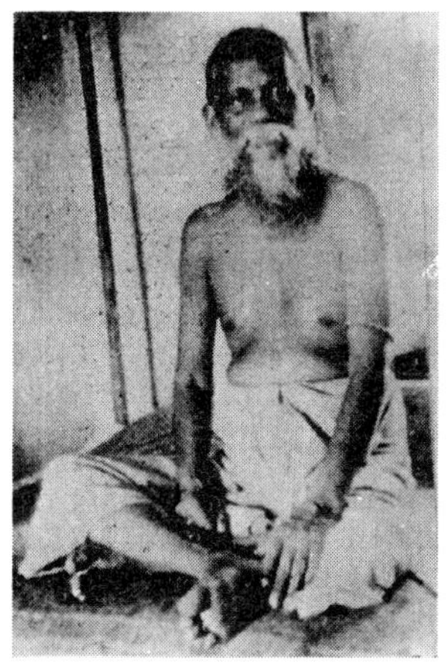

Swami Satyananda Giri Maharaj, President of Sevayatan,
Initiated by Hangsa Swami Kebalananda and
the chief monastic disciple of Swami Sriyukteswar Giri in India.

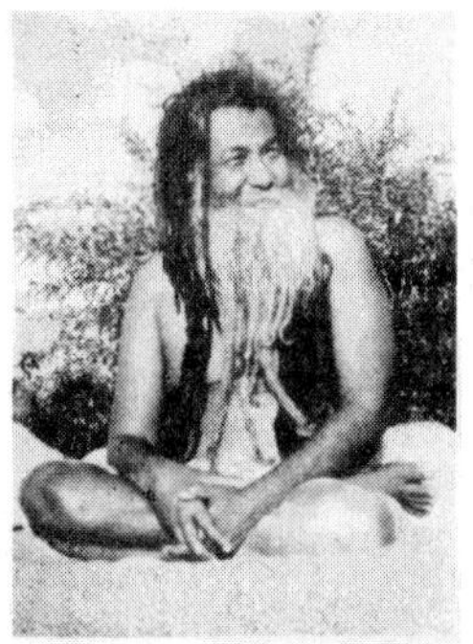

Swami Hariharanada,
Disciple of Swami Satyananda

Swamiji Maharaj was traveling from the Uttarkasi, Himalayas, on the way to Calcutta to attain a meeting with Sister Daya, President of SRF; the local authority of Yogoda Yogananda's organization had arranged the meeting to see if Swamiji can work with them. Swamiji knew it was impossible to work out. On the way he stopped at Bindudham Yogasram at Barharwa, S. P. Bihar.

Swami Satyananda told Swamiji that Hariharananda's *Kalipuja* (worshiping Goddess Kali) was unique since he learned *tantra* from Tara Khepa (the direct disciple of Bama Khepa) before he met Swami Satyananda. That was one attraction to drop by there as *Kalipuja* was near.

Swamiji stayed there almost twenty days. Surprisingly he saw two friends from Bengal: Chira Ranjan Panja, visiting his *Guru*, and Prof. Mahabir Maji, a personal friend of the author who a was disciple of Swami Satyananda. Swamiji learned from them that they had come to convince Hariharananda to be brought to their village asram which Sriyukteswar founded in 1813. Nobody was in charge of that asram. More surprisingly, Hariharananda suggested to them to take Swamiji to Khukurdaha. Swamiji said that Swami Satyananda had suggested this once, and politely but firmly he had rejected the idea then and Swamiji's position was not changed. (The reason for Swami Satyananda's interest was to avoid Sriyuktesar's forecast of litigation over the hermitages using Swamiji's legal background). However, Swamiji promised to them that wherever he would be in life, he would remember the people of Khukurdaha village on the day of the full moon in the month of February when Sriyukteswar founded that asram in 1813.

All of a sudden *Brahmachari* Bhubaneswarananda, disciple of Hariharananda, told Swamiji that his Baba may be moving from Bindudham Yogasram. Usually he stayed at one place for twelve years and then moved to another place never to return again. In spite of his suggestion that Swamiji be taken to the asram at Khukurdaha, for some unknown reason, Hariharananda was interested to take Swamiji with him wherever he was planning to move to his next place and that happened to be a beautiful place at Jaipur, Rajasthan.

Hariharananda found out that Swamiji was going to see Sister Daya, president of SRF & YSS in Calcutta. Learning this he became a bit uncomfortable and asked why Swamiji had to meet her? Swamiji said that they have made an appointment, so he has to go see her. It was then just a formality. Swamiji did not think he could work with them. Hariharananda felt a bit uncomfortable with the comment. However, Swamiji still could not figure out where Hariharanada's interest was in Swamiji. Many years later Swamiji found out that Satyananda once told Hariharananda that Swamiji would deliver him a message. Swamiji did not know this till Mahamuni Babaji told Swamiji to deliver a message. On Hariharananda's part, he thought it would be from Satyananda himself. That was the reason he was keeping an eye on Swamiji's. movement.

Swami Hariharananda was a good friend and a colleague of Swamiji.

Swamiji visited Swami Hariharananda at Jaipur, Rajasthan, to deliver the message from Mahamuni Babaji which Swamiji just received from him in the Himalayas and for which Hariharananda was keeping an eye on Swamiji. It was in 1975 before Swamiji undertook a world lecture tour at the instruction of Mahamuni Babaji.

Hariharananda was very surprised with the message. He originally thought it would be from his Guru Baba, Swami Satyananda, since he told him a message would be delivered to him by Swamiji.

Just after Swamiji arrived to Jaipur, *Brahmachari* Bhubaneswarananda, disciple of Hariharananda, arranged Swamiji's staying there at the hermitage, in which room he would stay, etc. Then he entered the room again and said that a foreigner wanted to see him. Swamiji said how a foreigner could know Swamiji was here. Swamiji suggested perhaps *brahmachari* was making a mistake; it could be the foreigner wanted to see his own Guru Baba, Hariharananda. Then *brahmachari* said "no sir;" he was not making a mistake; he asked the foreign visitor whom he wanted to meet and the visitor said that he would like to meet with Swami Satyeswarananda. Swamiji said, "then send him".

The foreign visitor happened to be a young research scientist. He was living in India for a while to complete his research on the subject of "brain waves." The visitor, not losing any time, introduced his interest to record the conversation on tape. Swamiji, also losing no time, said *Kriya Yoga* was not for commercial use and so he could leave the room and shut the door when he was leaving. The visitor was stunned at the quick response. His experience was quite different with the other Indian Yogis and sages. They welcomed him when he visited them and had recorded some conversations. Swamiji said, "Sorry. All yogis are not the same."

While writing these pages it reminded Swamiji that when he was leaving India for his world lecture tour to Italy, first he arrived at Delhi from Calcutta. Just before the day Swamiji had to fly, three Japanese girls entered his room in the evening with the hotel manager who mentioned that these girls were looking for him. The moment the manager left the room one of the girls started talking about how they looked for Swamiji in Bengal in many hermitages but could not find him. Finally, at Burdwan, Bengal, someone informed them that Swamiji just had left to Delhi from where he would take a flight to Europe. Losing no time they arrived at Delhi and found Swamiji. Sometimes it amazed Swamiji how the people got information so quick. They needed Original *Kriya*. Swamiji initiated them into *Kriya*. One of the girls was a social science graduate.

Hariharanandaji after receiving the message left his body in 1976.

A Non-Bengali Indian *Kriyanwit's* Perspective

A Handwritten letter by a Non-Bengali Indian *Kriyanwit* (Dr. B. P. Srivastava) to the author

From:- Dr. B. P. Srivastava
Associate Professor of Political Theory,
Deptt. of Political Science,
University of Raj
Jaipur (Raj)

7 Jha 26, Jawahar Nagar
Jaipur
Oct 21st 1985

Revered Shri Shri Swami Satyeshwaranandji Giri,

The set of books so assiduously and painstakingly written & so kindly sent by you to the Ashram here has been read by us with unflinching interest. It is needless to say that you have made a remarkable contribution and it is the continuation of a worthy tradition that you yourself had set, long ago, by publishing a brochure on Kriya yog.

Ever since the publication of Paramhans Yoganand's Autobiography an interest in "kriya" was aroused both among the intellectual elites and general masses but, despite there being a dire need, no effort by any body was made to quench the thirst. Thus the curious ones owe a debt of great gratitude to you for your publications.

Shri Shri Swami Yoga Nand was commissioned to write a book on Shri Shri Lahari Mahasaya. He worked on it but the book was not produced; Shri Shri Swami Satyanandji wrote but it could remain confined only to Bengali knowing people. Shri Bhattacharyaji made an earnest effort but the result was perfunctory. For the first time there is a comprehensive biographical sketch of the Mahasaya along with the many unravellings of the Kriya-mystery. Both the initiated and the non-initiated shall stand to gain by it.

One could think of book on the Mahasaya; but one could only wish & not think of a book on Shri Shri Maha Avtar Babaji Maharaj. Here a wonder has been done. I wonder if anyone else living has been so actively and intimately in touch with Him. In view of your living, continuous and constant contact with Him, wouldn't it be in the fitness of things to let devotees have His Darshan through a photograph which you alone can get printed. Some say that the one available through the Autobiography is not the authentic one. Would you be so pleased as to throw some light on this? The other books in their interest, absorbing capacity & fruitfulness are no less significant. I feel that some elaborate arrangement for their sale in India through right agencies should be made. And, you are more than capable of getting it done.

All those associated with Shri Shri Pahari Baba & Shri Shri Bhubneshwara Nandji offer their humble obeisance to you.

With humblest regards

Yours

B.P. Srivastava

A Non-Bengali Indian *Kriyanwit's* Perspective

From: Dr. B. P. Srivastav
Associate Professor of Political Theory,
Dept. of Political Science,
University of Rajasthan,
Jaipur (Rajasthan)

7 *Jha* 26, Jawahar Nagar
Jaipur
Oct. 21st, 1985

Revered Sri Sri Swami Satyeswarananda Giri

The set of books so assiduously and painstakingly written and so kindly sent by you to the ashram [hermitage] here has been read by us with unflinching interest. It is needless to say that you have made a remarkable contribution and it is the contribution of a worthy tradition that you yourself had set long ago, by publishing a book on *Kriya yoga*. [*The science of Self Realization – Kriya Yoga* in 1974; later, *The Kriya Sutras*].

Ever since the publication of Paramhansa Yogananda's Autobiography an interest in "*Kriya*" was aroused both among the intellectual elites and general masses but, despite there being a dire need, no effort by any body was made to quench the thirst. Thus the curious ones owe a debt of great gratitude to you for your publications.

Shri Shri Swami Yogananda was commissioned to write a book on Sri Sri Lahiri Mahasaya. He worked on it, but the book was not produced; Shri Shri Swami Satyananda-ji wrote but (it) could remain confined only to Bengali knowing people; [Non-Bengali Indian *Kriya* followers have no access to the original *Kriya* literature, written only in Bengali]; Shri Bhattacharya-ji [Sri Sri Panchanan Bhattacharya, the chief disciple of Lahiri Mahasay] made an earnest effort, but the result was perfunctory [as he was not destined to do it].

For the *first* time there is a comprehensive biographical sketch of the Mahasaya along with the many unravelings of the *Kriya* mystery. Both the initiated and the non-initiated shall stand to gain by it.

One could think of book on the Mahasaya [Lahiri Mahasay]; but one could only wish and not think of a book on Shri Shri Mahavatar Babaji Maharaj. Here a wonder has been done. I wonder if anyone else living has been so actively and intimately in touch with Him [Mahamuni Babaji, the Divine Himalayan Yogi].

In view of your living continuous and constant contact with Him wouldn't it be in the fitness of things to let devotees have His *Darshan* through a photograph which you alone can get printed. Some say that the one available through the Autobiography is not the authentic one. Would you be so pleased as to throw some light on this?

[Being asked by Swamiji, Mahamuni Babaji did not reveal his name. It is not possible to take his photo without his permission and he would not permit it; besides, Swamiji Maharaj had no camera with him at his hut in Dunagiri Hill, Himalayas].

The other books in their interests, absorbing capacity and fruitfulness are no less significant. I feel that some elaborate arrangement for their sale in India through right agencies should be made. And you are more than capable of getting it done.

All those associated with Shri Shri Pahari Baba [Swami Ushananda Giri, later known as Swami Hariharananda Giri [not to be confused with Swami Hariharananda Giri of Puri] and Shri Shri Bhubaneshwarananda-ji Giri [disciple of Hariharananda] offer their humble obeisance to you.

With humblest regards,
Yours
B.P. Srivastav

[Dr. B.P. Srivastav, disciple of Swami Hariharananda (disciple of Swami Satyananda)].

Typed Letter of Acharya Bubaneshwaranand, disciple of Swami Hariharananda

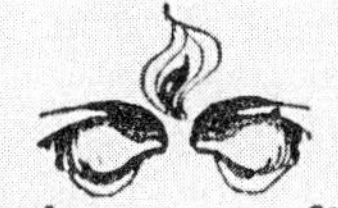

Bhubaneshawranand
Acharya

Satyayatan Ashram
Kala Mahadev,
Amber Road
Jaipur-302002
dated 15th Dec 91

To

Swami Shri Shri Satyeshawranand Giri
P.O.Box 5368
San Diego
C A 92165
U.S.A.

Revered Shri Shri Swamiji,

Sadar Jai Guru,

I am extremly grateful to you for placing me permanently on your mailing list.The latest pack of arrival contains Shri Shri Lahari Mahasaya's **The Gita, Lahari Mahasaya** Vol II,Shri Shri Yukteshwar Giri's **The Gita** and your**Kriya: Finding the True Path.**

Your gigantic project to publish the complete works of the Mahasaya should prove an epoch-making contirbution.Hitherto his works were published only in Bengali and were, therefore,rare documents of restrictive use.By translating them into English,with your profuse annotations,often emphasising a point over and over again with changing contexts,you have flung them open to the mass of English Knowing people,who,I believe,shall evoke the deserved interest in them. You have alreay published four volumes in the"**Commentary Series**"and the seven volume publication of his works in the"**Complete Works Reorganised Series**" is,happily,well under preparation.We wish you Sad-Guru speed in your venture.Your four-volume publication inthe "Biographies

Series"provides,**inter alia**,the needed & valuable preparatory background to the reader .

The Mahasaya's **The Gita** is a core Kriya work combining the ideational/conceptual and operative components of the Kriya.The like interpretations of other scriptures by the Mahasaya focuss on the Kriya as**the**principle and practice in the perspective of man's grandiose purpose and goal of life. The publication of Shri Shri Yukteshwar Giri's **The Gita** is purposive.Your **Kriya:Finding the True Path** is a mine of information.Particularly the fourth chapter on"The Kriya Science"is illuminating and the last chapter on " The Righteous Way " is quintessential.Your emphasis on the **Guru-Shishya-Parampara** is not anachronistic. In fact it is as modern and scientific as any process of learning and acquiring knowledge and practice-much more so to a seeker who can not enter the unchartered(for him)realm of sprituality without a Guru- the Guide.

Your's is a one man stupendous mission to disseminate the Kriya,on the authority of the Mahasay's works,in its prestine purity.Here I strongly feel that, since you are the recipient of incessant blessings of Maha Muni Babaji,have vast fund of knowledge and experience and your own inimitable realisation, your visit/visits to India is needed so that you may hold Kriyavan Sammelans(to be attened by the Kriya Masters as well as Kriyavanwitas) for the benefit of both the conformist as well as those deemed to be the deviationist.The former shall be illumined,get an oppurtunity to share experiences and evolve a commonly agreed formulation and pattern to promote the original Kriya.The latter shall be enabled to evolve a consensus that although,at one time,compulsions of the exegencies of the Western conditions & life situation might have brought about some experimental modifications and in the process got,perhaps unintentionally, diluted, such are the principles,practice and potential of the origional Kriya that the different life situation of a weatern seeker does not militate against them.Later the attempt can be replicated in the States. This shall ensure the uninhibited grace of the Sad-Guru(Sri Shri Lahari Mahasaya's)-the **Sad-Guru-Kripa** on all.

Kindly permit me to bring to your kind attention the predicament of the Indian reader to whom the prices of your published works are prohibitive.(They are all right in a country like the United States).To make the prices permissive,I wonder whether you can condescend to arrange with some Indian publisher to bring out their Indian Economy papaer back editions.

With humblest regards,

Yorus reverentially

(Bhubaneshwaranand)

Letter of *Brahmachari* Bhubaneshwarananda, disciple of Swami Hariharananda (disciple of Satyananda)

Bhubaneshwarananda
Acharya

Satyayatan Asram
Kala Mahadev,
Jaipur - 302002 Phone: 45100
Dated 15th Dec. 91

To
Swami Shri Shri Satyeswarananda Giri
P.O. Box 5368
San Diego
C.A. 92165
U.S.A.

Revered Shri Shri Swamiji, *Sadar Jai Guru,*

I am extremly grateful to you for placing me permanently on your mailing list. The latest pack of arrival contains Shri Shri Lahiri Mahasay's *The Gita*, *Lahiri Mahasaya* Vol. 2, Shri Shri Yukteswar Giri's The *Gita* and your *Kriya: Finding the true Path.*

Your gigantic project to publish the complete works of the Mahasaya should prove an epoch-making contribution. Hitherto his works were published only in Bengali and were, therefore, rare documents of restrictive use. By translating them into English, with your profuse annotations, often emphasising a point over and over again with changing contexts, you have flung them open to the mass of English knowing people, who, I believe, shall evoke the deserved interest in them. You have already published four volumes in the "Commentary Series" and the seven volume publication of his works in the "Complete works Reorganized Series" is, happily, well under preparation. We wish you *Sad-Guru* speed in your venture. Your four-volume publication in the "Biographies Series" provides, inter alia, the needed and valuable preparatory background to the reader.

The Mahasaya's The *Gita* is a core *Kriya* work combining the ideational/conceptual and operative components of the *Kriya*. The like interpretations of other scriptures by the Mahasaya focus on the *Kriya* as the principle and practice in the perspective of man's grandiose purpose and goal of life. The publication of Shri Shri Yukteswar Giri's The *Gita* is purposive. Your *Kriya* : *Finding the True Path* is a mine of information. Particularly the fourth chapter on "The *Kriya* Science" is illuminating and the last chapter on "The Righteous Way" is quintessential. Your emphasis on the *Guru-Shishya-*

Parampara is not anachronistic. In fact it is as modern and scientific as any process of learning and acquiring knowledge and practice-much more so to a seeker who can not enter the unchartered (for him) realm of spirituality without a Guru - the Guide.

Yours is a one man stupendous mission to disseminate the *Kriya*, on the authority of the Mahasay's works, in its pristine purity. Here I strongly feel that, since you are the recipient of incessant blessings of Maha Muni Babaji, have vast fund of knowledge and experience and your own inimitable realization, your visit/visits to India is needed so that you may hold *Kriyaban Sammelans* (to be attended by the Masters as well as *Kriyavanwitas*) for the benefit of both the conformist as well as those deemed to be the deviationist. The former shall be illumined, get an opportunity to share experiences and evolve a commonly agreed formulation and pattern to promote the original *Kriya*. The later shall be enabled to evolve a consensus that although, at one time, compulsions of the exigencies of the Western conditions and life situation might have brought about some experimental modifications and in the process got, perhaps unintentionally, diluted, such are the principles, practice and potential of the original *Kriya* that the different life situation of a western seeker does not militate against them. Later the attempt can be replicated in the States. This shall ensure the uninhibited grace of the *Sad-Guru* (Sri Sri Lahiri Mahasay's) - the *Sad-Guru-Kripa* on all.

Kindly permit me to bring to your kind attention the predicament of the Indian reader to whom the prices of your published works are prohibitive. (They are all right in a country like the United States). To make the prices permissive, I wonder whether you can condescend to arrange with some Indian publisher to bring out their Indian Economy papaer [paper] back editions.

With humblest regards,

Yours reverentially

(Bhubaneshwaranand)

The Handwritten Letter of Dr. M.L. Sharma, Secretary Satyayatan Ashram

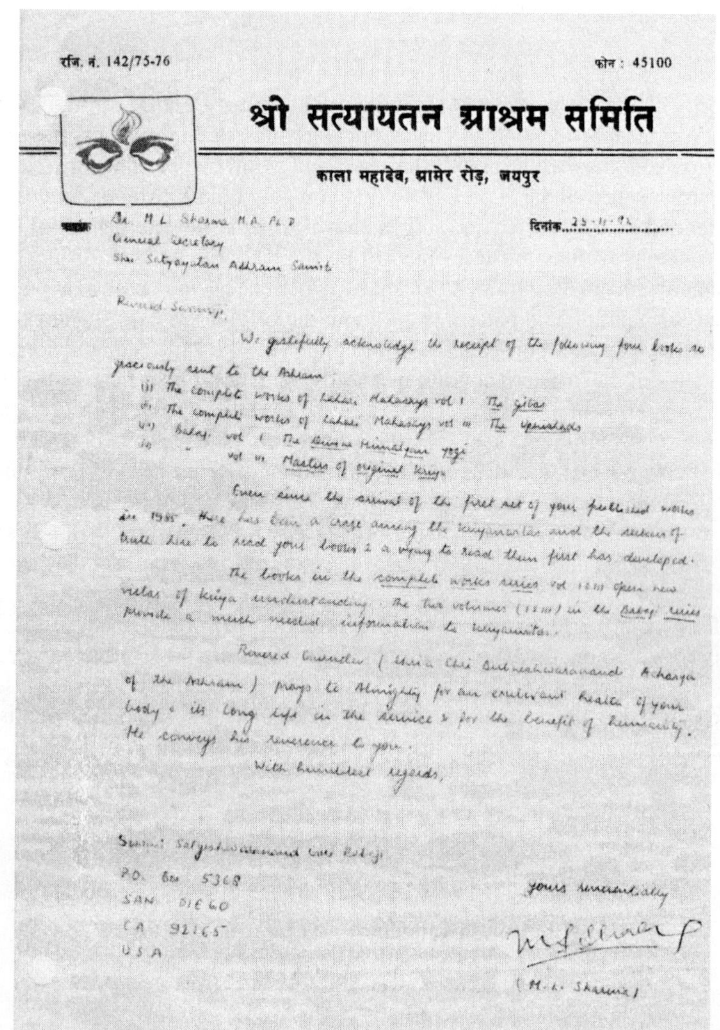

रजि. नं. 142/75-76 फोन : 45100

श्री सत्यायतन आश्रम समिति

काला महादेव, आमेर रोड़, जयपुर

Dr. M L Sharma M.A. Ph.D
General Secretary
Shri Satyayatan Ashram Samiti

दिनांक 23-11-92

Revered Swamiji,

We gratefully acknowledge the receipt of the following four books so graciously sent to the Ashram

(i) The complete works of Lahiri Mahasaya vol I The Gitas
(ii) The complete works of Lahiri Mahasaya vol III The Upanishads
(iii) Babaji vol I The Divine Himalayan Yogi
(iv) " vol III Masters of original Kriya

Ever since the arrival of the first set of your published works in 1985, there has been a craze among the Kriyavantas and the seekers of truth here to read your books & a vying to read them first has developed.

The books in the complete works series vol I & III open new vistas of Kriya understanding. The two volumes (I & III) in the Babaji series provide a much needed information to Kriyavantas.

Revered Gurudev (Shri Shri Bubneshwaranand Acharya of the Ashram) prays to Almighty for an exuberant health of your body & its long life in the service & for the benefit of humanity. He conveys his reverence to you.

With humblest regards,

Swami Satyeswarananda Giri Babaji
P.O. Box 5368
SAN DIEGO
CA 92165
USA

Yours reverentially

(M.L. Sharma)

Dr. M. L Sharma's Letter

Dr. M.L. Sharma M.A., Ph.D.
General Secretary
Shri Satyayatan Ashram Samiti

Revered Swamiji,

We gratefully acknowledge the receipt of the following four books so graciously sent to the *ashram* (hermitage).

1) The Complete Works of Lahiri Mahasay Vol. 1 *The Gitas*
2) The Complete Works of Lahiri Mahasay Vol. 3 *The Upanisads*
3) *Babaji* Vol. 1 *The Divine Himalayan Yogi*
4) *Babaji* Vol. 3 *Masters of original Kriya*

Ever since the arrival of the first set of your published works in 1985, there has been a craze among the *Kriyanwitas* and the seekers of truth here to read your books and a vying to read them first has developed.

The books in the complete works series Vol. 1 & 3 open new vistas of *Kriya* understanding. The two volumes (1 and 3) in the Babaji series provide a much needed information to *Kriyanwitas*.

Revered *Gurudev* (Sri Sri Bhubaneshwarananda Acharya of the ashrm) prays to Almighty for an exuberant health of your body and its long life in the service and for the benefit of humanity. He conveys his reverence to you.

With humblest regards.

Yours reverentially,

(M. L. Sharma)

The Hindu Way of Life

This explanation is for the Indian and the Western seekers of truth. It is felt to write for some obvious reasons; so that people can educate themselves and learn the proper way to write the appropriate words in the appropriate place.

The Vedic culture is *Sanatan Dharma*, and is popularly called Hinduism . In the Hindu way of life starting from the cutting of umbilical cord several rites are celebrated with worship conducted by the family priest. Like having a family doctor each Hindu family has a priest and the priesthood is hereditary for the family.

For the average Hindu people the last rite is funeral worship. The sons of the deceased person make the funeral worship for seven generations paternal and seven generations of the maternal ancestors including the deceased parent.

For the spiritual life *sannyas* (renunciation) is the last rite. Since the *sannyasi* has no connection with the family anymore, he has to make funeral worship of the seven generations paternal and seven generations of maternal ancestors; then his own funeral worship for his self (soul) as there will be nobody to do it for him later.

As mentioned before all these rites are observed and celebrated with ritualistic worship conducted by the family priest. The principal rites of the Hindu way of life are as follows.

1) *Nadichhedan* - Cutting the umbilical cord,

2) *Namkaran* - Giving a name to the baby,

3) *Sasthi puja*, Worshipping Goddess Sasthi (on the Sixth day) for the baby's welfare and future fortune,

4) *Mukhebhat* - Starting to give hard food within six months in addition to mother's breast feeding milk,

5) *Upanayan sanskar* - The boys are given sacred thread (*Yagyapabit*) only between 8 to 12 years of age in the *brahmana* family, between 12 to 16 in the *Khatriya* and *Vaisya* family. The *Sudras* are not given sacred thread. It is comprised of three, six or nine threads made of cotton. Three counts symbolically are the *Ida*, *Pingala*, and *Susumna* (spinal cord).

Having the sacred thread, the boys will be twice born (*dwija*) and start their spiritual life, practicing Vedic *Pranayam* with the *Gayatri mantra* thrice a day (morning, midday and evening) each time at least 12 *Pranayam* before taking their meals. Without practicing *Pranayam* they are not allowed to eat. The mothers usually supervise their young boys for their practice.

The Hindu way of life is divided into four parts:

a) *Brahmacharya* (the Student life, the first 25years).
b) *Garhastha* (the household life, the second 25 years),
c) *Vanaprastha* (the forest recluse, the third 25years), and
d) *Sannyas* (the renunciate life, the fourth 25 years).

a) The Student life - *Brahmacharya asram*:
Traditionally, the *Brahmachari* boys after the sacred thread is given are sent to *Guru's* asram for their education. The parents choose the teacher based on the conviction of the teacher, whether he believes in monism (the absolute Self) or dualism (the devotee and the Lord - that is, worshiper and the worshiped). The parents take the boy to an able Yogi or Swami who takes care of the boy providing everything including lodging and food. Parents are not allowed to visit or see them anymore until they are 25 years of age when the asram life finishes and the *Guru* makes convocation (*samavartan*). Thereafter, the boys are taken back home.

Brahmacharya vow - At this point some take *brahmacharya* vow under their Guru to advance the spiritual life and do not return home.

Many householders in India are not aware of all of the etiquette of the Vedic culture in details.

As in the West, the tradition is to write Mr., Miss, Ms, and Mrs. before the first name, so, is in India as for example - *Sri* (also can be spelled as *Shri*, *Shree*, *Sriyuta*, *Sriman*, and *Srimati,* the reason will be explained later),

While *Sri/Shri/Shree* is connected with the first name with a gentleman; for example, Sri Shyama Charan Lahiri, and Sri Manmatha Nath Mukherjee. In this context, the word *Sri* indicates that it is a masculine word. In case of a female, it will be like *Srimati/Shrimati/ Shreemati*, for example, Srimati Kasimoni Lahiri.

Sometime people drop their last name and use the spiritual style name; as for example, Lahiri Mahasay used and signed as Sri Shyamachan Devsarman, instead of Lahiri; in case of a female, like Srimati Kasimoni Devi (*Devi* is feminine word for *Dev*)

When a gentleman enters into a *Brahmachari* (celibate vow) order of the spiritual life, his *Sri* part is dropped and the new name is given by his *Guru* or Master depending on his Master's *sannyas* order (renunciate group out of ten groups Called *Dasnami*). *Dasnami* (ten) *Sannyasi* groups are as follows:

1) Giri,
2) Puri,
3) Bharati,
4) Saraswati,
5) Tirtha,
6) Ban,
7) Aranya,
8) Parvat,
9) Sagar, and
10) Nath.

For example, if the master is from the Giri order, he would give the name of his *Brahmachari* disciple as *Brahmachari* Sadananda. The "*ananda*" (means bliss) part will be towards the end of the name.

If the *Guru* is from Puri order, then he would give the name of his *Brahmachari* disciple as *Brahmachari* Siva *Chaitanya*. He cannot give *ananda,* instead will give *Chaitanya* (means consciousness).

When one takes a *brahmachari* vow and enters into the order of *Brahmachari*, he begs for food stuff and not the prepared meals from the householders. A *brahmachari* by rule must prepare his own food (called *Swapak* - *swa* means "himself", and *pak* means "preparation of food"). The reason is to maintain the purity of his breath with which he has to practice *Pranayam*, and to keep him healthy as well.

A *brahmachari* cannot use any of the above mentioned ten groups of Swami order names at the end of his name since he has not yet entered into the *sannyas*. For example, *Brahmachari* Kesavananda (who hails from a Banerjee *brahmana* family), a disciple of Lahiri Mahasay, once sought Lahiri Mahasay's permission to enter into the order of Swami. Lahiri Mahasay said, "You want to shave your head to be free of your heavy locks of hair." Kesavananda considered the comment as a negative answer. He did not enter into order of Swami. Again, another disciple of Lahiri Mahasay, Priyanath Karar (later, Swami Sriyukteswar Giri) hailing from a non-*brahmana* family, observing the situation of

Brahmachari Kesavananda (who was from a *brahmana* family) did not venture to seek permission, considered he had no chance. So he entered into the order of Swami later after Lahiri Mahasay had left the body. Only Sri Manmathanath Mukherjee, a disciple of Lahiri Mahasay, was permitted to enter into the order of Swami by Lahiri Mahasay. His given name was Swami Pranabananda Giri.

The next second 25 years begins.

b) *Garhastha* (The household life, the second 25 years),

6) *Bibaha* - the marriage. The parents bringing back their boys from the hermitage, get them married for the householder life. Having seen the grandson who can continue the lineage, the grandparents retire to the forest for the third stage.

c) *Vanaprastha* (the forest recluse, the third 25years),

7) *Vanaprastha* - Preparing for spiritual life, the husband and wife leave for forest or to the Hills, take shelter in some *Vanaprastha asram* and live there collecting alms from the nearby locality for the third 25 years of life.

d) *Sannyas* (the renunciate life, the fourth 25 years, often called the fourth *asram*).

8) *Sannyas* - The renunciate life. After completing the *Vanaprastha* life the husband and wife separate and the husband renouncing all (*sarba*) enters into *Sannyas* life which is the last rite.

The rules of *sannyas asram* are very strict. A few of them are narrated here.

Only the Hindu male of three classes (*Brahmana* - priest class, *Khatriya* - military class, and *Vaisya* - trade and agricultural class) can enter the *Sannyas asram* or into the Swami order. The female of all classes including the man of the *Sudra* class and the Non-Hindus are prohibited to enter into the order of Swami. according to the Vedic rules and tradition.

A Swami usually begs alms from the householders who maintain the three classes (*Brahmachari*, *Vanaprasthi*, and *Sannyasi*) people of the Vedic society. Therefore, there is a tremendous responsibility upon the householders life style in the Vedic society. The householder is supposed to prepare at least one extra meal for a guest. The lady of the house or a representative of her, another female (not a male member of the family) since, lady of the house is in charge of the home front, clearly defined in the Vedic culture as her division of responsibility, is supposed to give alms to the guest.

Generally, a Swami, around 12 o'clock seeing the smoke of the chimney of the householders from the hill or the forest, comes to the door and utters: *Bhabati bhikhang dehi,* "Please give me alms." He is not supposed to enter the house. After waiting for a while, if he gets food, then he should move on. He is supposed to beg only a definite number of doors (which he had decided before). If he does not get anything, he is not supposed to beg alms at more doors than what he had previously decided. He should go back to his niche and drink water, considering that is the day for him according to his providence the Lord had decided, and engage in his meditation.

It should be mentioned here that a *brahmachari* is supposed to prepare his own food by himself (*swapak*), on the other hand, a renunciate Swami renounces all including the fire, so he cannot start a fire and prepare his food; he begs alms, the prepared food.

The *Sri* part of his name is dropped when man enters into the order of Swami. Example, Sri Narendranath Dutta became Swami Vivekananda Puri. He belonged to the Puri group, though he did not use it.

The word *Maharaja* means "the great king". A renunciate Swami is called *sahangsa*, all in all, so he is called Maharaj, dropping the last letter "a" to be distinguished from a great king.

Finally, during the *sannyas* vow, to enter into the Swami order, the name is given not to the person but to the body to be identified in the society. A Swami is the representative of Lord Narayan, for that reason, he is His Holiness. Although a decent Swami does not care for that; he considers: "He is nothing and he has nothing". He is a naked fakir.

All rules are broken nowadays, in the age of individualistic freedom. Even a western woman enters into Hindu style of Swami order and uses the term Swami which is a masculine word.

In this connection, it should be pointed out here that according to the Vedic Culture, there are four *Yugas*. As the conventional belief that the *Yugas* operate one after another starting orderly from - *Satya* to *Treta*, then to *Dwapara*, and finally to the *Kali*. The human being loses one fourth of their intelligence in each *yuga*. The *Kali Yuga* being the last one, the human beings possess only one fourth of intelligence. The popular belief is that we are in *Kali*

Yuga when we have only one fourth intelligence; as this *Kali Yuga* is moving to the end; and so eventually there will be total annihilation of the entire manifestation. Naturally, the individual freedom, disorder, and the chaotic situation are bound to happen towards the end. The four *Yugas* make a *Kalpa*. After the annihilation the new *Kalpa* will start with full intelligence again.

However, spiritually speaking from the realization point of view, in each moment all the four *Yugas* are present; as in a big circle several small circles can be accommodated or drawn.

Not knowing all the rules and appropriate use, the devotional householders use these terms inaccurately considering by doing so that they are showing respect. The devotional people do not know how to hold the balance; they always seem to be carried away.

Now about the use of *Sri/Shri/Shree*. The Sanskrit alphabet contains twelve vowels and thirty nine or forty (some counts) are consonants. Among these consonants, there are three *sa*, two *na*, and two *ba*.

1) *Sa* - (*talabya Sa* - get the help of palate),
2) *Sa* - (*murdhana Sa* - get the help of top of the head), and
3) *Sa* - (*danta Sa* - get the help of dental).

1) *Na* - (*murdhana Na* - get the help of top of the head), and
2) *Na* - (*danta Na* - get the help of dental).

The first Sa - (*talabya Sa*), some people use extra "h" with it which makes it *Shri*; some use two *ee* for "i" to make it *Shree*.

The University of Calcutta, where Swamiji was alumni, dropped the letter "h".

With this explanation, in the conclusion, at the suggestion of a Western seeker of truth who happens to be an attorney, Swamiji leaves those inaccurate uses as they are in the original letters. He pointed out that spelling Sibmoy or Sivamoy of the same person's name will be confusing to the Western readers. In the Sanskrit alphabet there are two letters *ba*. People write either *ba* or *va,* for that matter both are correct.

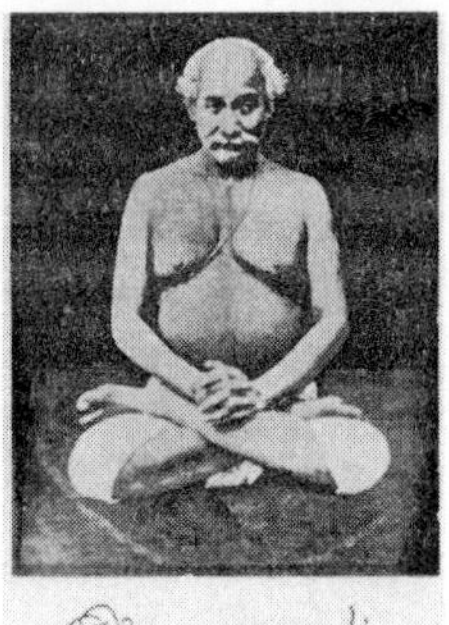

Yogiraj Sri Sri Shyama Charan
Lahiri Mahasay

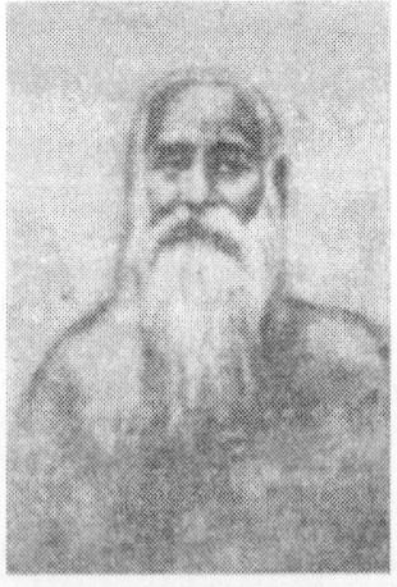

Tinkori Lahiri, eldest son of
Lahiri Mahasay

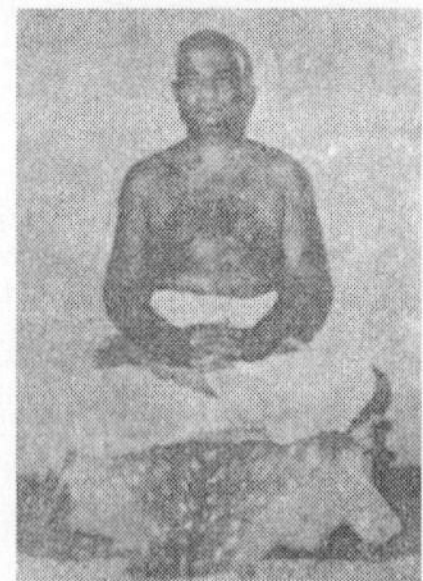

Satya Charan Lahiri,
Son of Tinkori Lahiri

The Handwritten First Letter of Sri Shibendu Lahiri,
Son of Satya Charan Lahiri (grandson of Lahiri Mahasay)
to Swami Satyeswarananda

ওঁ ১১ জুলাই ১৯৯২

শ্রদ্ধাভাজনেষু,

চাক্ষুস সাক্ষাৎ না হলেও যে আত্মিক টান ও যোগ বিদ্যমান, তার জোরেই এই পত্র লেখায় উৎসাহ ও প্রেরণা পেলাম। আমার পরমারাধ্য পিতা ৺ সত্যচরণ লাহিড়ী মহা-শয়ের নিকট হতে আপনার কথা শুনেছিলাম। January 1987 এ পিতা ইহলোক ত্যাগ করেন। একমাত্র পুত্র, তাই কর্ম্মত্যাগ করে সত্যলোকের পরম্পরা অব্যাহত রেখেছি। বাবা 1960 তে আমায় প্রথম দীক্ষা দিয়েছিলেন। 1978 এ সকল Stage এর সব গুলি ক্রিয়া সুসম্পন্ন হয়। Inner wholeness & holyness was not vitiated by the outer humdrum of the family and working life. হালে জানলাম — আপনি আমার ওপর খুব রেগে আছেন। আমার সকল অপরাধ আপনি নিজ-মহিমায় ক্ষমা করবেন।

9th Aug. থেকে 9th Sept. 92 পর্য্যন্ত আমি ও আমার স্ত্রী U.S.A. তে থাকব। ওই সময়ে আপনার দর্শন ও সৎ-সঙ্গ লাভ করতে পারলে অনুগৃহীত হব। জানিনা, আপনার ভক্তেরা সে ব্যবস্থা করতে পারবে কিনা। যদি তারা চায়, তাহলে Roy Eugene Davis, Centre for Spiritual Awareness, Lake Rabun Road, P.O. Box 7, Lakemont, Georgia - 30552 (Tel. no. — (706) 782-4723) এর সাথে Contact করে আমাদের উভয়কে দু'এক দিনের জন্য আপনার

हवाई पत्र
Aerogramme

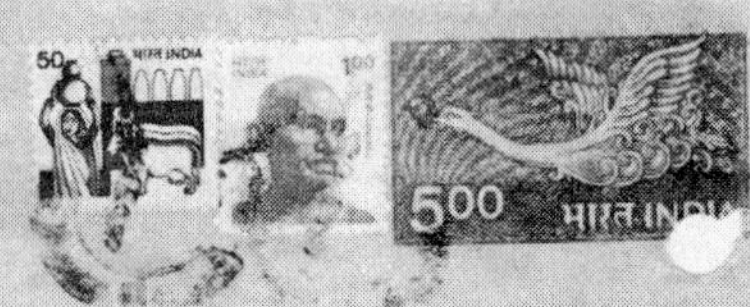

Swami Satyeswarananda Giri
P.O. Box 5368
San Diego
CA 92165 (U.S.A)

Sender's Name and Address

Shibendu Lahiri
D22/3, Chousatti Ghat
"Satyalok", Varanasi-221001
[India]

No Enclosures Allowed

স্থানে নিয়ে যাওয়ার ব্যবস্থা করতে পারে। দেখা
হলে অনেক কথা হবে। আরও কয়েক স্থানে যেতে
হবে। Roy সব Co-ordinate করছেন। তাই ওঁর
সাথে পরামর্শ করে San Diego programme ও
fix করা যেতে পারে। আপনি যা ভালো বুঝবেন,
করাবেন। আন্তরিক শ্রদ্ধাপূর্ণ প্রণতি জানাই। ইতি।
বিনীত, স্নেহাকাঙ্ক্ষী,
শিবেন্দু লাহিড়ী

The English Version of the Handwritten first letter of Shibendu Lahiri, Son of Satya Charan Lahiri (grandson of Lahiri Mahasay)

OM July 11, 1992

Respectable (*Shradhabhajanesu*),

I received the strength and courage to write this letter although I have not seen you with my own eyes, yet there is the relation (*atmic tan*) and the connection.

I learned about you from my supremely worshipable father, Satya Charan Lahiri.

[Swamiji does not know what Satya Babu told his son about him. But what *sat sanga* had transpired between Swamiji and Satya Babu will be written after this letter].

In January 1987, this father left this world. Being the only son, giving up the job, have returned to Satyaloka [home] and to maintain the tradition. My father gave me the first initiation in 1960 and in 1978 all the *Kriyas* of all the stages were performed. Inner wholeness and holyness was not vitiated by the outer humdrum of the family and working life. Recently learned that you are very angry at me. Kindly forgive me all offences with your own glorious qualities.

[Before this letter, Swamiji only heard about Shibendu Lahiri from his father that he had a son who was working in the state of Maharastra. Both Swamiji and Shibendu never met. Shibendu had done nothing wrong to Swamiji. So why would Swamiji be angry at him? There was no reason. In fact, Swamiji has no malice against the whole world. It was Shibendu's imagination only or perhaps, he wanted an affectionate reply from Swamiji drawing attention writing this line. Swamiji was surprised to read that line].

I and my wife will be in the U. S. A. from the 9th Aug. to 9th Sept. 92. I will be obliged if I could meet you and have your *sat sanga* at that time. I do not know if your devotees could arrange that meeting. If they want then they can contact Roy Eugene Davis, center for Spiritual Awareness, Lake Rabun Road, P.O. Box 7, Lakemont, Georgia - 39552 (Tel. No. (706) 782-4723) and they can make arrangement to take both of us for a day or two to your place.

[Swamiji could not request anybody as per Shibendu's request to fulfill his travel plan. Swamiji by nature never imposes anything upon anyone. He learned it from Swami Satyananda who never imposed anything on anyone.

Swamiji had seen this quality of Swami Satyananda; also he never criticized anyone in his life. Swamiji had observed this saintly quality for twenty years; never heard him criticizing anyone. One day, it came up and Swamiji was remarking to him that he did not impose anything upon anyone. Then he surprised Swamiji mentioning that sometimes he did impose and as an example he added saying "In your case." Swamiji was as if falling from the sky listening to his statement and waiting for the rest of the story.

[Then Satyananda said, "Although you were a good student yet you did not like to prosecute your studies since the eighth grade (Class VIII) and you wanted to go away from your studies to the Himalayas as a *brahmachari* seriously to meditate. I sent you back to studies."

[Swamiji was totally surprised to hear that and it never crossed in his mind; the example was very personal and irrefutable].

There will be long discussion. We shall visit some other places. Roy is co-ordinating. So consulting with him a programme can be arranged for San Diego. Do as you feel good. With heartfelt respect and *pranati* (bowing).

Humbly, expecting affection,

Shibendu Lahiri

Swami Satyeswarananda's *Sat Sanga* with Satya Charan Lahiri, the grandson of Lahiri Mahasay

Swamiji did not know what Satya Charan Lahiri told his son, Sibendu Lahiri, about him.

However, what was with Satya Charan Lahiri and Swamiji should be mentioned here. Swamiji knew Satya Charan Lahiri for a long time. He was a decent person and perfect gentleman. Whenever Swamiji arrived at Benares he used to visit the original house of Lahiri Mahasay at Garureswar and then Satyalok at Chousatti *ghat* and meet Satya Charan Lahiri.

Once, Swamiji was traveling from Vrindavan to Benaras while he was in continuous silence.

While staying in Vrindavan, Swamiji used to stay on the bank of Yamuna River. Similarly, at Benares, he chose the bank of the Ganges River. It was the month of June, so the water level of the Ganges was down and the bank was dry. The first day arriving there as was his usual routine, he took a bath at Dasaswamedha *ghat*, visited Lord Biswanath temple, then went to Garureswar to pay respect to Lahiri Mahasay in his original house; then visited Satyalok and then sat on the bank of Ganges at the Chousatti Yogini *ghat* facing the Ganges. Swamiji chose this *ghat* (steps to the Ganges) as Lahiri Mahasay used to bathe everyday in the Ganges at this *ghat*. One day, Babaji Maharaj giving *darsan* to Lahiri Mahasay near the Chousatti Yogini (sixty four *Yogini* - female Yogi) Temple corrected his negative feeling towards a Sadhu (renunciate) who used to stay near the temple.

All of a sudden a thought generated in the mind of Swamiji that there was a proverb that in Benares, the place of Lord Biswanath (Lord Siva), there was his consort, Annapurna (the Divine Mother of food), as a result, nobody remained hungry in Benares. For no reason, the idea came to test the proverb. Swamiji sat on the bank with the intention not to get up for a long time.

All of a sudden a vast storm began to blow. The people started to rush back into town for shelter. Swamiji remained sitting there. The strong storm blowing the dry sand covered his body. It was terrible. The wind struck his face. In a few minutes the bank became empty. Swamiji, being a Yogi, did not want to move so soon as he had settled to sit for a long time. After a long time the storm passed. A gentleman near the *ghat* from the third floor was watching Swamiji from the very beginning of the storm. When Swamiji did not move it surprised him. He was moved and brought food for Swamiji. He said, "Maharaj! *prasad payiye* which means "Maharaj, kindly accept some food."

Swamiji was grateful to Ma Annapurna, making *pranam* mentally at the heart and accepting the food from the devotee.

Swamiji was a month at Benares. He used to stay during the day at the Chousatti Yogini *ghat*; sometimes meditated near the *ghat* where there was a hole in the wall of a building starting towards the steps to the Ganges and where there is a Siva temple too. At night, he rested near the Asi *ghat*. During the month three things happened:

1) One day, *Brahmachari* Amulya Kumar, disciple of Swami Abhedananda (closest friend of Swami Vivekananda, vice president of Ramakrisna Math and Mission) who was living at Lahiri Mahasay's area, Garureswar, Benares, found Swamiji sitting in the hole when *Brahmachari* was going to take a bath in the Ganges. He was very surprised and concerned about Swamiji being in continuous silence. He practically forced Swamiji to spend one night with him.

We knew each other from Sevayatan. *Brahmachari* was living there at Sri Ramakrisna Kutir at Sevayatan. We used to make *Sat Sanga*. *Brahmachari* was a *Sastri* and a Vedantist like Swamiji. Swamiji had to agree with *Brahmachari* and spent a night with him. He prepared food and fed Swamiji. It was he who continued talking almost the whole night. Swamiji was just a listener being a *akhanda mouni* (one who is continuousy silent).

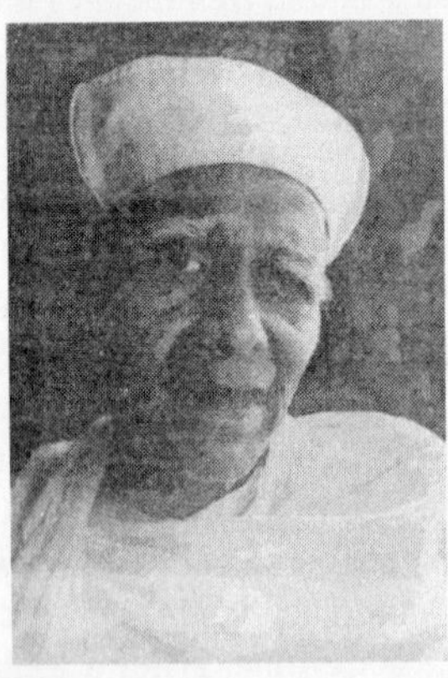

Brahmachari Amulya Kumar,
Disciple of Swami Abhedananda

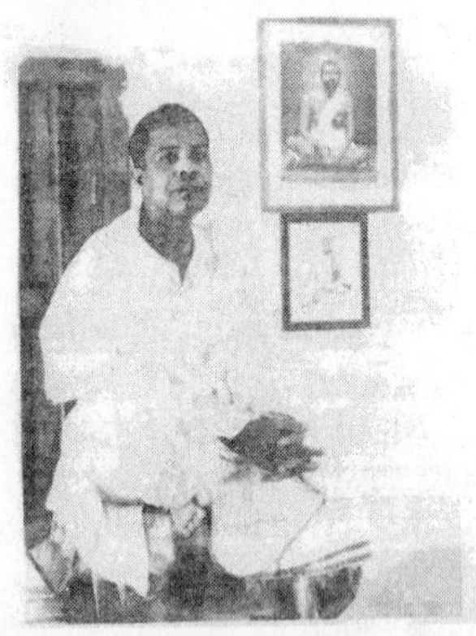

Brahmachari Narayan,
Disciple of Swami Abhedananda

Brahmachari Amulya Kumar as well his younger brother *Brahmachari* Narayan Chandra (also disciple of Swami Abhedananda) were good friends of Swamiji.

2) One day, Swamiji was sitting on the Chousatti Yogini *ghat*, and five Italian seekers of truth met him. They were looking for Lahiri Mahasay's house but could not find it. They said, "We read in a book about Lahiri Mahasay and his place is near Chousatti Yogini *ghat*, but we cannot find it." Swamiji gestured to them that he would show them the original place and another place.

Accordingly, Swamiji showed them the house of Lahiri Mahasay and Satyalok. At Satyalok, Satya Charan Lahiri, at first could not recognize Swamiji, since he was wearing an outfit of jute made cloth from the mid section to the knee and furthermore, he was observing continuous silence. When he found out that the Italians were with Swamiji he was curious and later he recognized Swamiji; then he requested him to come the next day because he wanted to talk about something.

Among the five Italians one was a medical graduate, Massimo. He knew English and the rest did not know English well. So Massimo helped his other friends in communicating while interviewing the Indian people. When Satya Charan Lahiri requested Swamiji to come next day, Massimo heard it and became very curious. They wanted to talk to Swamiji about *Kriya Yoga*. They wanted to know where they could find Swamiji next time. Swamiji gestured at which *ghat* they could find him.

3) The following day Swamiji arrived at Satyalok. Satya Babu, after the evening prayer, took Swamiji to the top floor in a small room which was his personal prayer room. Generally, he did not take anybody to that special room.

After entering the room when we settled down Satya Babu began his life's story starting from the very birth. He said that one of his regrets was that he was born to such a famous Yogi's family but he could not meet him [Lahiri Mahasay] because he was born eight years after his grandfather left body. Then he mentioned how he purchased the house, the Satyalok.

The house actually belonged to the Royal Dutta Family of Hutkhola (in the Howrah district of W. Bengal). It was a vacation house in Benares at the holy place of Chausatti *Ghat* for them. It was a single-story building. Later, sometime in the early 1940's, Satya Charan Lahiri, one of the eight grandsons of Lahiri Mahasay, bought it for Rupees 6,000.00.

Satya Babu said, "On the fifteenth day after I purchased the house, a non-Bengali business man offered me fifteen thousand rupees, an offer which I rejected. Then he gradually increased his offer to Rupees 92,000.00. I started praying to my grandfather that he not tempt me any further lest I will succumb when the offer reached Rupees 100,000.00. I did not understand why the gentleman was so eager to buy that particular piece of property. Then I researched the two Siva *Lingam* which were located on the property. The experts said that they were worth a fortune. I informed the business man that I had no intention of selling the house." Satya Charan Lahiri later made the house three stories.

(We find a strange coincidence, Ramtanu Bhattacharya, the grandfather of Panchanan Bhattacharya, was the royal priest of the Dutta family. The King was involved in the import and export business. A good many British gentlemen used to call on the King. Since they came for business reasons they were received by the royal family accordingly, and were served wine and liquor in accordance with British taste.

(One year, during Durga *Puja* - the worship of Goddess Durga, the Divine Mother, on the day of *Vijoya* - Victory day of Divine Mother, on the tenth day of the lunar cycle of a bright fortnight of October, a celebration party was held there. Suddenly, Ramtanu Bhattacharya, the dynasty priest, was shocked to see that the King was drinking liquor with his English guests. Thereafter, he walked out and left the royal family. In his mind he abandoned them.

(Later, the king visited Ramtanu Bhattacharya at his Ahiritola residence and apologized to him requesting him not to abandon the royal family. Ramtanu Babu commented frankly, "You drink and you will not be able to give it up. Therefore, I shall not set my foot in your house again."

(Later, at the request of the king, Ramtanu Bhattacharya said, "If my son, Thakurdas, wants to render service to your family he will be allowed to do so. It is entirely up to him."

(Thus, Thakurdas Bhattacharya, the father of Panchnan Bhattacharya, agreed to continue the role of dynasty priest for the royal Dutta family with the condition that it would not be his only profession. He accepted this role simply because they had been the disciples of his father.

(Nevertheless, it was a matter of loss of prestige for the royal family to have their priest engaging in a job elsewhere. According to custom, they must provide for the priest's family and the priest should be dedicated solely to them with the sole exception for his own family and personal worship. But Thakurdas did not agree in spite of repeated requests from the royal family. He had a full-time job and the salary was Rupees 200.00 a month, at a time when less than a rupee could purchase about eighty pounds of rice.

(So Thakurdas Bhattacharya continued to serve as the dynasty priest of the Dutta royal family even though they were uncomfortable with his being engaged in another job).

Satya Babu then moved on to tell about his family. He said that he became a widower long time ago. His only son was working in the state of Maharashtra, his elder daughter was married and the younger one just passed M.Sc. in Chemistry and found a job in the local Intermediate college. When he would be able to get her married then he would be free of worldly responsibilities.

Swamiji was in continuous silence so he was a patient listener to Satya Babu. In the meantime, from the Ganges side very close to Satyalok a group of devotional people started chanting. It was a bit loud. Satya Babu mentioned that recently, a Sitaramdas Omkarnath group bought a house and every evening they made *kirtan* (a group chanting). He mentioned Sitaramdas Omkarnath was initiated in *Kriya* by Ram Dayal Mazumder. Swamiji nodded his head, giving an indication that Swamiji was aware of that.

Satya Babu moved to another subject. He mentioned that once four Sankaracharyas were here at Benares. He met them and particularly was interested to ask one question. He said he selected Sankaracharya of Sarada Math, he appeared to be more wise and learned.

Before posing his question to *Jagatguru* Sankaracharya, Satya Babu said that he made an introduction disclosing that he was a grandson of Lahiri Mahasay and he did not want to hear an intellectual answer, rather an answer from the personal experience.

Satya Babu said that the learned Sankaracharya did not open his mouth at all. Then Satya Babu requested him again but still the learned seer did not budge. Satya Babu said if he could not get an answer from Sankaracharya himself then where would a person like him go for an answer? Sankaracharya remained silent. Satya Babu said perhaps his demand of an answer from personal experience placed a condition on Sankaracharya that prevented him from answering the question and so he was trying to be honest to Satya Babu by not saying anything. Then he posed the question to Swamiji if he has any answer to his question. Swamiji simply smiled. As a matter of fact, Swamiji had the same issue, however, Swamiji made an answer or explanation to himself.

Then, slowly, Satya Babu moved to his most interested subject for which he wanted this meeting. He said that ten years before in 1962 there was held an International *Kriya* Conference at Mandar Hill, Bhagalpore, Bihar, for the occasion of the celebration of Sri Bhupendranath Sanyal Mahasay's leaving the body in *Mahasamadhi.* Swami Hariharananda of Bindudham Yogasram, Barharwa, S. P., Bihar, as a convener made an elaborate arrangement. He made his Guru, Swami Satyananda, president for the entire week's conference and Satya Babu as chief guest, and both were put in one room for the stay.

Satya Babu said that during that period, one day, Satyananda requested Satya Babu for his own behalf and on behalf of millions of *Kriya* followers round the world to start in his place an evening prayer, *sat sanga*, a kind of discussion on *Kriya*, as many *Kriyanwits* visit Benares as a *Kriya* pilgrim place; especially since there is no asram or center there, either at Garureswar (in the original house) or in Satyalok.

Satya Babu said it touched his heart; he replied that he would think on the subject. So returning from the conference he started making arrangements for evening prayer and *sat sanga*. He hired a local Bengali *brahamana pandit* (priest) to conduct it. The old *brahamana* priest started it and it went well for a few weeks; then one day, Pandit Mahasay did not come and he did not earlier notify Satya Babu either. So he became nervous. Quickly, another Pandit Mahasay was brought to handle the situation. Then the first *Pandit* Mahasay showed up and apologized for his sudden absence. He said that his back pain was so bad he could not move. For a while it was good; then again, Pandit Mahasay was absent. Satya Babu said on that day he thought he has to try to handle the situation. He said to Swamiji that all knew his education had limitation. Yet, he sat on Vyasa's seat and reading Sanyal Mahasay's elaborate interpretations on the *Bhagavad Gita* and *Ramcharitmanas* of Goswami Tulasidas managed the evening. The very next day, he did the same. Satya Babu said that he got the confidence that he could continue to conduct the evening prayer in that manner.

Ten years passed and now he became tired. He wanted to retire. He said to Swamiji that since it was the request of Satyananda and since Swamiji has a master's degree in Philosophy and was an advocate (attorney) and was associated with Satyananda for twenty years, plus now being a renunciate, that it was Swamiji's job to conduct this evening prayer and take over at this *Gurusthan* (place of *Guru*). He could stay at Satya Babu's place free and receive alms at any *khestra* (charitable institutions at Benares) as a renunciate. It was good on Satya Babu's part; he made it clear. It did not cost him anything.

At this point, Swamiji gestured to have a piece of paper and a pen to answer Satya Babu in writing. Immediately, Satya Babu provided pen and paper. When Swamiji got them, he wrote that he was an unbounded wandering person and would feel suffocated within the four walls of Satyalok. Sorry, he could not accept the proposal.

Satya Babu said, "Let us both think for a week on the proposal." Swamiji wrote again that as for him, the answer was the same. Our meeting ended, Swamiji left Satyalok.

The Italian seekers approached Swamiji for *Kriya* initiation. Through medical graduate Massimo's help in English they were initiated.

(After four years Swamiji received a post card from Satya Babu at Dunagiri Hill, Himalayas. He kept his eyes focused on Swamiji's movement. He found Swamiji was in the Himalayas most often where Lahiri Mahasay met Babaji Maharaj. Satya Babu wanted to know how far one could travel by car in the hill and how far one has to walk on foot to visit the cave where Lahiri Mahasay was initiated. He expressed his desire to visit the holy place. Swamiji replied that since he was there he would do what would be required if Satya Babu visited the hill. However, ultimately, Satya Babu could not make the trip to the hill.

(It is interesting that Satya Babu wanted to take the risk of going out of Benares when once he refused his only son's, Shibendu's, invitation to visit him for only fifteen days at his place in the state of Maharastra where he was working. Shibendu related this information to Swamiji when he visited the author. He said that his father refused to visit him, telling him that Satya Babu lived at Benares all his life and he wanted to die at Benares so that he could attain the state of *Sivattva* - the essence of Lord Siva. In other words, entering into Lord Siva. There is a legend that whoever would die in Benares would go to Sivalok, the sphere of Lord Siva since Benares is one of the twelve *Jyotilingams*, the seat of Lord Biswanath (Lord Siva).

The Handwritten the second Letter of Shibendu Lahiri to Swami Satyeswarananda

ॐ 21 Jan. 1993

Revered Swamiji,

It was indeed a joy to have your kind letter dated July 22, 1992 as also the parcel containing your valuable books on Kriya and Lahiri-lore. By your grace, I have the following books: 1) The Mahabharata 2) The Bibles 3) Hidden Wisdom 4) Inner Victory 5) Kriya 6) Bhagavad Gita 7) Babaji (Volume II) i.e. Lahiri Mahasay (The Polestar of Kriya). My gratitude knows no bound. I wonder if I may request you to kindly send your other books and publications to Satyalok as your loving presents in due course of time. Many good things are happening in Satyalok — not because of myself, but inspite of myself. Satyalok is the abode of truth, tranquility, trance and transformation.

Myself and my wife were taken to various places in U.S.A., England and Australia by Devotees and disciples. It was a rewarding experience. Lectures, discourses, dialogues, satsangs, seminars were arranged. There was a lot of energy and enthusiasm and euphoria. People were almost taken by a Lahiri-storm. Bliss and benediction was evident. We had no finance of our own and thus we had to depend on the arrangements made by our sponsors. Hence we were not able to visit San Diego to see your esteemed self, although we would have very much loved to do so.

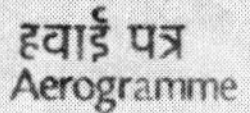

Swami S. Giri
P.O Box 5368
San Diego
CA 9 (U.S.A)

दूसरा मोड़ SECOND FOLD

भेजने वाले का नाम और पता -
Sender's Name and Address

Shibendu Lahiri
D22/3, Chousatti Ghat
"Satyalok", Varanasi-221001
[India]

इस पत्र के अन्दर कुछ न रखिये
No Enclosures Allowed

पहला मोड़ FIRST FOLD

Our elder daughter is a Eye-Surgeon, the only son is an Engineer and the younger daughter is a budding Doctor (studying M.B.B.S.). They are on their own and thus we are free to move from place to place as and when required. Devotees look after the religious & spiritual work at Satyalok during our absence from here. Apart from Initiations, Vedic ceremonies & mass feedings are conducted from time to time at this holy shr[ine] as per the established tradition.

With warm regards,

yours affectionately,

[signature]

(SHIBENDU LAHIRI)

The Handwritten Second Letter of Shibendu Lahiri to Swami Satyeswarananda

OM

January 21, 1993

Revered Swamiji,

It was indeed a joy to have your kind letter dated July, 22, 1992 as also the parcel containing your valuable books on *Kriya* and Lahiri lore. By your grace, I have the following books:

1) The Mahabharata,
2) The Bibles
3) Hidden Wisdom,
4) Inner Victory,
5) Kriya,
6) Bhagavad Gita
7) Babaji (Volume II) i.e. Lahiri Mahasay (The polestar of *Kriya*)..

My gratitude knows no bound. I wonder if I may request you to kindly send your other books and publications to "Satyalok" as your loving presents in due course in time.

Many good things are happening in Satyalok - not because of myself, but inspite of myself. Satyalok is the abode of truth, tranquility, trance and transformation.

Myself and my wife were taken to various places in U.S. A.. England and Australia by Devotees and disciples. It was a rewarding experience. Lectures, discourses, dialogues, *satsanga*, seminars were arranged. There was a lot of energy and enthusiasm and euphoria. People were almost taken by a Lahiri - storm. Bliss and benediction was evident. We had no finance of our own and thus we had to depend on the arrangements made by our sponsors. Hence we were not able to visit San Diego to see your esteemed self, although we would have very much loved to do so.

Our elder daughter is a Eye-Surgeon, the only son is an Engineer and the younger daughter is a budding Doctor (studying M.B.B.S.), They are on their own and thus we are free to move from place to place as and when required. Devotees look after the religious and spiritual works at Satyalok during our absence from here. Apart from Initiations, Vedic ceremonies & mass feedings are conducted from time to time at this holy shrine as per the established tradition.

With warm regards,

Yours affectionately. signed (SHIBENDU LAHIRI)

A letter from Prem Sudha, disciple of Satya Charan Lahiri. A non-Bengali resident of Benares she appreciates having the opportunity to read the English translation of Lahiri Mahasay's work.

Dear Sir,

I have gone through the book Vol I written by you, which is an explanation based on Lahiri Mahashaya's versions. I am really pleased to read it. You have translated altogether 26 books in English. We believe that you have done a great job and a favour to the people who believe in Kriya Yoga. This book is not available in Kashi or elsewhere, as far as I know.

Yogi Prakash Shankar Vyas is placed very high ranking in Kriya Yoga, who was very near and dear and was initiated in yoga by Yogiraj Satya Charan Lahiri a grandson of Lahiri Mahashaya. Yogi Prakash Shankar Vyas initiates Kriya Yoga to the able disciples and imparts training in Asana of Hath Yoga to foreign nationals and Indians as well. He has also taught Yoga for three years in Benaras Hindu University, Varanasi. He is a right and able yoga trainer. Lot many foreigners come every year to see him for Yoga and get benefited. He also maintains books in his library on Yoga and spritulism written by Indian and foreign writers as well. Every body has a easy access to these books. We know that Sri Shivendu Lahiri also have all these kinds of books, but due to his regular foreign entourage he is XXXXXXXX usually away from India. Secondly, he keeps all the books under lock and keys, hence a common interested man does not have a easy access to these books.

Devotees and followers of Lahiri Mahashaya are unable to read the books and the literature of his own, as all the literatures are written in Bengali language. Every Indian do not understand or read Bengali. A general Indian can read and/or understand Hindi and English.These books are not available in Hindi too. The devotees and followers of Lahiri Mahashaya have inspired and have a great pleasure to know that you have published his commentories in English. We all feel obliged to you for this deed.

We, who have been initiated in Kriya Yoga, shall be pleased and feel obliged if you could send one set of all those 26 books translated in English for the library of Yogi Prakash Shankar Vyas, but not to any body else. From where we can read and assimilate the thoughts once expressed by Lahiri Mahashaya. Once again we ask your extended help for this noble cause. Thank you in an anticipation .

I am a principal in a local women college named as Kasturba Inter College, Varanasi and I was initiated in Kriya Yoga by Yogiraj Satya Charan Lahiri. I personally believe that more and more people who have a faith in Kriya Yoga and spritualism shall welcome these literatures by their depth of heart, as most of them can not afford to buy expensive books. Hence, this request.

Books and periodicals can be addressed to;

Yogi Prakash Shankar Vyas
"Yoga clinic & centre for meditation"
D 16/19 Man-Mandir
Dasaswamedh, Varanasi 221 001 (India)

Regards,
Prem Sudha
Mrs Prem Sudha
Principal
Kasturba Balika Intermediate College
Orderly Bazar, Varanasi 221002 (India)
Dated . 27.8.97

A letter from Prem Sudha, disciple of Satya Charan Lahiri. A non-Bengali resident of Benares, Principal, Kasturba Balika Intermediate College. Being Non-Bengali, she appreciates having opportunity to read English Translation of Lahiri Mahasay's work.

Dear Sir,

I have gone through the book Vol. 1 written by you, which is an explanation based on Lahiri Mahasay's versions. I am really pleased to read it. You have translated altogether 26 [twenty six] books in English. We believe that you have done a great job and a favour to the people who believe in Kriya Yoga. This book is not available in Kashi [Benares] or elsewhere, as far as I know.

Yogi Prakash Shankar Vyas is placed very high ranking in *Kriya Yoga*, who was very near and dear and was initiated in yoga by Yogiraj Satya Charan Lahiri a grandson of Lahiri Mahasaya. Yogi Prakash Shankar Vyas initiates *Kriya Yoga* to the able disciples and imparts training in Asana of *Hatha Yoga* to foreign nationals and Indians as well. He has also taught Yoga for three years in Benaras Hindu University, Varanasi. He is a right and able yoga trainer. Lot many foreigners come every year to see him for Yoga and get benefited. He also maintains books in his library on Yoga and Spiritualism written by Indian and foreign writers as well. Everybody has a easy access to those books. We know that Sri Shivendu Lahiri also have all these kinds of books, but due to his regular foreign entourage he is usually away from India. Secondly, he keeps all the books under lock and keys, hence a common interested man does not have a easy access to these books.

Devotees and followers of Lahiri Mahasaya are unable to read the books and the literature of his own, as well the literatures are written in Bengali language. Every Indian do not understand or read Bengali. A general Indian can read and/or understand Hindi and English. These books are not available in Hindi too. The devotees and followers of Lahiri Mahasaya have inspired and have a great pleasure to know that you have published his commentaries in English. We all feel obliged to you for this deed.

We, who have been initiated in Kriya Yoga, shall be pleased and feel obliged if you could send one set of all those 26 books translated in English for the library of Yogi Prakash Shankar Vyas, but not to any body else. From where we can read and assimilate the thoughts once expressed by Lahiri Mahasaya. Once again we ask your extended help for this noble cause. Thank you in an anticipation.

I am a principal in a local women college named as Kasturba Inter College, Varanasi and I was initiated in Kriya Yoga by Yogiraj Satya Charan Lahiri. I personally believe that more and more people who have a faith in Kriya Yoga and spiritualism shall welcome these literatures by their depth of heart, as most of them can not afford to buy expensive books. Hence, this request.

Books and periodicals can be addressed to:

Yogi Prakash Shankar Vyas
"Yoga clinic & centre for Meditation"
D 16/19 Man-Mandir
Dasaswamedha, Varanasi, 221 001 (India)

Regards,

Mrs. Prem Sudha
Principal
Kasturba Balika Intermediate College
Orderly Bazar, Varanasi 221002 (India)
Dated 27/8/97

One month passed in Benares. Swamiji was not able to concentrate well each day because one particular asram of Bengal was surfacing in his mind. Swamiji felt to check out what was happening there and why it was hitting to his mind the entire month. As Swamiji mentioned this to the Italians they bought a ticket for Swamiji for Bengal and they headed towards Himachal Pradesh.

Back to Swamiji's travel; he arrived at Bengal from Benares and visited the hermitage. Swamiji was observing silence and he was wearing a jute cloth. Having seen this, one boy informed the lady principal, a disciple of old Swami Bidyananda Giri (disciple of Yogananda). When the lady principal came, she understood Swamiji was observing silence. Immediately, she asked the boy to bring an exercise book and a pen. When Swamiji wrote who he was to answer her question, she went inside to inform her Guru, Swami Bidyananda. Listening to the information, Swami commented, "He is god sent." Bidyananda told her that she must arrange for Swamiji's stay and he would meet him later. When Bidyananda met Swamiji he said that he was praying to his *Guru* almost a month to send somebody to help him. Under the circumstance, he was not able to help the girl's high school situated in the same hermitage campus.

There, Bidyananda had started a boy's high school earlier, also a bit far from the hermitage campus. The boy's school was administered by a managing committee. It was running well. The principal was Hiralal Chand, an advanced *Kriya* disciple of Swami Satyananda. Because of Hiralal Babu's involvement as principal, the boy's school did not need Bidyananda's help but recently started the girl's high school which needed his service.

Hiralal Babu was a *Khecharisiddha* household *Kriya* Yogi, like his very good friend, Sailendra Bejoy Dasgupta (disciple of Sriyukteswar). In fact, Swami Satyananda in a handwritten letter, dated January 16, 1956, instructed the author to show the letter to Hiralal Babu and ask him about the instruction of the *Khecharimudra* and practice accordingly. The portion of Satyananda's handwritten letter is as follows:

[illegible]

The above document says, "Please ask Hiralal Babu how one takes the tongue into the *Khecharimudra* in *Kriya* practice and practice according to the instruction."

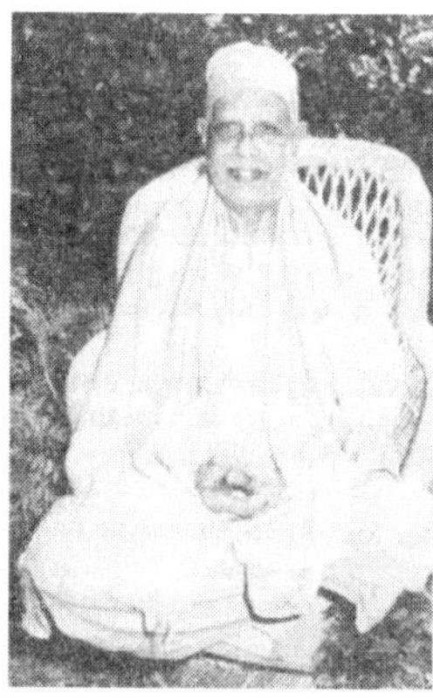

Swami Bidyananda Giri,
Disciple of Yogananda

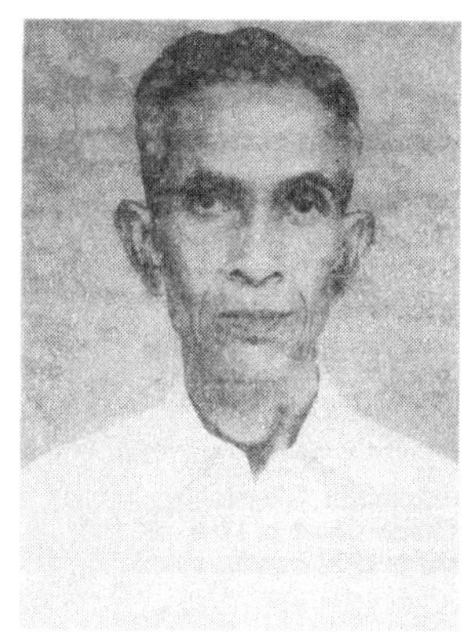

Hiralal Chand, Principal, Vidyapith
Disciple of Satyananda

Then the old Swami added something which was interesting. Bidyananda had a fancy small silence room outside his house. Whenever he would please to observe silence he entered in the room and stayed the whole day inside. But he was praying in silence the entire month in a different small hut to his *Guru* to send somebody. This thatched hut was named "Satyananda Kuti." In 1939, Swami Satyananda had laid the foundation stone of the hermitage. That is why in his honor the hut was named Satyananda Kuti (hut). Satyananda was the founding general secretary of Yogoda Sat Sanga (YSS). He came there from Ranchi to start the hermitage in 1939.

Then it became clear to Swamiji why at Benares that hermitage was surfacing in his mind. It was Swami Bidyananda's prayer in Satyananda Kuti.

The old Swami Bidyananda had an eye operation at that time, as a result, he could not help in administering the girls' high school attached to the campus.

It should be remembered that Swamiji did not take any vow of silence; it just happened in Vrindavan. Since then he was continuing, but under the circumstances here, to help the school and the hermitage, Swamiji had to break his long continuous silence at this hermitage.

After some months when Bidyananda recovered his health at a function, he announced that Swamiji would be the next "Asram Swami". It was a total surprise to Swamiji. Bidyananda did not consult or get his consent before making the announcement.

Swamiji heard from the lady principal and the vice principal of the girl's high school that they needed Swamiji to stay here. They needed him. Swamiji learned hints from them that Bidyananda was having trouble with the American administration of Yogoda from Ranchi.

That explained why Bidyananda announced hurriedly that Swamiji would be the "Asram Swami."

Swamiji silently observed the situation and decided in his mind that he had to leave that hermitage soon, before something else was thrust upon him. Soon, Swamiji left the asram stopping at Benares, Vrindavan and Haridwar, returning back to Dunagiri Hill, Himalayas.

It would be appropriate to provide an explanation here.

***Sat Sanga* with Swami Bidyananda Giri, disciple of Yogananda**

When Swami Yogananda returned to India in 1935/36 many people were initiated by him; and after the initiation he would say that the rest of the discipline they could learn from Swami Satyananda, since Yogananda would go back to the United States.

Among the newly initiated people by Yogananda the following three later became renunciate Swamis and one, Krisna Chandra Dutta, under Swami Satyanada's guidance, became an advanced *Kriya Yogi*. The author personally knew all these four people. The three renunciate swamis were :

1) Girindra Chandra Dey (Swami Bidyananda),
2) Anil Kumar Bose (Swami Satchidananda),
3) Sadananda Mukherjee (Swami Sadananda).

Girindra Chandra Dey was a college graduate. He was working in a publishing house at Calcutta editing a popular magazine. He was a good friend of Sailesh Mohan Mazumder (Swami Suddhananda, brother of Swami Satyananada) and also a good friend of Panchkori Dey (*Brahmachari* Shatnanada). That is how he came in contact with Yogananda.

Girin Babu was a follower of Mahatma Gandhi. He was a strict nationalist and a patriot.

When he started the boy's school in 1939 and the hermitage, fortunately, he got help getting the school's recognition from the government through Sachindralal Dasvarma, the District Inspector of schools (DI) who happened to be the classmate and good friend of his Guru, Yogananda.

Girindra Chandra Dey was a very good organizer and a good administrator.

In 1936 Yogananda founded Yogoda Sat Sanga Society of India with Satyananda, Ananda Mohan Lahiri, and Panchkori Dey. In 1941 these founding members had to leave Ranchi because Yogananda sent Swami Binayananda back to India making him acting president over these founding members.

Actually, just in 1939 at the request of Yogananda to send some worker, Swami Satyananda made Mr. Sachindranath Chakraborty a *brahmachari*, named Premeswarananda and sent him to America. On the same occasion, Satyananda made Anil Kumar Bose a (*Brahmachari* Animananda) and also Sadananda Mukherjee (*Brahmachari* Sadananda). In that sense Swami Binayananda was a *brahmachari* disciple of Swami Satyananda.

Within a short period of time, Yogananda made him a swami and sent him back to India. Let us see how Mr. Chakraborty came in contact with Yogoda.

Before Yogoda (YSS) was founded in 1936, in Calcutta as early as 1925 a "Students Home" was run by Swami Satyananda and others. The purpose of running the Student Home was to recruit good dedicated workers from the educated students. In the Student Home, in fact, shelter was given to those good students who came from the countryside to Calcutta to study in the University of Calcutta. A program of asramic lifestyle was introduced with morning and evening prayer there to build good character.

An ex-Ranchi graduate student, Jatindranath Banerjee (disciple of Yogananda), was in-charge of running the Students Home. When Yogananda asked Satyananda to send some worker, Satyananda made Jatindranath Banerjee (a *brahmachari* Jatin) and sent him to America in 1928. Thereafter, the Student Home was run by Sailesh Mohan Mazumder (later, Swami Suddhananda) and his assistant Sailendra Bejoy Dasgupta (disciple of Sriyukteswar). Yogananda visited in 1936 several times and liked the Student Home. Let us see what Mr. Dasgupta wrote about Swami Binayananda.

Binayananda send back to India

"The change in the mode and direction of works at the main center in Ranchi necessitated new workers to join the organization. At this time, a young man named Sachin Chakraborty began working for Yogoda Satsanga. Although he was not highly educated, he had worked in Bharat Sevashram for a while, which gave him some general familiarity with the ways and needs of a spiritually oriented institution. But behind it all, the man's main reason for joining Yogoda Satsanga's workforce was to be a part of an internationally powerful organization, and his primary and ultimate goal was to go to America. When he came into contact with the writer in Calcutta, Sachin Chakraborty immediately asked about the possibilities of working with the Ranchi center, as well as bringing up the subject of traveling to America several times. *Paramhansa Swami Yogananda – Life-portrait and Reminiscences* by Sailendra Bejoy Dasgupta, [private secretary of Yogananda in 1935-36], page 113, Chapter 6 - The Last Act.

"Swami Yogananda's youngest brother Bishnu Charan went with his future son-in-law Buddha Bose to Swamiji's ashram in America. Within only a few days Bishnu Charan saw many incidents of unbecoming and suspicious behavior by Vinayananda [can be spelled Binayananda] and made Yoganandaji aware of these, after which Yoganandaji's perception of Vinayananda completely changed. Vinayananda then became a problem for Yoganandaji. The open-hearted and love-filled Yoganandaji did not have an easy time when he had to make harsh and stern decisions against someone. At the same time, he also could not take the chance of a troublesome Vinayananda causing problems for him in America. In the end, Vinayananda was sent back to India with the title of 'President' for the Yogoda Satsanga in India. This way, the American part of the organization was free of any more complications from the situation. However, this arrangement certainly caused noticeable discontent to rise in the Indian part of the organization which eventually resulted in the formal resignation of several distinguished members [founding members of Yogoda like Satyananda, Panchkori Dey and others] of the workforce of Yogoda Satsanga in India." *Paramhansa Swami Yogananda – Life-portrait and Reminiscences* by Sailendra Bejoy Dasgupta, private secretary of Yogananda in 1935-36], page 114, Chapter 6 The Last Act.

Panchkori Dey, who had been made *Brahmachari* Santananda by Yogananda and who was a disciple of Hangsa Swami Kebalananda (Kebalananda was a disciple of Lahiri Mahasay), and a founding member of Yogoda related the situation to the author, "On Satyananda's part, he wanted to see that Yogananda's desire be fulfilled, that is, to see that the change took place peacefully. So he advised us to find jobs outside and gradually move out from Ranchi. It took time for us to find jobs. So Satyananda stayed on at Ranchi to see that the change took place without any unpleasant events.

"Binayananda lost all sense of proportion that Satyananda had been his teacher; that it was Satyananda himself who had made him *Brahmachari* Premeswarananda from Sachindranath Chakraborty; that in this respect, Satyananda was his *Guru*, or Master, as well, and lastly, that it was Satyananda himself who had sent him to America to help Yogananda.

"Meanwhile, Binayananda became nervous and desperate, because Satyananda's staying at Ranchi put him in a handicapped situation, so that he could not implement his ideas. Besides, nobody was obeying him. He wanted Satyananda to leave as soon as possible.

"Binayananda misinterpreted Satyananda's delay and seemed to conclude that we had written to Yogananda requesting that his position be revoked and that we were only waiting for Yogananda's reply. He suspected that we were buying time.

"So he could not stand this delay. The power hungry man becoming desperate, he made threats on Satyananda's life. He insisted that Satyananda leave right away."

At this point, Binayananda appointed *Brahmachari* Prakas Das as Yogoda's secretary, in place of Swami Satyananda. (*Brahmachari* Prakas Das Yogoda's new secretary, who became Swami Atmananda, will be discussed later).

So in the mid 1940's at the residential school, *Brahmacharya Vidyalay* Ranchi, the student strength came down to only about nine from about one hundred twenty. It was a very miserable situation. Why did it so suddenly become such a bad situation?

One reason must be mentioned here, that Ranchi *Brahmacharya Vidyalay* was a residential high school in the state of Bihar (currently, Jharkhand) which is a Hindi speaking state. The school was registered under the University of Calcutta making an exception for Calcutta University to have a school registered from outside the state of Bengal. Thus the instruction in the school was in the Bengali language and residential students were all from Bengal. No local Hindi speaking students were in the school. Thus, because of the change to come under the authority of Yogoda and the leaving of the Principal and Secretary, Swami Satyananda, as well as the *Brahmacharis* Santananda and Sadananda and the bachelor grandson of Lahiri Mahasay, B.A. (classmate and good friend of Satyananda), the parents of Calcutta students and the Bengali parents living outside Bengal did not like to send their boys to the Ranchi school.

Having heard this information Yogananda immediately wrote to Girindra Chandra Dey (later, Swami Bidyananda) and advised him to go to Ranchi asram and revive it. As mentioned before, Girindra C. Dey was a very good organizer. Taking charge Mr. Dey contacted old and good acquainted people of Ranchi to get help to revive his Guru's school and asram. One of those people was barred from entering the Ranchi campus.

So *Brahmachari* Prakas Das, the newly appointed secretary of Yogoda by newly appointed president Binayanada, wrote to Yogananda about it. Mr. Prakas Das had a habit to write to Yogananda against Swami Satyananda and wanted to be the secretary of Yogoda, and his dream was fulfilled when Binayananda appointed him secretary of Yogoda which made a partner of his team.

Swami Bidyananda told Swamiji that he got a letter from his *Guru*, Yogananda, that he should not allow a particular gentleman from the Ranchi town to enter Ranchi campus. Having this letter, Bidyananada wrote to Yogananda in reply that he had sent him to revive Ranchi; so let him decide who would be helpful and from whom he should seek help. Bidyananda wrote that the concerned gentleman was really a good person. Yogananda replied back that Bidyananda should go ahead and work with the person concerned as well. Bidyananda worked hard ten years at Ranchi.

In the meantime, in 1952 Yogananda left body.

In 1953, Bidyananda, having revived Ranchi to its glory, handed over the administration to *Brahmachari* Animananda (disciple of Yogananda) and left to his place to look after the hermitage and boy's high school which he founded.

In the mid 1950's, Bidyananda started a girl's high school (*Kanya Vidyalay*) attached to the hermitage campus.

On the Ranchi side, the school again started deteriorating. They changed the registration of the school from Calcutta University to Bihar Higher Secondary Board and made the medium of instruction in Hindi to increase the admission of local boys, yet it did not improve.

In 1955, *Brahmachari* Prakas Das and the Vice president of Yogoda, Pravash Chandra Ghosh, Yogananda's cousin, visited the United States. Prakas Das said they found a paper which Yogananda had written before leaving the body that *Brahmachari* Prakas would be Swami Atmananda and *Brahmachari* Animananda would be Swami Satchidananda. Accordingly Prakas *Brahmachari* became Swami Atmananda. Returning to India, when it was told to *Brahmachari* Animananda, he did not like it. He had his doubts. Once, he expressed his sentiment to Satyananda that he would like to receive his *sanyas* (Swami order) directly from Yogananda. Once, Satyananda mentioned it to Swamiji. So when Animananda did not have the chance to receive *sanyas* directly from Yogananda, he thought that he would remain as *Brahmachari* and would not become Swami. At that point Atmananda began to pressure him, or else, meaning that he might be discharged from Yogoda. If *brahmachari* Animananda did not accept it, then it would create a question mark as to the authority of Atmananda's own order of Swami as well. So he created more pressure on *brahmachari* Animananda. Finally, Animananda had to accept it and became Swami Satchidananda.

In 1958/59, Sister Daya arrived as president of Self Realization Fellowship (SRF) and Yogoda Sat Sanga Society of India (YSS), for the first time to India with young and dashing *Brahmachari* Kriyananda and two other Americans. Swamiji saw them in different asrams. She was very enthusiastic, although a bit sad seeing her *Guru's* asram at Ranchi.

In 1958, Mr. Binay Narayan Dube a widower, associated with the Anandamoyee Ma group. He could not make a place for himself in the group since in the group of Anandamoyee Ma there were big people like the Prime Minister Indira Gandhi and her cabinet ministers. So Mr. Dube happened to read *Autobiography of a Yogi* just six months before Sister Daya arrived in India. When they met, it instantly clicked like love at first sight for several reasons. Because Mr. Dube was born in a royal family in the state of Uttar Pradesh. He was about six feet tall, as was Daya. Mr. Dube had a European white complexion: very impressive looking. Nobody could tell he was Indian born until someone knew the details of his birth. He lost his father when he was just eight years old. The King of Mahisadal from Bengal who was his father's good friend had between them a verbal agreement to help each other in bad times. Thus Mr. Dube was brought to Bengal and was brought up there. As a result, he knew Bengali. Eventually, he was given the king's daughter in marriage and he had two daughters.

After meeting Sister Daya he drove his car to accompany her. Instantly being impressed, Sister Daya appointed him, an outsider and householder, as secretary of Yogoda, bypassing those associated lifelong like Swami Bidyananda, Swami Satchidananda and Swami Hariharananda of Puri. All of these Swamis were Yogananda's disciples and associated with Yogoda since the very young days; and above all they were good, dedicated whole time workers and organizers with a renunciate background.

When Sister Daya for the first time met Swami Satyananda, all her preconceived impressions about Satyananda completely disappeared instantly. She realized in him how much he had unconditionally loved Yogananda. Both had loved Yogananda unconditionally, and so it did not take time to realize that, and understand each other.

During that time, Satyananda brought up Binaya Narayan Dube's appointment as General Secretary for Yogoda. He wanted to make her aware about the rules of the Vedic culture and specially pointed out that in the Vedic culture a swami could not serve under a householder.

Satyananda reminded repeatedly Yogananda himself, in that respect, when Yogananda, in the usual course, crossed the line of Vedic culture. Once, Yogananda informed Satyananda that he was thinking of making his American disciple, Mr. James J. Lynn, as Yogoda's president. In reply, Satyananda wrote he would be the first person to leave his organization; however, if Mr. Lynn would enter into some kind of renunciate order then he would have no objection to serve under him.

On another occasion, Satyananda repeatedly reminded Yogananda that the word "Yogoda" is grammatically wrong, that the correct word would be "Yogad". Yogananda said, "For us everything is okay". Since Yogananda used it in the United States as Yogoda Sat Sanga of America, now, he did not like to change it to expose his Sanskrit weakness.

There was another occasion where Satyananda did not agree with Yogananda and turned down his request. Yogananda said to Satyananda, "Why don't you exhibit a bit of miracle and when people would be attracted, then serve them." Yogananda did exactly this in his life. In the world of real Yogis, this style is called *tuktak*, "cheap shot".

Satyananda said, "Nothing is impossible by the Lord. Who am I to do this? Please don't request me on the subject."

Two different personalities: one is emotional and the other is rational.

Daya's answer to Satyananda was: "I need this man to revive Guruji's school and Ranchi asram".

He also pointed out to her that they should give some responsible job to Satchidananda who was very sincere and dedicated to his *Guru*.

Mr. Binaya Narayan Dube dropped his last name "Dube" and added before his name "Yogacharya" which means "the teacher of Yoga."

In her second visit in 1963, Binay Narayan thought the Sister Daya name is not that high; most spiritual women in India are Mata or Mother, like Anandamoyee Ma with whom Mr. Dube was associated. So he made her Daya Mata. Since then she was Daya Mata.

In 1963, the Yogoda administration, during their international president Sister Daya's visit, removed Swami Binayananda for his misconduct. They locked him out from the Calcutta Dakshineswar center (Registered head office of Yogoda). They also removed Secretary Swami Atmananda who could not appropriately account for three hundred thousand Indian rupees (Rs.300,000.00) sent to Yogoda from the United States in U.S. dollars. A house was bought with the money in Calcutta in the name of Mrs. Bela Bose. In fact, Swami Atmananda also had behavior unbecoming of a swami and for that reason he did not like to live in the headquarters at the Dakshineswar center, instead, he lived at the Barahanagar center. That was convenient and comfortable for his unbecoming Swami lifestyle.

Both of them wrote to Swami Satyananda. Swamiji was there with Satyananda. After reading the letters he handed them over to Swamiji who read them too.

Binayanada complained that Yogoda did not even allow him to take his furniture away. He begged help of Swami Satyananda. This was the man who practically created a terrible situation causing Satyananda to leave, in Satyananda's language, the "blood built" asram and school (so called because Satyananda was Principal for Ranchi *Brahmacharya Vidyalay*, a high school, and did not take his salary. Every month it used to go directly to the general fund of the asram. He did not see or touch the money). He wrote a brief reply:

"Sorry for the situation you are in. What can I do? As you know I am not officially connected with them. Who will obey my instruction?"

In a letter, Atmananda, too, complained about Yogoda. Previously writing letters to Yogananda with his complaints against Satyananda, Atmananda had fooled Yogananda; now he tried to fool Satyananda. He requested Satyananda in the letter, "You have founded with Sriyukteswar all those branch centers [now, the branch centers are as many as thirty five] in the Midnapore district. Why don't you convert the centers of Midnapore district from Yogoda to Sat Sanga Mission under you? I am behind you in this matter."

Satyananda sent a postcard with a note in reply to Atmananda's letter. Satyananda wrote in the note. "I do not see any need to change the status of these centers. The centers of Midnapore district are doing fine. There will be no change as long as I am alive."

This was the man who used to write to Yogananda against Satyananda and wanted to be secretary in Satyananda's place. He succeeded but temporarily.

One day, at Sevayatan, an unusual thing was witnessed by Swamiji. He was returning to the thatched hut of Satyananda where he shared the hut's only very small room with him with his kind permission. Satyananda was shouting at the top of his lungs against a lady devotee who was visiting the asram for a few days. She was walking around another small tin roofed house close to Satyananda's hut, where Swami Sadananda who was teaching at the Sevayatan Vidyalay (high School) lived. Satyananda was saying that she must leave the asram the next day.

Later, Satyananda shared something related to the incident. Swamiji was totally surprised because generally Satyananda's personality was that of a very reserved man. He was very honest and shared lots of things like Puri asram's history, which Swamiji did not like to hear, yet Satyananda forcibly told him commenting, "You have grown up. You should know these things. It would be necessary in future." But this was a very different event than other displeasing infights of asram life.

Due to Swami Atmananda's, unbecoming of a Swami, behavior the lady devotee who was Satyananda's disciple and a widowed school teacher, already with an eight year's old son, conceived. Satyananda told Swamiji that somehow she was sent to Bangladesh to clean her. Satyananda did not want to see that same thing happen again in his backyard with Swami Sadananda who used to love his students and sometimes visited their homes, and thereby there was a rumor about his reputation.

After putting on the Yogacharya title, Mr. Binaya Narayan looked at the list of Yogoda centers in the Self Realization Magazine, and to his utter surprise at the Ranchi office, he did not find any legal documentation of affiliations to Yogoda from many branch centers. Occasionally, he used to drive with his American colleagues like Swami Shantananda who was in charge of finance from Ranchi to Calcutta via Sevayatan visiting Swami Satyananda. Binaya Narayan, since he was a newcomer to the organization, had a lot of respect for Swami Satyananda, the founding life member of YSS. He wanted to learn the past history of the organizations and some *Kriya* as well. In one such visit Swami Satyananda asked Swamiji to take Shantananda for a walk in asram's big campus so that Binay Narayan would have privacy to talk about something personal with Satyananda. Shantananda, while walking with Swamiji in the asram premises in the evening, asked Swamiji about Satyananda's schooling; where Satyananda went to school? The question surprised Swamiji. The American gentleman by then was living in India in the very same asram five or six years but did not know one of the founding fathers of the organization. They simply did not care except about Yogananda who they probably never even met. Swamiji in reply said in Calcutta of course and he was an honors graduate in philosophy from the Calcutta University. We returned to the hut after a while. They resumed their journey to Calcutta. Binay Narayan was in the driver seat; he loved to drive.

Satyananda told Swamiji that Binaya Narayan told him, "Swamiji! I am administering Yogoda with a sword in hand; if somebody raise their heads, I will chop off their heads".

Then Satyananda said to Swamiji, "He is the right person under the circumstances."

Binay Narayan learned from Satyananda how these branch centers were started:

To his utter surprise, Binay Narayan heard from Satyananda that the centers were not affiliated. Then Satyananda told him how those centers had been started and who had founded them.

Satyananda said, "The centers were started by the local *Kriya* devotees of Sriyukteswar, Bhabananda, Paramananda, and myself. In fact, the local devotees contributed their money, labor and donations in building *asrams* and schools.

"For that reason, we formed everywhere a local committee. Generally, in the committee some of us renunciates were included having the honor of the office of the president [as the founder], a few members from the donor family who donated the land were also included, as well as some members from the villagers who were interested in education and spiritual life.

"Everywhere the donor, the rich man or his family, transferred the land to the local committee by registered deed. So, thereafter, legally the local committee became the owner. Since everywhere the local devotees were the organizers, the local people and their children were the beneficiaries, so, we did not feel to affiliate the centers with YSS, but rather, we left these centers independent, and that was a democratic gesture.

"In fact, these are not branches in the technical sense. Legally, they are separate, independent centers, *asrams* and schools.

"Everywhere, the local committee had to accept the rules of the State Board and the Government when an asramic school became affiliated with and received the sponsorship of the State Board of Education. As you know, the State Government provided finances, once the schools got affiliation from the Board of Education of each respective State.

"Accordingly, the previous local committee acted as 'Asram Committee' and formed a separate committee by the name of school 'Managing Committee' to facilitate and abide by the rules of the Government. If a center ran more than one school, then more managing committees or governing bodies were formed, according to the rules of the State Government and the Board of Education.

"So, in addition to the permanent members from founder's representatives and donor's representatives, there were one Government nominee, two teachers' representatives, two representatives from the students' guardians, one local medical doctor, and a person interested in education, in the school Managing Committee.

"The common links between the different centers were the fellowship of brotherhood through *Kriya*, and we, the *Kriya* advisers, the founders. That's why you did not find any documents. The Asram Committee remained as the authority of the center.

"Legally, these centers are independent and have nothing to do with your listing in *Yogoda magazine*, or *SRF magazine*."

Having consulted his lawyer and good friend, Mr. Banamali Das (whom he recommended to the Americans to appoint as the future secretary for Yogoda) at Calcutta and returning to Ranchi, Binaya Narayan drafted a *proforma of application* (legal document applying for a position or business relationship) for affiliation and sent it to all the secretaries of the branches asking them to convene meetings at their centers and to make resolutions to the effect that they wanted to be affiliated with the YSS as branch centers. They were told to send back the applications after being duly filled out, with copies of resolutions.

Mr. Dube wanted to legalize the relationship between the center and the branches through this back door process. This attempt in the 60's created a stir in the *Kriyaban* circles everywhere. The local people understood the legal impact of the proposed affiliation, so it created divisions among the *Kriya* followers.

Many of the centers which run the schools under the hermitage wanted to apply for affiliation. Some school teachers had spread the rumor that if the centers became affiliated then there would be a possibility of receiving generous donations from the U.S.A. which could be utilized for the development of the village or the center.

Of course, some villagers, especially the old *Kriyabans*, disciples of Sriyukteswar, Satyananda and Bhabananda (disciple of Sriyukteswar) did not like to be affiliated, understanding that they would then have to abide by the organizational rules of YSS in addition to the present rules. They did not like to lose control to YSS in managing the schools of their respective centers. After all, they themselves had built these.

They also raised questions about what would happen if YSS did not like Satyananda coming over to the centers to give *Kriya* instruction as he had done since Sriyukteswar's time? From whom would they get their *Kriyas* checked every six months as per Lahiri Mahasay's rule? Was there any competent *Kriya* teacher in YSS? They did not know of anyone; they had known only Satyananda and Bhabananda since Sriyukteswar's time.

The other centers which had no schools associated with the asram only acted as meditation centers, and they did not want to be affiliated with YSS.

Some said, "We have been conducting our meetings since Sriyukteswar's time in the name of Yogoda Sat Sanga Sova. What benefit would the proposed affiliation bring us? The only benefit would be losing our control."

Many old *Kriyabans* were disciples of Sriyukteswar who pleaded that they had known only Satyananda since Giri Maharaj-ji's [Sriyukteswar's] time. So they wanted to discuss the matter with Satyananda first before taking any decision.

When the devotees arrived at Sevayatan from many centers, they talked with Satyananda on the subject; but Satyananda sent some of them to discuss the subject with Swamiji, the author.

The author sent them back to Satyananda informing them that he was not in any way connected with these asrams and schools. After all, it was Satyananda who had been connected from the very beginning, so it was Satyananda's jurisdiction to advise them.

Swamiji told them that as a legal expert and an attorney he had nothing more to add to what they had already found out by that time from many other lawyers.

Later, the author learned that Satyananda had told them, "Let not there be any change; rather, maintain the status quo if possible."

But it was not possible for some centers to remain neutral and to maintain the present status. So some applied for affiliation, especially those which ran schools. Many centers did not apply.

During this period, Yogoda started a new center of their own in this Midnapore district and spent money there.

Affiliated centers were called branch centers. They did not receive any money as they had expected. Nobody had given them any assurance. This had simply been their fantasy.

Meantime, two or three years passed, and they were told every time they approached Ranchi YSS that YSS had no money to spare for them.

So the authorities of the affiliated branches realized that they had brought upon themselves nothing but trouble. Sometimes, the principal of the school had to go all the way to Ranchi, Bihar State to consult with the joint secretary YSS.

In addition, many *Kriyabans* of the affiliated branch centers felt ashamed to contact Satyananda for *Kriya* check up or advice. Some of Sriyukteswar's disciples went to see Satyananda anyway. Gradually, the others too discovered that their branch's affiliation with YSS Ranchi did not make any difference to Satyananda. Then slowly they reestablished their *Kriya* relationship with Satyananda.

Mr. Dube (Binay Narayan), newly appointed secretary to Yogoda, learning the history of the organization from Swami Satyananda, used to praise Swami Bidyananda who was sent to Ranchi by Yogananda himself to revive Ranchi in difficult times in the forties and early fifties. But conflict was inevitable between the two well experienced organizers.

Once, Bidyananda told the author, "I did not like Mr. Dube's dictation. Of course, in the eye of a *sanyasi* [Swami] every woman is mother; but Daya is my *Guruji's* disciple, and naturally is my sister. What's wrong with addressing my sister as 'dear sister'? No. Mr. Dube would not accept it. So I said to him I have nothing to do with you."

(It should be mentioned here that Girindra Chandra Dey was working with the Yogoda organization twenty three years by then, since 1936, when he was initiated by Yogananda; yet he did not enter into renunciate life. He was a bachelor; so Sister Daya in 1958 approached and advised him to enter into the Swami order.

(At this Mr. Dey said, "From whom I can take *sanyas*? There is nobody in the organization through whom I can enter into Swami order. I can take *sanyas* from Swami Satyananda but you would say 'he is not in our organization.'

(So Sister Daya managed to arrange for Mr. Dey's *sanyas* with *Jagatguru* Sankaracharya of Puri Gobardhan Math at Sriyukteswar's Puri Karar Asram. He became Swami Bidyananda Giri. At that time *Brahmachari* Robindra Narayana also entered into the Swami order; his name changed to Swami Hariharananda Giri.

(Sankaracharya told, "I am giving this *sanyas* as the representative of Swami Yogananda Giri and hence, I am giving them the "Giri" order from the ten group (*Dasanami*) and not from my own "Bharati" group.

(It is the tradition that no Sankaracharya of India out of four ever has set foot on foreign soil. However, the only exception was the Sankaracharya of Puri Gobardhan Math, Swami Krisnatirtha Bharati, perhaps, in exchange for this service he rendered to Yogoda. Yogananda's organization sponsored his trip to the United States).

So Swami Bidyananda, being frustrated with the American administration of Yogoda through Mr. Binaya Narayan Dube, being a very independent person announced that Swamiji would be the next "Asram Swami" of his hermitage.

As mentioned before, Bidyananda in the young days worked in a Publishing Co. at Calcutta to edit a very popular magazine. He also wrote several small books on Yogananda in Bengali and in English.

What really made Bidyananda mad was in the Bengali version of the *Autobiography of a Yogi* (the Bengali title is *Yogikathamrit*) that Binaya Narayan (Mr. Dube) added a chapter, a small biographical sketch of himself, and after publishing, sent several copies to the girl's high school, advising to distribute them among the girl students.

When Bidyananda came to know this, he instructed the lady principal of the girl's high school to tear off the chapter which was added at the back portion of the book.

Bidyananda told Swamiji that "Mr. Dube had the audacity to pollute my Guru's *autobiography,* such a beautiful book".

Sris Chandra Banerjee (Master *Mosai*), disciple of Bhupendranath Sanyal Mahasay:

One day, just after the day of *Maha Sivaratri* (auspicious day for Lord Siva), Sris Chandra Banerjee joined in our *sat sanga*. Bidyananda knew him before since Sris Banerjee was a freedom fighter against the British Rule. So he was visiting Bidyananda. The three of us were having our *sat sanga* under the *bel* tree. Leaves of a *bel* tree are absolutely necessary to worship Lord Siva, since Ma Parvati used to live eating only the leaves of a *bel* tree before getting Lord Siva as her husband. She even had to give up eating the *bel* leaves to convince Lord Siva. At that time her name became famous as Aparna (*A* means "no", and *parna* means "leaf" so Aparna means "one who lives without eating leaves").

The day before was *Siva Ratri* (night for Lord Siva), and there was a small Siva temple near the *bel* tree where the residents of the hermitage worshiped at night. Naturally our *sat sanga* was centered around Lord Siva, his path of renunciation.

About Sris Chandra Banerjee, he was a freedom fighter in early days, a lifelong bachelor, a high school principal. He used to teach in the school where a king had requested him to tutor his young son who was one of his students in the school. One day, while Sri Babu was tutoring him, the young prince started smoking in front of Sris Banerjee who slapped the young prince very hard. The prince went inside the palace. The incident was reported to the king. Some people thought Mr. Banerjee would lose his job in the school. The next day, the king sent a man to inform Mr. Banerjee to see the king. When Sris Babu arrived, the king asked a man to bring the young prince. When the prince arrived, the king ordered Sri Babu to slap the young prince very hard on the other cheek. Sris Babu did not hesitate to strike the other cheek. Then the king said to his son, "Never, you smoke in front of your teacher." Since then Sri Chandra Banerjee became famous as "Master Mahasay."

Sris Babu was a disciple of Bhupendranath Sanyal. He had his own principles and lifetime routine; he used to close the day's business at sun down; no more worldly work for him. It was time to practice *Kriya* and rest at night. He maintained his principles very sincerely and honestly the entire life.

He asked Swamiji two questions : How do you know your man of the mind (heart)?

In reply Swamiji said, "If you love and respect someone and you have to live with him witnessing ups and downs and in different circumstances, with different odd situations, his actions and responses, yet your love and respect continue to increase. Then you know that you have met your man of the heart."

Sris Babu commented, "Pretty good. Exactly what I was thinking." Then Sris Babu said, next question : "I am told you have been practicing *Kriya* for a long time. Any comment about *Kriya*?"

Swamiji said, "This one I don't know how to reply; but I will try. It seems to me that practicing *Kriya* for a long time, my thoughts are reducing. Before, there were many thoughts intruding upon me, but now they are less and less and gradually even further narrowing. That is all I can comment."

Master *Mosai* said, "You are in the right direction."

Swamiji asked, "Did I pass?"

This time both Bidyananda and Sris Babu said, "Sure you do,"

Swamiji knew that he had earned their affection.

In the crisis period of Bengal in the sixties to serve the people, Sri Chandra Banerjee contested the election and became M. L. A. (Member of the Legislative Assembly) of West Bengal like our Panchkori Dey.

How Swami Satyananda trains Swami Satyeswarananda

In the beginning of their relationship once Satyananda told the author, "Do not hesitate to speak out if you think you are right and if it is contrary to the view of what I have said."

Nevertheless, in Vedic culture, it is conventional wisdom for everybody to relate to a situation or to speak after having considered three things:

1. *Sthan*, "place,"
2. *Kala*, "time," and
3. *Patra*, "person."

Before one opens one's mouth to say something, one is required to consider these three things: where one is standing or sitting, that is, whether it is the right place for saying something; what time it is, that is, whether the time is appropriate for speaking something; lastly, one must consider with whom one is to communicate, that is, whether one is in contact with the right person for questioning or talking.

Satyananda in training the author was very honest and provided every opportunity to grow truly according to his principles and idealism. He never imposed anything upon the author, instead, he let him know the whole situation and draw his own conclusion according to his principles.

Once Satyananda commented to another devotee, "He [the author] is very upright; his sword of righteousness is kept open from the clip always, so that he can cut immediately what is wrong or unrighteous."

On another occasion, he said to some other devotee who was a high court judge who came to see Satyananda during vacation time, who seeing the author posed the question why this boy had not gone home on the vacation.

Satyananda replied, "He [the author] is my Sankara [Lord Siva]."

Satyananda was so honest in his training that he once invited the author to accompany him to Puri Asram to attend the annual celebration in March, in spite of the fact that the author had refused his request to look after Puri asram.

Satyananda knew what was going to happen there, yet he wanted the author to witness the event.

Unfortunately, the author was busy at that time in Calcutta and had prior commitments to some projects that he had been asked to look after.

On another such occasion, Satyananda took the author with him and attended the annual meeting at Dakshineswar, YSS Calcutta. The moment both arrived at YSS Calcutta, they saw that many people were already there. Both moved to the open ground where the meeting would be held in the open air on the bank of the Ganges. Both were noticed by Pravas Chandra Ghosh, vice president of YSS; besides Satyananda, Mr. Ghosh was the only founding member of YSS there at that place.

Among the audience, some had been Satyananda's students at Ranchi, *Brahmachari* disciples, and some had joined the organization after Satyananda had left Ranchi, so they did not know Satyananda's position.

Satyananda as the president of Sriyukteswar's organization, Sadhu Sova, appointed Mr. Ghosh as secretary. So they had served together in that organ-ization closely. As a matter fact, they had been good friends since their college days.

Mr. Ghosh, cousin of Yogananda, then a retired old man, noticed Satyananda and managed to bring him to the platform. The author followed him. Many did not like it. Mr. Dube, secretary of YSS, happened to know that Satyananda's name was on the list of the speakers.

Later, one of Satyananda's students at Ranchi, among the organizers, asked the other who was holding the list, also a student of Satyananda, to strike off Satyananda's name. He was saying it in such a loud voice that it was within the hearing of many, including Satyananda and the author.

One of them asked, "Satyananda's name? But Mr. Ghosh, the vice president [of Yogoda], has included it."

"So what? Don't you remember what happened at Puri? Satyananda's connection is not required here; in fact, he is not even invited here. So don't worry. You had better strike off his name."

The other organizer struck off Satyananda's name in front of us.

On the way returning from the meeting, both the author and Satyananda boarded a rickshaw [paddy cab] and headed toward the bus stop. The author commented, "You were not invited and you have come here uninvited."

Satyananda replied saying, "I do not need any invitation to attend where the Lord's name is chanted. Besides, I had to show you what the life of a *sanyasi*, or Swami is."

The author felt like crying within: What humiliation in the hands of his own students and *Brahmachari* disciple Satyananda had to go through for providing training to the author. For this reason, the author is ever grateful to the egoless, realized yogi.

Both were silent for a while. Then breaking the silence, the author asked, "What happened at Puri?"

Satyananda did not like to answer. The author repeated the question, but still he preferred to remain silent. Meanwhile, both arrived at the bus stop. Satyananda said, "I shall tell you later." Both remained silent all the way back to Ballygunge, Calcutta.

One day, the author was visiting the hermitage of Swami Bidyananda and spent some time with him. He told the author, "In the annual meeting celebration of Puri asram one year I attended. Did you know what happened in that meeting?"

The author said, "No, I don't know. Would you like to share what happened?"

Bidyananda said, "Well! I was asked to say something on *Kriya*, but I felt sorry, observing Satyananda sitting in the back in the midst of attending ordinary devotees and not on the dais. In fact, I had learned that he was not even invited. I was so upset that I could not check myself. My conscience was bothering me.

"My God! Satyananda was the direct disciple of Sriyukteswar, the founder of the hermitage, the founder of the organization and Sriyukteswar appointed Satyananda as the '*asram* swami ('monk of the hermitage', long ago in 1919) and above all, at the present time, Satyananda is the third president of Sadhu Sova. That meeting was the annual meeting as well as the foundation day celebration of the hermitage, and the organizers did not invite him. If Satyananda chose to assert his legal right he could drive away everybody.

"I learned that in some previous years he was invited. He usually attended three day annual meetings in the month of March, because he had been asked by Sriyukteswar to look after the hermitage and the worship in the *Annapurna* Temple (Divine Mother of wealth) at the hermitage. So he felt an obligation to carry out that responsibility and duty regardless of his being invited or not; that is why he was there even uninvited.

"(Possibly, that is the reason why specifically Satyananda had asked the author to accompany him that year to the Puri asram).

"So I focused my address after the initial introduction and drew the attention of the audience towards Satyananda saying, 'We who are assembled here have no elementary decency or courtesy to invite the president of this organization and the monk of the hermitage, that is Satyananda, appointed by the founder himself (Sriyukteswar). Look there in the back! He is sitting there among the devotees. He has come uninvited here as I understand.

"What authority do we have on earth to lecture on *Kriya* when the organizers of this meeting failed to invite him?

"I will not lecture on *Kriya*, instead, I will lecture on the history of this hermitage. I was continuing my address to the audience, but meantime, I got many slips to sit down. I told them I was not going to sit down till I finished narrating the history of the hermitage.

"Mr. Sailendra B. Dasgupta, Sriyukteswar's disciple, Satyananda's student at Ranchi, from the midst of the audience loudly said, 'Bravo Bidyanandaji.'

"I completed my speech in brief. In the meantime, a murmur grew to an uproar in the audience. Hurriedly, the organizers ended the meeting."

The author noticed that Bidyananda's hands were trembling when he narrated the event; he generated excitement.

The author said to him, "I am sorry! If I caused you suffering. I am grateful to you for sharing the event with me."

Returning from there, some days later, once again, the author confronted Satyananda saying, "You did not tell me what had happened at Puri".

He looked into the eyes of the author and gently and briefly narrated the event in his way always focusing on the good side. He did not mention that he had not been invited; he also left out Dasgupta's cheering of Bidyananda, but he added that after coming out from the meeting that he had said to Bidyananda, "Which kind of gentleman are you? I was doing fine in the back in the midst of all. Your drawing the attention of the audience and focusing their attention on me, put me in such an embarrassing situation that neither was I able to stand up and walk out, nor could I continue to sit there."

The author asked, "Is this all that happened there?"

Satyananda said, "Yes, as far as I remembered. Have you heard this before from someone? Did I miss anything?"

He asked two questions without waiting for the author to reply, which was very unusual.

The author then said, "You missed to mention Dasgupta's cheering of Bidyananda.

Satyananda looked into the eyes of the author and asked, "From whom did you hear this?'

The author said, "From Bidyanandaji, of course. He also missed one part. He did not mention what you said to him after the meeting outside."

Satyananda's style of training the author was unique: he never imposed anything against the author's will; he gave him freedom to think independently; unconditional love was the essence of the relationship.

One day, Suddhananda wrote to the author in the Himalayas that Pravas Chandra Ghosh had sent a money order of five hundred rupees (Rs.500,00) to appropriate the amount for Satyananda's *samadhi* temple and he wrote a note: It said, "Satyananda lived with us so closely his entire life, but we could not recognize him."

What Mr. Ghosh meant was that they had been friends since their college days. Satyananda was a philosophy honors student in the City College under Calcutta University while Mr. Ghosh had graduated from Presidency College and had enrolled as a student of philosophy (M. A.) in the Calcutta University. They were the founding members of YSS.

Satyananda was the third president of Sriyukteswar's organization, Sadhu Sova, when Mr. Ghosh was appointed as secretary, and they served together.

It was Pravas Chandra Ghosh who had witnessed Satyananda's life having many twists and turns. Having been involved in the administration of these organizations, he witnessed these from the very inner circle.

The author remembered the last meeting at Ballugunge, Calcutta, between Satyananda, Mr. Ghosh and the author. Mr. Ghosh whispered into the author's ear, "He [Satyananda] is so egoless and saintly, but we could not recognize him. Also we have failed to honor him."

It should be noted here that the *Sat Sanga Mission* had been founded in 1953. In this matter, Satyananda told the author, "One day, Sailendra Bejoy Dasgupta commented that I seemed to have a very soft heart for Yogoda, and that I could even merge Sevayatan with it if I have a chance. Sailen asked me about his observation.

"I confessed and said, 'Remember! I told you all in the beginning that I would write to Yogananda that he was my dear friend, and that you could not object to it. Yes, if I had the chance I would like Sevayatan to work with Yogoda.'

"Thereafter, Sailen Bejoy told his seniors, Suddhananda, Panchkori and others, 'Don't trust Satyananda. He is Yogoda. We must form our own registered organization.' They founded the Sat Sanga Mission and appointed me [Satyananda] as its President."

At the age of over hundred years, Bidyananda left body.

About Binaya Narayan, Sister Daya was able to make him a *sanyasi*, Swami Shyamananda Giri; the ceremony was held in the United States. He could not resist. By that time he was so deeply indebted to them.

Mr. Kanta Banrejee, a Bengali *Brahmana* (priest class), a student of Yogananda and Satyananda at Ranchi school, joined the Bihar Police Force.

After his retirement, Binaya Narayan found him and brought him to the asram to manage the boy's hostel. When Binay Narayan was back in India as Swami Shyamananda Giri, Kanta Banerjee was stunned. When Swamiji was in Ranchi for a month before meeting Daya at Calcutta, Mr. Kanta Banerjee, who contacted Swamiji first and then their secretary, made the appointment. During that one month at Ranchi, Mr. Kanta Banerjee personally told Swamiji that he posed a question to Binaya Narayan saying, "*Dada* [means elder brother]! Being a *brahman* yourself, you take *sanyas* [enter the order of Swami] from a Christian lady?"

Then Kanta Banerjee commented it was so shocking to him, that thereafter he did not live long. He died in 1971. As Binay Narayan suggested to Yogoda, they created the posts of joint general secretaries and his friend, Mr. Banamali Das, an eminent lawyer, was appointed one of them, a kind of silent partner so that they could get free legal advice. The other active real joint-general secretary was Shantanada, an American.

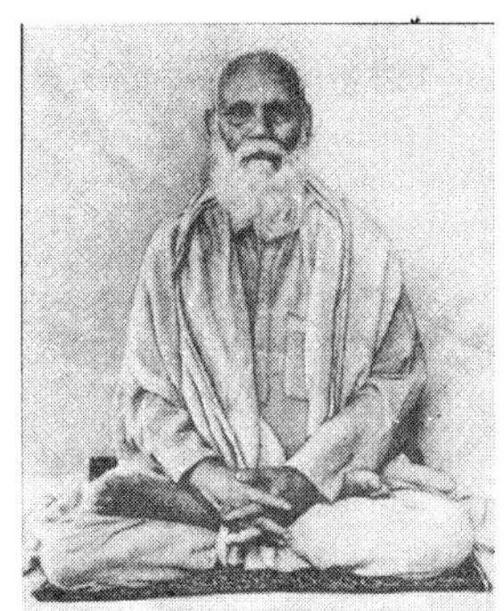

Swami Suddhananda, Disciple of Swami Satyananda, initiated by Hangswa Swami Kebalananda

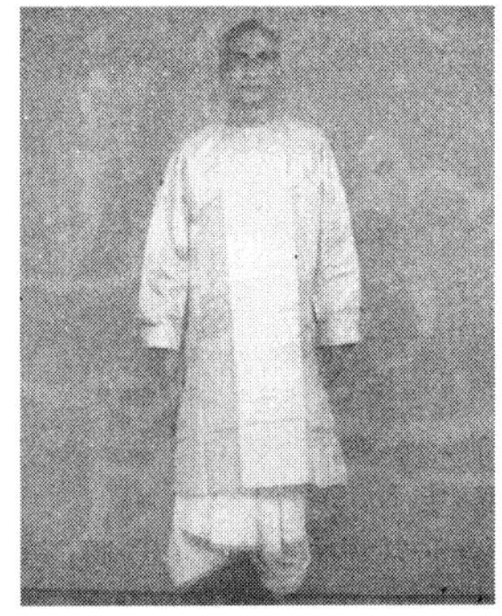

Prof. Amarendranath Bhattacharya Disciple of Swami Satyananda, and A good friend of the Author

The Handwritten Letter of Professor Amarendranath Bhattacharya, disciple of Swami Satyananda, to Swami Satyeswarananda

Amarendranath Bhattacharyya
Retired Lecturer, Sevayatan Sikshan Mahavidyalaya
Debendra villa
Santinagar
HOWRAH - 711109
India

Dated, Howrah, the 10 th March, 1997

My dear Swami Satyeswaranandaji,

Perhaps you remember me, I have retired from Sevayatan Sikshan Mahavidyalaya on the 31 st Oct, 1996 and I have been residing at my Howrah residence. Swami Virajananda Giri of Sevayatan Ashram has presented a set of books written by you and sent by you to him recently. I have gone through these books and I highly appreciate these books.

Swami Virajanandaji has presented your books to Sri Siddhartha Sankar Roy, ex- Ambasador of India to America. Sri Roy has visited Sevayatan recently. Swami Virajanandaji presented your books to several High Court Judges and other notable persons of India.

However I am very much happy to know that you have been writing other books also.

May you live long with good ~~health~~ health.

With my regards and best wishes,
Sincerely yours,
Amarendranath Bhattacharyya

The letter of Professor Amarendranath Bhattacharya,
disciple of Swami Satyananda to Swami Satyeswarananda

Amarendranath Bhattacharyya,
Retired Lecturer, Sevayatan Sikshan Mahavidyalaya
Debendra Villa
Santinagar
Howrah - 711109
India

Dated, Howrah, the 10th March, 1997

My dear Swami Satyeswaranandaji,

Perhaps you remember me. I have retired from Sevayatan Sikshan Mahavidyalaya on the 31st Oct. 1996 and I have been residing at my Howrah residence.

Swami Virajananda Giri of Sevayatan Ashram has presented a set of books written by you and sent by you to him recently. I have gone through these books and I highly appreciate these books.

Swami Virajanandaji has presented your books to Sri Siddhartha Sankar Roy, ex-Ambasador [Ambassador] of India to America. Sri Roy has visited Sevayatan recently. Swami Virajanandaji presented your books to several High Court Judges and other notable persons of India.

However, I am very much happy to know that you have been writing other books also.

May you live long with good health.

With my regards and best wishes,

Sincerely Yours,

Amarendranath Bhattacharyya.

The Handwritten letter of Swami Virajananda Giri in Bengali
to Swami Satyeswarananda

ওঁ

Swami Virajananda Giri
VILL + P. O. – SEVAYATAN
DIST.—MIDNAPUR
W. B.—721514.

Ref. No.......... Dated ৪।১১।৯৯

পরমপূজনীয় স্বামীজী মহারাজ,

ওঁ নমো নারায়ণায়

আপনার বইগুলি পড়ে খুব আনন্দ পেলাম। আপনি এত সুন্দরকরে সেবায়তনের মহিমা প্রচার করে চলেছেন; সেজন্য আপনাকে সাধুবাদ জানাই। আপনার সাথে আমার পরিচয় নেই। আমি এই আশ্রমে নবাগত। আপনার বইগুলি পড়ে অনেককিছু জানতে পারলাম। অশেষ ধন্যবাদ। সেবায়তনের বয়স ৮৫ বছর হলো। আসন্ন উৎসব। এই উৎসবে আসার জন্য আপনাকে আমন্ত্রণ জানাই। পত্রে সাষ্টাঙ্গ প্রণাম নিবেন। ইতি

শুভাকাঙ্খী—
স্বামী বিরজানন্দ গিরি

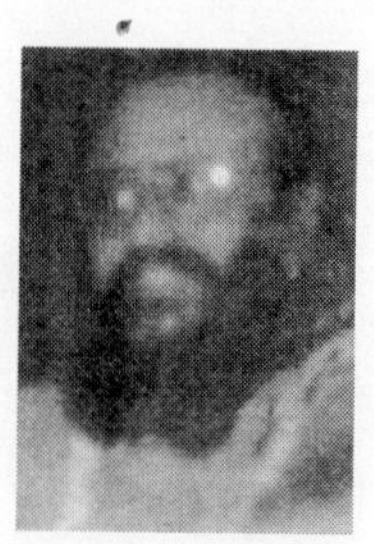

Swami Virajananda Giri

The English Version of the Handwritten letter of Swami Virajananda Giri

Swami Virajananda Giri
Vill & P.O. Sevayatan
Dist. Midnapore
W.B. 721514
Dec. 4, 1991

Parampujaniya Swamiji Maharaj,
[Supremely worshipable Swamiji Maharaj],

Om Namonarayanaya [Bowing to Lord Narayana],
I have tremendous joy reading the books written by you. You have described so nicely the glories of Sevayatan [Hermitage of Swami Satyananda]. Thank you for that.

I have no acquaintance with you.

[The reason is Swamiji had left the hermitage, Sevayatan in 1971, after twenty years association, and Virajanandaji joined Sevayatan recently after many years later; so there was no acquaintance].

I am a newcomer here. I have come to know many things [from your books]; countless thanks for that reason.

The age of Sevayatan becomes forty eight years (48). There is the annual celebration (*utsab*). I invite you to come to the forthcoming celebration.

With this letter please accept my sincere regards.

Swami Virajananda Giri

NOTE - Swami Satyeswarananda left Sevayatan after a few months just after Swami Satyananda left body since he gave word to Swami Satyananda that he would stay with him to help him till his last breath.

Long after twenty years Swami Virajananda joined Sevayatan and that was the reason he did not know many things and acknowledged learning many things reading Swamiji's books.

Typed Letter of Swami Virajananda Giri
to Swami Satyeswarananda

STD-03221 PHONE: JHARGRAM-55024

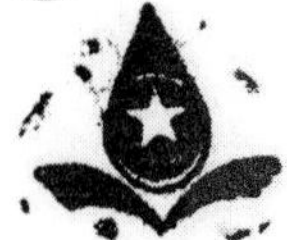

SATSANGA MISSION

Certificate of Registration of Societies Act XXI *of* 1860

No 22597/335 *of* 1955-1956

P.o. SEVAYATAN Via-JHARGRAM (Midnapore)pin-Code 721514 (W.B.)

No ....

Dated 22/8/96

Dear Swami Satyeswaranandaji,

It gives me ample pleasure to inform you that we are going to celebrate the birth centenary of Swami Satyananda Giriji, the first Acharya of Sevayatan. We are organising an International Kriya Yoga conference to be held on 28th and 29th Sept, 1996 at Yuba Bharti Krirangan (Salt lake), in Calcutta. Hon'ble Governor of West Bengal will inangurate the function. The Kriya Yogis, from different parts of the World, are expected to participate in that function. You are cordially invited to attend the Ceremony.

I would like to request you to donate at least hundred Copies of the biography of Swami Satyananda Giriji written and published by you. Any other donation from you may be thankfully received.

Please intimate us about your date of arrival in calcutta.

With kind regards,

Yours faithfully.

Swami Virajananda Giri

President

SATSANGA MISSION

Sat Sanga Mission,
Sevayatan, Jhargram (Midnapore)

Dated, August 22, 1996

Dear Swami Satyeswaranandaji,

It gives me ample pleasure to inform you that we are going to celebrate the birth centenary of Swami Satyananda Giriji, the first Acharya of Sevayatan.

We are organizing an International Kriya Yoga Conference to be held on 28th and 29th Sept.,1996 at Yuba Bharti Krirangan (Salt Lake), in Calcutta. Hon'ble Governor of West Bengal will inaugurate the function. The Kriya Yogis, from different parts of the world, are expected to participate in that function. You are cordially invited to attend the Ceremony.

I would like to request you to donate at least hundred copies of the biography of Swami Satyananda Giriji written and published by you. Any other donation from you may be thankfully received.

Please intimate us about your date of arrival in Calcutta.

With kind regards,

Yours faithfully

Swami Virajananda Giri,
President, Sat Sanga Mission

Chapter 5

The Ancient and Pure Original *Kriya*

NOTE - The present author has written and published a book, the title is: *The Original Kriya* (ISBN # 1-87785-43-5). This chapter is a very small excerpt regarding "*Kriya* at a glance" from the book.

There is another book by the present author the title *The Kriya Sutras* which is the "Aphorism of the *Atma Kriya* of the *Aryya* civilization".

The purpose of this excerpt on this chapter is to act as an introduction for the better understanding of the following chapter (The Modified *Kriya*). The special features mentioned on the current chapter should be kept in mind while the reader is going through the next chapter.

Fundamental Features of the Ancient and Pure Original *Kriya*

First, let us remember some of the fundamental features of the Ancient and Pure Original *Kriya* before going into the alterations, modifications, disintegrations, dropping some essential *Kriya*, and changing the whole process from the very beginning of initiation to the end of teaching the fourth *Kriya* without teaching the essential precondition of the *Khecharimudra* or the *Talabya Kriya*.

The following are the special features of the ancient and the original pure *Kriya*. If these are not observed then one must know that *Kriya* and the practice are not according to Mahamuni Babaji and Lahiri Mahasay.

1. The Original *Kriya* Tradition is *Guru-Param-Para*, that is, the disciple receives *Kriya* initiation personally from his or her *Gurudev*, the Master. The initiate learns the *Kriya* discipline having a personal relationship with his or her *Gurudev* or the Master, that is, *Guruvraktagamya*, "learning from the living lips of the *Guru*."

2. There is an INJUNCTION from Mahamuni Babaji, the Divine Himalayan Yogi, which is "Not to develop organization around the teaching of *Kriya*."

3. So the Original *Kriya* Tradition is free from an organizational way of teaching. It is free from organizations. The teaching is based upon one on one.

4. *Kriya* initiation is given in private and in strict confidence, personally and secretly, behind closed doors and not in public or in a group. The *Kriya* initiation ceremony is neither a public affair nor a matter of public display.

5. **Most importantly**, the *Kriya* practitioners must "abandon the expecta-tion of the results of the practice."

In the language of Lahiri Mahasay, *Phala-kangkha-rahit* ("abandoning the expectation of the results"). This is the true **SPIRIT** of the *Kriya* discipline.

As a matter of fact, without this feature of abandoning the results, any spiritual discipline becomes short of NOTHING.

6. The *Kriya* initiate has to have his or her *Kriya* practice checked every six months personally by the Master. If the disciple misses two consecutive check-ups he or she would be treated as a non-*Kriyanwit*. This rule was introduced by Lahiri Mahasay.

7. Lahiri Mahasay initiated his disciples personally on a one to one basis. Only in a few cases did he initiate husband and wife together. In such a situation, if either of the spouses required additional *Kriya* which the other did not, then he initiated that *Kriya* separately.

8. Original *Kriya* is practiced in strict secrecy. Occasional practice among the close *Kriyanwits*, the followers of *Kriya*, is the exception. Group *Kriya* practice in public is prohibited.

9. Although Babaji himself is a renunciate Swami, in fact, there is no necessary connection that one has to be renunciate to practice *Kriya* discipline.

The ancient original pure *Kriya* is suited for both renunciates and householders. It is so scientific that people from different religious faiths can benefit from the practice of the *Kriya* Science, as it is based on "breath" which is the universal ground of life and religion.

Lahiri Mahasay, the polestar of *Kriya*, became the role model of the house-holder *Kriyanwits*, while Babaji remains the role model of the renunciates.

The Ancient and Pure Original *Kriya* at a Glance

How to Attain eternal Realization of the ultimate Self?

Can thirst be quenched by merely shouting the word "water"?

Certainly not! Shouting only worsens the situation. The uttering of words does not produce the desired results as some devotees advocate and propagate.

Can a person learn how to swim simply by talking to the instructor while standing on land?

Obviously not. It is ridiculous to think to have eternal Realization simply by talking about and not practicing meditation. The nature of the ultimate Self may be understood through intellectual speculation, but eternal Realization comes only through "**actual**" practice.

Can hunger be satisfied by the thought of food?

The answer is no. Thoughts and reason leave us at a point quite indecisive; they cannot go beyond. "Dissolve thoughts or the mind (the restless breath) in the very Source by any means."

Realization is relative when the seeker tries to realize something outside himself without "**first**" realizing the truth behind himself. Relative realization, or relative knowledge, arises from relative existences.

Inquire who is the knower. When the seeker knows himself (the knower), this is absolute Knowledge from One Existence, which is both subject and object of knowledge.

To hold onto the quest "**Who am I**?" undistractedly with efforts is practice; when the same becomes effortless and natural, it is Realization.

Absolute Realization is simply being the ultimate Self spontaneously.

What is love?

It is Oneness between the seeking self (son) and the ultimate Self (father) **within**. When one achieves it **within**, one knows that the whole world is the reflection of his self.

This is the only "**right**" way to grow into divine Love and attain eternal Realization.

"... *O Father, glorify thou me with thine own self with the glory which I* ***had with thee before the world was.*** " John 17:5

"*God is a spirit* [the word Spirit comes from the Latin word *Spiritus* which means "**breath**". So it can safely be said that God is a definite state of breath, that is, "**Tranquil Breath**"]: *and they that worship him must worship him in spirit* [through Breath, that is through the practice of *Pranayam* or *Kriya* with the help of *Sthirabayu*, or "tranquil breath"*] and in truth* [Tranquility]." John 4:24

"*The kingdom of God* [Tranquil Breath] *is "**within**" you* [inside the physical body in Oneness between the seeking self and the ultimate Self of the seeker]." - Luke 17:21

What is Grace?

It is pure Consciousness of the ultimate Self, which is "**internal**". It is always there in everybody and never out of operation. If it were external - coming from someone from outside, then it would be useless, as it would not be permanent. What comes, goes. What appears, disappears. So all "**visions**" (including inner visions, or revelations) are "**secondary**" and impermanent.

"*No man hath seen God at any time.*" 1 John 4:12

So, "**being**" God, not seeing God, is inner Realization, and "**being**" the ultimate Self, not seeing the ultimate Self, is eternal Realization.

"*Brahmabid Brahmaiba bhabati* ("One who knows Brahma, becomes Brahma").

Truth (*Satya*) is permanent, hence its Realization must be eternal.

"Above all, be true to yourself": Be one with the ultimate Self.

The Path :

The *Kriya* Path is: Attaining eternal Tranquility by practice of *Pranayam* and continuing meditations on the Formless, i.e. Tranquility.

Increasing the practice of *Kriya*, doing all works "**without expectations**" for the results thereof, the path aims at achieving Tranquility, observing everything which is revealed in *Yonimudra* (Beatific-Inner-Revelation-*Kriya*), and terminating all desired expectations, renouncing every desire before it originates, being freed from all thoughts.

It is meditating on the thoughtless state of Consciousness, especially holding that state of Consciousness where there is no sun, moon, light of fire; still everything is seen eternally.

One bright, dazzling star of Consciousness is seen very secretly in between the eyebrows, and the unmanifested state of Consciousness is revealed.

Thereafter, whatever sentiments one possesses can be seen in "**vision**" in the inner Self ("***Kutastha***"). Thereby believing the advice of the Master, five states of vibrations (earth, water, fire air and ether), mind, intelligence, ego and Supreme Being are seen, resulting in the steadfastness of mind towards inner Consciousness.

When all the three qualities are harmoniously together in one rhythm inside the Spinal Cord, then the supreme Being is revealed, going beyond the sentiments of discrimination between good and bad.

Having the pure Love and reverence, when the breath is tranquil or still, the seeker attains ***Sthirattva*** ("**eternal Tranquility**", or Peace).

"*Be still* [attain the state of tranquil Breath by the practice of *Pranayam*], *and know that I* [the seeking self] *am God* [Tranquil Breath, that is Spirit]." Psalms 46:10

"*Peace be still. And the wind* [breath] *ceased, and there was a great calm* [Tranquility]." Mark 4:39

The Keys of the *Kriya* Path :

1. To attain the tranquil state of breath in natural course by practicing *Pranayam*.

2. To see in *Yonimudra*.

3. Placing the tongue in the head [*Talabya Kriya*].

4. Holding onto the divine Spot and listening to the sound of *Om* [*Brahmayonimudra*].

5. Holding the bright star at the forehead from the throat.

Requirements for *Kriya* :

1. The person must be honest and not a liar.

2. The person should not smoke and drink.

3. The person should read some portion of the *Bhagavad Gita* every day.

4. The person should lose self-importance to destroy his or her ego.

5. He should treat all women as his mother, except his wife, and she should treat all men as her father, except her husband.

6. The person should sit a little lower than his or her *Gurudev* or Master's seat and offer everything to him.

7. The person should practice *Kriyas* every day in strict accordance with the instructions personally received from his or her *Gurudev*.

How to be in the Path?

The ultimate Self, being pure Consciousness, is beyond sensation, concept, thought, and intellect. A definite mode of action to make the mind inward and dissolve it is called *Kriya*.

The *Kriya* path is the "**righteous way**" to realize the ultimate Self.

Having true *Kriya* depends on three points :

1. The initiate must receive *Kriya* personally from the mouth of the Master.

2. He must receive "*Kriya* of *Aksara*, or letter," and

3. He must receive "*Kriya* of the inner *Aksaras*, or letters."

In Sanskrit the word *Aksara* can be scanned into two words: (*A* means "No," and *ksara* means "transitory"; Thus, the word *Aksara* also means "eternity". The Sanskrit *Aksara* is a letter which is part of a word, e.g. A, B, C, etc. A letter by itself has no meaning.

What does "*Kriya* of the letters" mean?

When the Master utters a letter, of course, it has sound although it does not by itself represent a concept, meaning or thought. So, "*Kriyas* of the letters" obviously means "**sound**" and "**vibrations of Eternity**" [the ultimate Self], free from concepts, thoughts and meanings.

"*Kriya* of the inner letters" means vibrations of "**inner sound**" (*Om/Aum. Amen*) resonating from the ultimate Self.

When the Master utters a letter, the vibrations of the sound of the letter come directly from the enlightened state of mystic Energy (***Kundalini***), and penetrate the ear of the initiate, resulting in true initiation to the *Kriya* path.

Vibration of Sound is the means of communicating *Sakti*, or energy.

It should be pointed out here that the odd number of the Sanskrit alphabet carries "**less**" number of atoms of the inner Light and the inner Sound; while the even number of the alphabet carries "**greater**" number of atoms of the inner Light and the inner Sound.

As a result, a "**word**" carries a composite vibration of the inner Light and the inner Sound depending on the basis of how the word is formulated by how many numbers of letters and from which location (the odd or the even from the alphabet) of those letters are chosen.

Thus, following the vibration and the inner Sound to transcend concepts, thoughts, and the intellect, the initiate can find the true Path.

Unfortunately, many seekers do not know this "**subtle point**" and they try to understand the advice through "**preconceived**" concepts, thoughts, and meanings and find the intellectual path (full of meanings, instead of vibration) which is the negative way.

The scriptures support the righteous way, *Guruvraktagamya* - "learning from the living lips of a *Guru*"; and through the *Guru-param-para* way, from the *Guru* or the Master to the disciple, having a personal relationship with the *Guru*

"... *I have need to be baptized of thee, and cometh thou to me*? Matthew 3:14

"... *Suffer it to be so now: for thus it be cometh us to fulfill all righteousness*" Matthew 3:15

".. *Except a man be born again* [attain the state of tranquil Breath, thereby, vibrations and rhythms of inner Light and inner Sound], *he cannot see the kingdom of God.*" John 3:3

Initiation is "**essential**". It must be received personally and in a righteous way.

List of the Pure and Original *Kriyas*

1. ***Mahamudra*** (Great *Kriya*) :

"*And as Moses lifted up the serpent in the wilderness, even so must the Son of man be lifted up*." John 3:14

2. ***Navi Kriya*** (Electronizing *Kriya*) :

"*My little children of whom I travail in birth again until* ***Christ be formed*** *in you*." Galatians 4:19

3. ***Talabya Kriya*** or ***Khecharimudra*** (Inner-Outer-Space- *Kriya*) :

"*... I have meat to eat that ye know not of.*" John 4:32

"*The nobles* [the realized ones] *held their peace* [Tranquility], *and their tongue cleaved* [*Khecharimudra*] *to the roof* [at the forehead] *of their mouth.*" Job 28:10

4. ***Pranayam*** (Equilibrium *Kriya*) :

"*Peace, be still. And the wind ceased, and there was a great calm.*" Mark 4:39

"*Be still, and know that I am God.*" Psalms 46:10

Sthir Bayur Kriya

("*Kriyas* of the Tranquil Breath")

According to the Pure *Kriya*, Lahiri Mahasay taught that after the successful *Khecharimudra* or *Talabya Kriya,* the *Sthir Bayur Kriyas* are introduced. It is a "**precondition**" in the Pure *Kriya*.

In other words, after the successful *Khecharimudra* the *Sthir Bayur Kriyas* (*Kriyas* of the tranquil Breath), that is *Kriya* such as, *Thokar/ Thokkar, Omkar Kriyas,* and the *Uchcha Kriyas* are introduced.

If these *Kriyas* of the tranquil Breath are introduced before one has achieved the success in *Khechari*, it will be a **violation** of the Pure *Kriya* and the practice will bring no good result. The simple reason is that the practice is missing its life, the "**Tranquil Breath**".

How do you practice the *Kriyas* of the Tranquil Breath when your breath is not tranquil? It is a strange practice of the ridiculous teaching.

It will be counterproductive; instead of helping the seeker, it will harm the practitioners.

On the one hand, It will develop a sense of egoism that the person is practicing higher *Kriyas* and so he is an advanced *Kriyaban*.

On the other hand, as far as his teacher is concerned, clearly he is a violator of the rules of Pure *Kriya* and he is an ambitious, egotistic, emotional, immature, irresponsible, non-permitted and self style *Kriya* master. Beware of them. They can say and do anything to increase their followers. Receiving *Kriya* from them is not actually receiving *Kriya* rather some unauthorized information.

5. **The first *Omkar Kriya*** (Electromagnetizing *Kriya*) :

"*That he would grant you, according to the riches of his glory, to be strengthened with might by his Spirit in the inner man*." Ephesians 3:16

6. **The second *Omkar Kriya*** (Cosmo-electromagnetizing *Kriya*) :

"*Thou fool, that which thou sowest is not quickened, except it die*."
1 Corinthians 15:36

7. **The third *Omkar Kriya***

"*...I die daily*". 1 Corinthians 15:31

8. **The fourth *Omkar Kriya*** (Spontaneous transmigrating *Kriya*):

"*... When ye have lifted up the Son of man, then shall ye know that I am he...*" John 8:28

9. ***Yonimudra*** (Beatific-Inner-Revelation-*Kriya*) :

"*The light of the body is the eye: if therefore thine eye be single* [one-pointed]*, thy whole body shall be full of light.*" Matthew 6:22

10. ***Brahmayonimudra*** (Spontaneous Tranquility) :

"*He that hath an ear, let him hear what the Spirit* [Tranquil Breath] *saith unto the churches.*" Revelation 2:7

11. ***Purna Kriya* (Eternal Tranquility) :**

"*... I AM THAT I AM*". Exodus 3:14

Kriyas are the "**keys**" to eternal Realization of the ultimate Self.

The Original *Kriya* Science (The Psycho-physical Discipline) The eightfold :

1. ***Yama*** : regulation on compassion, truthfulness, honesty, inwardness and self-sufficiency.

2. ***Niyama*** : Regulations on purity of body and mind, contentment of heart, sincerity, adhering to the sound of *OM*, merging the mind in pure Consciousness.

3. ***Asana*** : Steadfast sitting at ease.

4. ***Pranayam*** : Breathing exercises to dissolve the mind and intellect by attaining naturally the still state of breath from the operation of *Prana*, *Apana*, *Smaman*, *Udana* and *Byana*.

5. ***Pratyahara*** : Interiorization of senses - smelling, touching, tasting, seeing and hearing.

6. ***Dharana*** : Glimpse of eternal Tranquility.

7. ***Dhyana*** : Meditation, merging the mind in Tranquility.

8. ***Samadhi***: Attunement in Oneness between the seeking self and the ultimate Self to attain eternal Tranquility.

Yama, *Niyama* and *Asana* (1-3) are the "**container**"; *Pranayam* and *Pratyahara* (4-5) are the "**process**"; *Dharana*, *Dhyana* and *Samadhi* (6-8) are the "**means**"; and eternal Tranquility (*Sthirattva*) or Peace of the ultimate Self is the "**content**."

For dissolving concepts, thoughts, mind and intellect The Dissolving of the Five States of breath:

1. ***Prana*** : Appropriation - and

2. ***Apana*** : Elimination or ejection - The First *Kriya*; First, Second and Third *Omkar Kriyas*

3. ***Samana*** : Assimilation - *Navi Kriya*

4. ***Udana*** : Regeneration and

5. ***Byana*** : Distribution - *Mahamudra*

For Dissolving sensation:

1. Smelling : Nose and

2. Touching : Skin and

3. Tasting : Tongue - *Talabya Kriya*

4. Seeing : Eyes, visions and

5. Hearing : Ears, sound - *Yonimudra*

The four *Yugas* of the Vedic culture :

1. The *Satya Yuga* - The age of first step of a *Kalpa* (a day of Brahma, the Creator).

2. The *Treta Yuga* - The second step of a *Kalpa*.

3. The *Dwapara Yuga* - The third step of a *Kalpa*.

4. The *Kali Yuga* - The fourth step of a *Kalpa*.

The four *Yugas* in the light of *Kriya* as follows :

1. The *Satya Yuga* is to hold onto the *Kutastha*, or the inner Self.

2. The *Treta Yuga* is to see the *Kutastha*.

3. The *Dwapara Yuga* is to generate Happiness through *Kriya* practice.

4. The *Kali Yuga* is to initiate into *Kriya*." *Manusanghita* 1:86

Commentaries by Lahiri Mahasay.

However, spiritually speaking from the realization point of view, in each moment all the four *Yugas* are present; as in a big circle several small circles can be accommodated or drawn.

The four *Asram* (stations of life) in the Vedic Society :

According to Vedic culture, a Hindu's life is to be divided into four parts, covering a lifespan of one hundred years. The sequences are as follows:

1. **The Student (*Brahmachari*) Life** is called *Brahmacharya asram/ashram*. The first twenty-five years are to be dedicated to spiritual learning as a student (*Brahmachari*) boy.

2. **The Householder Life** is called *Grihastha asram*. The second twenty-five years are to be spent as a spiritual householder.

3. **The Forest Recluse Life** is called *Vanaprastha/Banaprastha asram*. The third twenty-five years is to be the period spent in retirement, that is, one retires to the forest.

4. **The Renunciate Life** is called *Sanyas/Sannyas asram.* The fourth twenty-five years are to be years of renunciation from all.

The four divisions (*Varna*) in the Vedic Society :

The Vedic Society is divided into four classes. The scriptural reference is as follows:

Chaturvarna maya sristang guna karma bibhagasa.
Tasya kartaramapi mang bidhyakartaramabyayam. Bhagavad Gita 4:13

Lord Krisna said, "I myself made the four classes based on the nature of the *Guna*, 'quality' and *Karma*, 'action' of the person." *Gita* 4:13

The following are the four Classes (*Varnas*):

1. ***Brahmana*** The priest class whose profession it is to worship for them-selves and others.

2. ***Khatriya***: The warrior or military class whose duty is to rule or govern the country and to defend it against the enemies. Also to donate to the *brahmana* on charity.

3. ***Vaisya***: The trade and agricultural class whose function is to cultivate and to carry on commerce and ensure monetary stability.

4. ***Sudra***: The servant class whose purpose is to serve the other three classes.

The four divisions (*Varna*) in the light of *Kriya* :

1. ***Brahmana***: He who is One with the supreme Self. In other words, who realizes *Brahma*, the ultimate Self, he is *Brahmana*.

2. ***Khatriya***: He who practices *Kriya Yoga* or meditation and witnesses inner Revelation between the eyebrows, and in whose practice there is no expectation of the results there from.

3. ***Vaisya***: He who is practicing *Kriya* or meditation with the expectation for results such as occult powers or Liberation. This expectation for results puts him in the trade or business mind and creates attachments.

4. ***Sudra***: He who is not aware of the true path. This type of person should serve others of the three classes by honest labor so that by righteous actions he will find the true path.

These are the features of the Original *Kriya* discipline in brief.

Although there is no room and scope for modifications to this "Ancient and Pure Original *Kriyas*", yet unfortunately, certain modifications are made to these Ancient and Pure Original *Kriyas*. So we will see them in the next chapter.

Like the auspicious 108 number, there are 108 steps of the original *Kriya*. Lahiri Mahasay received them from Mahamuni Babaji in Dunagiri Hill, Himalayas in 1861. Lahiri Mahasay condensed the 108 steps of the Original *Kriyas* and grouped (not modified) them into the following four divisions on the line of the four *Vedas* (*Rik*, *Sam*, *Yayur* and *Atharva*), on the four sides of the body (front, back, left and right), and the four directions (east, west, north and south). He took the responsibility strictly to maintain the tradition of *Parampara*, meaning, personally, teaching one on one (Master and disciple).

Group 1 It is comprised of the following *Mudras* and *Kriyas*:

Mahamudra (the Great *Kriya*); *Navi Kriya* (the Grand Center, the seat of the seeker – *Kriyanwit* or *Kriyanwita*); *Khecharimudra* or *Talabya Kriya*, the Aerial Mode or Inner-Outer-Space *Kriya*; First *Kriya* or *Pranayam* – *Sarab* (with sound), *Nirab* (without sound), *Manasik* (mental); and simple form of *Yonimudra* (Inner-beatific-Revelation-*Kriya* – this *mudra* must not be confused with *Jyotimudra* of modified *Kriya*).

Lahiri Mahasay once made a comment: Everything can be achieved by the First *Kriya* (What he meant by the First *Kriya* was the entire group 1 and not a particular *Kriya*). For example, Vrinda Bhakat, a postal peon (mailman) did not need more *Kriyas*. **Most people practice in this group of the original *Kriya* discipline.**

Group 2 Only after the successful *Talabya Kriya* or *Khecharimudra* was the second *Kriya* or *Thokar/Thokkar Kriya* introduced in addition to group 1. It is a "**Precondition**" in the Original *Kriya* system. This is called *sthir bayur Kriya* ("*Kriya* of the tranquil Breath"), in addition to group 1. **A few people are practitioners in this group.**

Group 3 At this higher stage, *Brahma Yonimudra* is introduced, and the greater dimension of *Thokar Kriya* also is advised, in addition to groups 1 and 2. **Very few practitioners are in this group.**

Group 4 This is also a higher stage, when all *Kriyas* are integrated, all four sides of the body are integrated, and all four *Vedas* are revealed and integrated into Oneness, eternal Tranquility or *Sthirattva* (Peace or *Brahma Nirvan*). This is a state of *Chira Mouna* (Eternal Silence···), in addition to groups 1, 2, and 3. **Extremely rare practitioners are in this group.**

Chapter 6

The Modified *Kriya*

A Note of Caution

Since Mahamuni Babaji, the Divine Himalayan Yogi, commissioned this body in the Himalayas to re-establish the ancient *Kriya* yoga discipline and sent him to the United States, it becomes imperative to highlight a few fundamental features of the ancient *Kriya* discipline; otherwise, this body could remain silent in the spirit of *Atmanyebaatmanatusta* (*Gita* 2:55), "Satisfied in the self by the self within."

"Srinnantu biswe amritasya putra." - Upanisad.

"Listen to this, *Oh*, the sons of nectar of the world!"

1. The ancient original *Kriya* is a pure and scientifically proven established discipline from the very ancient days. It has no room at all whatsoever to improve or modify as this is *Apta Vakya*, the Authority, the self-axiom. If someone says or does otherwise, one must know that is for accommodating their own limitations, weaknesses, egotistic, individualistic, petty commercial and vested interests. This is the simple truth.

They even dragged Lahiri Mahasay's name into their petty interests.

"Lahiri Mahasaya was the first to openly teach Kriya in modern times --- but he forbade his disciples to start an organization to spread the teachings of Kriya Yoga, because he knew that God and the Great Ones had assigned that task to Paramhansa Yogananda --- not only to spread the teachings of Kriya

Yoga throughout the world, but to keep those teachings pure." *Self-Realization Magazine*, Spring 1985, Page 24

This is written as if Lahiri Mahasay told this personally to the writer of the article (an American disciple of Yogananda) who was not even born before Lahiri Mahasay left body.

They also ridiculously commented "to keep those teachings pure," to protect their commercial interests; while liberal Yogananda modified at random not only the *Kriyas* but the whole process with mass initiation and the public teaching with the written lessons.

Violating the traditional principles *of Guru-param-para* and *Guru-vraktagamya* in the name of modern democracy (with commercial motivation) is just the state of a perverted mind. Therefore, the violators are not practicing pure *Kriya*. They are practicing something that is an unproven system.

Some of them put their personal thoughts and beliefs ridiculously to write: "I believe Lahiri Mahasaya also granted Higher Initiation to those who could not achieve *Kechari* [*Khechari*] *Mudra*. My belief is based on his attitude and his partaking in human suffering. I cannot conceive that the achievement of *Kechari* [*Khechari*} was intended to create a sharp division among people."

The individual (we do not want to mention his name) who we quoted above can neither spell *Khechari* nor pronounce it properly and brings the idea of modern democracy to comment ridiculously on the spiritual discipline.

It is true Lahiri Mahasay suffered for the fellow human beings, but that was his "big weakness" and for that his *Guru*, Mahamuni Babaji, the Divine Himalayan Yogi, helped him to overcome it by restricting him from initiating people at random so that he would not add bad *karmas* in his incarnation.

A few of Lahiri Mahasay's Personal Letters:

Some excerpts from the personal letters of Lahiri Mahasay to his *Kriya* disciples in Bengali with English translation are shown below. These letters will throw light about how to practice *Kriya* or else practice will be a farce.

1. *Anugrahapurbak bidhipurbak upadesmata karjya kariben nachet bidambana matra.*

"Kindly practice *Kriya* strictly according to the instruction, otherwise, all will be a farce."

Lahiri Mahasay was so serious about practicing strictly according to the instruction that he mentioned the following in one of his letters:

2. 5 [*panch*] *ghanta pranayam na kariya jahate bidhipurbak* 2 [*du*] *tio karite paren tahar chesta kariben, Sakaler eirup bidhipurbak kara uchit.*

"Without practicing five hours, if you can practice only two *Pranayam* strictly according to the instructions even that is GOOD. All should practice according to the instructions [personally given to them by the *Guru*, as he diagnosed the nature of the limitations of their present state].

3. *Upajukta byakti chhara kahakeo kriya dite pari na.*

"I cannot give *Kriya* until I find the right person."

[The Vedic scriptures mentioned about the qualification of a seeker's ripeness; it is called *Adhikari* (deserving person). It is absolutely necessary to consider who is *adhikari* and whose time is not ripe (*anadhikari*), and accordingly *adhikari* should be initiated and *anadhikari* (non-deserving) should not be initiated. If liberally *anadhikari* (non-deserving) is initiated, soon the person will develop confusion. It is injustice to initiate the person].

4. *Madhye madhye upadestar sahit sakshat na haile saba golmal haiya jai.*

"Frequently, if one (*Kriyanwit*) does not meet the advisor (Guru or the Master), then everything becomes confused."

(*Kriyanwit*/*Kriyanwita* respectively, male and female *Kriya* practitioner).

5. *Roger janya aneke Kriya len; pare aram hale ba na hale keha kayek din pare sab chhere den.*

"Some people used to take *Kriya* just for curing some diseases. After some days, whether diseases were cured or not, they stopped *Kriya* practice."

6. *Kriyate jader astha nei tader Kriya diber ichha nai.*

"I do not feel inclined to give *Kriya* to those who have no faith in it."

7. *Apnar ichha haile apni upades dite paren, jadi bhalo lok hay, prabanchak na hay.*

"If you so desire, you can give advice (*Kriya*) to others, if the person is good (honest), and not a liar or deceitful.

8. *Ami ar kata kariba? Amar, loker janya asukh haiyachhe.*

"How much can I do? I am ill for people."

Lahiri Mahasay on Detachment:

Total realization means total "**detachment**" in letter and spirit; no ifs, ands, or buts; for example, Lahiri Mahasay's sixteen year old married daughter when visiting her parents became sick and was dying, upstairs, while Lahiri Mahasay was listening to the *Bhagavad Gita* read by his chief disciple, Panchanan Bhattacharya and surrounded by other disciples downstairs.

Lahiri Mahasay's wife, Kashimoni Devi, came downstairs which was a rare event, and at her request, he gave her an herb and asked her to apply it; but while she was going back upstairs, a thought generated, if she applied the herb her in-laws might blame her (in case it was fatal) as to which kind of medicine she gave to her. So she did not apply the herb and the daughter died.

At a certain point Bhattacharya Mahasay stopped reading the *Gita*. Lahiri Mahasay said, "They are doing their works, you do yours." Panchanan Bhattachaya obeyed and resumed reading the *Gita*.

Then the crying became louder from upstairs; Bhattacharya Mahasay said, "I do not feel like reading."

Lahiri Mahasay said, "Then stop."

Such was the degree of **detachment** in Lahiri Mahasay.

Lahiri Mahasay expressed his realization in Bengali:

9. *Ami kichhu noi, amaro kichhu nai.*

It means, "I am nothing and I have nothing."

It indicates that his ego or the individuality is dead forever. Usually that happens when the person merges into Oneness pure Consciousness in the state of *Sthirattva*, the state of eternal Silence; his activities are in the line of *bichityra dasa* (mysterious state) of *bikarma* (*bigata* - dissolved actions - beyond the purview of Law of *Karma*, does not accrue any results to affect him. Only the realized person can function in the line of *bikarma* which is beyond *karma* and *akarma*.

In another letter Lahiri Mahasay wrote:

10. *Dekha karar janya eta byasta kena*? *Had mas* (*amar*) *dekhiya lav ki*? *Kutasthe lakshya rakhun, tahai amar rup, ami hadmas ba "ami" ei sabdao ami nahi, ami sakaler das.*

"Why are you so anxious to meet me? Seeing my physical body (which is made of bones and flesh) - what benefit can you have?

"Focus on *Kutastha*, that is my form, I am not bones and flesh, nor even the word "I". I am the servant of all."

Some people dragged him from such pure state of Consciousness to make him a human being which he dissolved a long time before.

Please be aware of these people in your search for *Kriya.* They are the polluters to the ancient and pure *Kriya*. Unfortunately, they are innumerable.

The *Kriya Yoga* discipline is psycho-physical: to qualify or to practice this discipline requires special anatomical constitution of the body. Certain *mudras* (*Kriyas*) like *Mahamudra* and *Khecharimudra* need a special type of body that one can get as per his providence.

Khecharimudra (not *kecharimudra* as some Westerners misspelled the word for lack of Sanskrit knowledge) in Sanskrit, *Khe* (not *Ke*) means 'sky', and *charan* means 'moving', or 'walking', moving or walking in the sky, that is why it is called *Khechari*; or *Gagan bihari*, *Gagan* means 'sky' and *bihari* means 'one who moves.' *Khechari* is a feminine word; its masculine counterpart is *Khechar* which also means "a bird" that flies in the sky.

In the light of Yoga, like *Khechari*, movement in the sky, there are other movements as follows:

Bhuchari, movement on the land (at the coccygeal center), all living creatures walking on the land, including the human beings are *Bhuchar* beings,

Chanchari, curled movement (at the sacral center),

Agochari, Invisible movement (at the dorsal center), and

Unmoni, absent-minded movement (at the cervical center).

This **ABSOLUTELY ESSENTIAL** *Khechari* is **PRE-CONDITION** to the higher *Kriyas*, and also it is not very easy to master.

Actually the *Talabya Kriya* or the *Khecharimudra* is "the aerial mode of meditation or practicing *Kriya*." The mode of conducting is as follows:

Kapala Kuhare jiohva, pravesita vipartaga,
Bhruvorantargata dristir, mudrabhavati Khechari.

"Putting the tongue in reverse order into the skull, and the sight, *dristi*, internally is focused between the eyebrows, is called the *Khecharimudra*."

Khechari is described from the point view of functionality:

Mana sthirang jatra bina abalambanam.
Bayu sthiro jatra bina aborodhanam.
Dristi sthira jatra bina abalokanam.
Sa eba mudra kathita tu Khechari.

"Where the mind is tranquil without adherence with any object;
"Breath or air is tranquil without obstruction;
"Sight or the eyes are tranquil without seeing;
"It is said to be the *Khecharimudra*."

In the perspective of pure practice of *Kriya*, Yogananda's teaching the higher *Kriya* without *Khechari* (*Talabya Kriya*) is not proper and the practice cannot be fruitful.

Since in the practice of higher *Kriyas*, like the *Omkar Kriyas*, the life of the practice, that is the "**Tranquil Breath**" is lacking,

These higher *Kriyas* are called ***Sthira bayur Kriya*** which means "***Kriyas* of the Tranquil Breath**", and so if one has not achieved the tranquil state of breath, to introduce these *Kriyas* under this circumstance, are meaningless. Moreover, they will not be fruitful.

Yogananda's big Deal with his Inner Circle Devotees:

Yogananada knew that his teaching of higher *Kriya* without *Khechari* would not bring results, and so he cut a deal with his inner circle devotees that they might not attain self-realization in this incarnation. They had to set aside their salvation in the present life.

A portion of the handwritten ten page letter of a former *Brahmachari,* of his organization, to Swam Satyeswarananda Maharaj is produced here.

> A high official of the Order once told me that probably none of us (in SRF) would achieve Self realization in this life — that we are pioneers, meant to sacrifice our salvation or set it aside in this life, in order to devote ourselves to bringing the Master's Teachings — missionary-like — to the world

The reflection of the big deal of the inner circle of Yogananda which was also found in Kriyananda's enclosures with the letter to Swamiji were printed (October 15, 1981) for mass distribution as an explanatory measure for understanding of Kriyananda's recent marriage with Rosanna Golia, a young Italian lady. Kriyananda called her Parameswari.

"My [Kriyananda] whole life has been offered to Master [Yogananda] for his work. Long ago I decided [Kriyananda did not decide, it was a deal from Yogananda himself for his inner circle devotees] it didn't even matter if my 'salvation was deferred', so long as I might serve him."

Physical fitness is essential in the primary stage. However, after the 5th step, *pratyahara* (interiorization), of eightfold Yoga, when a *Kriyanwit* seeker is successful, the three rest of the steps - *dharana*, *dhyana*, and *samadhi*, can be practiced on the mental plane: in this context, the mental plane means on the basis of the tranquil Breath. Since in *Kriya* Science, the mind is defined as restless breath; so tranquil Breath is tranquil mind. At this state the awareness becomes subtle and the physical body becomes immaterial, and so for some, it automatically levitates, (although the person is not aware of it).

Let us pose these questions: How does a dead person become *Guru*? How does the disembodied person get lips or mouth to give advice? The answers are obvious - they can't.

This ancient tradition is just, scientific, and reasonable. Violating the traditional principles *of Guru-param-para* and *Guruvraktagamya* in the name of modern democracy of human rights is just the state of a perverted mind.

Therefore, the violators are not practicing pure *Kriya*. They are practicing some unproven system.

The Life Style of a Swami

When the present author discussed with Swami Satyananda about entering into the order of Swami, he mentioned to the author that he must focus on the Sankaracharaya' *Mohamudgar* for a while day and night.

"Koupin banta khalu bhagya banta." Sankaracharya

One who is satisfied with only wearing a strip of cloth (*koupin*), he is a happy person.

Mohamudgar by *Adi* [First] Sankaracharya

"The club that strikes down attachment"

In the eighth century, the first Sankaracharya wrote *Mohamudgar* ("The club that strikes down attachment") for the renunciate Swamis. In it there is a stanza :

Arthamanrtham bhabaya nityam
Nasti tata sukhalesa satyam.
putradapi dhanabhajang bhiti
Sarbatroisa kathita niti.

The English translation by the present author of the above stanza is as follows:

Think always that money is the root of all troubles.
Certainly wealth can't deliver true happiness.
Even a wealthy man is afraid of his son.
This is the rule known to the world.

For a *sanyasi* (Swami), a renunciate, it is always good to live with alms and wear a piece of small cloth (*koupin*). That makes a person happy. A swami must always think that wealth is the root of all troubles. Wealth never gives happiness.

Being a Swami, Yogananda had forgotten the warning for a Swami by Sankaracharya that wealth is the root of all troubles for a Swami or renunciate.

Mahamuni Babaji's Injunction "Not to start Organization"

The great *Guru*, the Mahamuni Babaji had injunction on the *Kriya* - "Not to develop organization around the *Kriya* teaching".

His principal *Kriya* disciple, Lahiri Mahasay, the polestar of *Kriya*, upheld the injunction. Yogananda was fully aware of this injunction. He wrote it in his *Autobiography of a Yogi*:

"The great Master [Lahiri Mahasay] lived his sublime life in partial seclusion, and steadfastly refused to permit his followers to build any organization around the teachings." *Autobiography of a Yogi,* by Paramhansa Yogananda, 1979 Paperback edition, page 339.

Having known this injunction very well, Yogananda willfully violated the injunction and founded two organizations: Self Realization Fellowship Church (SRF in 1935) and Yogoda Sat Sanga Society of India (YSS in 1936).

One has to imagine in which degree one has to be confused to perform that kind of act of violation of injunction of the supreme *Guru*. Yogananda had to pay the price for such violation. He admitted this in his own handwriting.

Handwritten letter of Yogananda

Write to ...

SELF-REALIZATION FELLOWSHIP

MOUNT WASHINGTON ESTATES, LOS ANGELES, CAL.

Encinitas Calif
March 23rd 1937

[illegible]

[illegible] Mrs Sokolov [illegible] cash or check [illegible]

[illegible] Centre [illegible]

[illegible] gossip [illegible] Centre [illegible]

[illegible] public meetings [illegible]. Don't discuss anything publicly. Find out & feel if the Centre is worth having or not. [illegible] advertisement [illegible] meetings [illegible]

How many promised after Khagen advertized you. Did anybody come? Let me know at once. On your decision I will tell you to close or keep it open. Anyway write to me by air about your opinion — then I will promptly let you know about my decision. Don't tell anybody [illegible] till you hear my final decision.

[illegible] Yogananda

We will consider only the first two sentences from this document.

The very first sentence of the handwritten Bengali line in the document said, "*Kharacher jwalay pagal hoye gechhi*. 'It means for the expenditure, I have become mad.' "

Apat kale biporit buddhi
"In crisis, one's intelligence works in the reverse order"

There is a famous proverb it says, "*Apat kale biporit buddhi*, it means "at the time of crisis, one's intelligence works in the reverse order". As a result, the person cannot help himself, rather goes further in deeper trouble. That is exactly what happened to Yogananda. During the financial crisis his intelligence worked in reverse order. **He developed business plans.** He started teaching philosophy of material prosperity which is just the "opposite (reverse)" of the fundamental spirit of Pure original *Kriya*.

Lahiri Mahasay himself expressed it in one word in Bengali, *Phalakankharahit*, which means "Abandoning the expectation of the results of the *Kriya* practice".

In the crisis period, when the person intelligence works in the reverse order, person cannot think "right at that moment or period" what could help him in his situation. Instead, he would do what would bring him into deeper trouble.

The example, in this crisis period, instead of teaching the true spirit of *Kriya*, Yogananda's intelligence started teaching the reverse spirit of *Kriya* that is "the philosophy of material prosperity" to overcome the financial crisis which brought him to deeper trouble in the teaching of *Kriya*. Here it is in his own handwriting:

This place is losing $52 per day — from lack of organization — and since you think God will help us inspite of ~~at~~ our unreasonableness - let it be so Henceforth I will not exert ~~to~~ my will to work the laws of prosperity - and you will have to accept conditions as they come.

Yogananda's hand written letter says - " – This place is losing $52 per day – thru lack of organization - and since you think God will help us in spite of our unreasonableness – let it be so. Henceforth I will not exert my will to work **the laws of prosperity** – and you will have to accept conditions as they come."

To run everything smoothly for the teaching of philosophy of prosperity, he opened a "Prosperity Bank" for the program. Here it is in his own handwriting:

Will Please write to head quarters for prosperity banks like these enclosed -

The handwritten letter reads – "Please write to headquarters for **prosperity banks like these enclosed**."

By **teaching the philosophy of prosperity** Yogananda accumulated wealth as follows:

The proof of material success of the organization is the list of properties which the organization acquired and filed in 1971-72 at the Franchise Tax Board, Sacramento, California.

Thereafter, there were many more which have accumulated by now.

Property with addresses filed in 1971-72 by S. R. F. are as follows:

2 Bedroom House	4229 Camino Real, Los Angeles, CA 90065
5 Bedroom House	3980 San Rafael, Los Angeles, CA 90065
1 Story Steel Industrial Bldg.	2816-24 Newell St., Los Angeles, CA
Parking Lot	4874 Sunset Blvd., Hollywood, CA
6 Unit Apartments Bldg.	1433-35 No. Catalina, Hollywood, CA
8 Unit Apartments Bldg.	1427-29 No, Catalina St., Hollywood, CA
8 Unit Apartments Bldg.	1415-1417 1/2 No. Catalina, Hollywood, CA
8 Unit Apartments Bldg.	1414 No. Edgemont, Hollywood, CA
3 5 Room Apartments and	
1 3 Room Cottage	3040 - 72 First Ave, San Diego, CA 92103
3 Bedroom House	1800 W. Monroe St. Phoenix, AZ
1 Story Abode Cottage	72223 Juanita Rd., 29 Palms, CA
1 Story House on 7 acres of Land	10757 Fabian Lane, Beaumont, CA

Land	Andrew Ave at Sheridan, Leucadia, CA
House	17300 Sunset Blvd., Pacific Palisades, CA 90272
House	1153 Second St., Encinitas, CA 92024
House	4956 Genevieve Ave., Los Angeles, CA
House	Avenue 56, Los Angeles, CA
4 1/2 Story Apartment Bldg. (3 Stories are Apartments)	424-430 E Ocean Blvd., Long Beach, CA
9 Unit Apartment Bldg.,	416 So. Monroe St., San Diego, CA
2 Bedroom Residence, Apartments, Parking Shed, and 25 Acres Land	387050 Orchard St., Beaumont, CA
40 Acres Land	Valpariso, Ind.
Apartment Bldg.,	Long Beach, CA

Again, there is a proverb: If winter comes can spring be far behind?

When Yogananda accumulated such a great deal of wealth can lawsuits be far behind?

Yogananda himself and his organizations were involved in the lawsuits. The lawsuits will be listed later.

Now the second sentence in the document, *Okhane centre* (center) *kore ki gukhuri*.

It means. "Making center there have I done *Gukhuri*?"

The sentence should be with a question mark but he put a period (full stop). He always made this type mistake in Bengali in his own mother language because he studied in his childhood up to the seventh grade (Class VII) in Hindi medium school at Gorakhapur where he was born and then brought to Calcutta and studied there from grade 8 (Class VIII). That is why his grammar in Bengali as well as in English was very weak.

(With this comment, naturally the question may rise in the mind of the readers: How about the beautiful writing of his autobiography? The answer is simple, it was practically written by his dear disciple, a college graduate of Berkley University, L. V. Pratt (Tara Mata); Yogananda acknowledged her contribution as a copy editor but actually she was the shadow writer for him after Swami Dhirananda (Dr. Basu Kumar Bagchi, Ph.D.) his classmate and colleague and the former shadow writer left Yogananda in 1935. It was Dhirananda, Yogananda's first shadow writer who wrote his first book, *The Science of Religion*).

Yogananda's admission weak Knowledge of English

It is hard to believe that Yogananda with his poor grammar in English and weakness in Bengali, Sanskrit and English wrote such a beautiful book. Yogananda admitted his weaknesses about the English and Bengali in his book.

"The best mark I [Yogananda] could possibly score in that paper [English] would be 33-three points [33 out of 100] less than the passing mark of 36 [36 out of 100]." *Autobiography of a Yogi*, page 225, Eighth edition, published in1959.

[The university authority lowered the passing mark to 33 from 36; otherwise, Yogananda would fail in English, and have to sit for the examination again next year in all subjects as per the Calcutta University Rules].

The word *Gukhuri* is rarely used; as it is uncultured-slang which means "eating feces" according to *Sangsad Bangla Abhidhan* 14th Edition, 2000, on the page 200, a Bengali dictionary by Dr. Sasi Bhusan Dasgupta, Head of the Department of Bengali in Calcutta University, Ramtanu Lahiri Professor. Yogananda had used the word twice in his handwritten letters.

Observing Yogananda and his organizations, a dozen of others follow the same route.

There is a proverb in Bengali, *Ganga jale Gnaga puja,* which means "Worship the Ganges with the water of Ganges." Nothing is required from outside for worshiping the Ganges. The present author did the same, depicted him with the paper trail he left behind and used his handwritings. Nothing is required from outside.

What a mess! What a confusion! and what a plight! Once he set his feet on the slippery slope, it came down to this low level and got stocked in the mud.

This is the price he had to pay starting the organizations in violation of the **injunction** by Mahamuni Babaji and Lahiri Mahasay.

Yogananda was so obsessed or confused with organizations that he had developed a perception as if founding organizations instead of *Kriya* would bring him permanent peace. This understanding is an utter confusion because of attachment to the idea of being great.

The following handwritten letter would prove that sentiment.

October 22, 1937

Dear Mrs. Nerode,

... I will give up my Iness to create an organization. As I realize that's the way I will find reasonableness and the way to imperishable peace.

My deep blessings to you, Sri Nerode and Anil.

Ever yours
Very sincerely,
Swami Yogananda

If we impartially look at his handwritten letter (produced here) the following information can be observed:

1. Yogananda wanted to create another organization in October 22, 1937.

2. He admitted in the letter that his "Iness (individuality or ego)" was still in him on October 22, 1937. His admission is very **important** and

historical in Yogananda's life, as well as in the *Kriya* world since he claimed that his *Guru*, Sriyukteswar, "awarded" him the *Paramhansa* title in 1936.

We will produce an eye witness description of the event. As a matter of fact the eye witness was his own private secretary and Sriyukteswar's disciple.

3. Yogananda considered that all of his previous organizations (two registered and three unregistered) were not reasonable. He did not define his sense of the word "reasonable," or what he meant by reasonableness. Only he knew what he meant by the word reasonable.

4. He admitted that by this way he would find "reasonableness" and his "imperishable peace."

It is amazing that his understanding is to achieve imperishable [permanent] peace through an organization which he characterized as reasonable.

On the other hand, Mahamuni Babaji and Lahiri Mahasay had already made abundantly clear to the *Kriyanwits/Kriyanwitas* not to start any organizations (which is a means of hindrance to *Kriya* practice as well as to achieving eternal realization of the absolute Self).

In that perspective, it can be called a great misunderstanding on the part of Yogananda. The word "reasonable" comes from the word "reason" and the verb "reasoning" is from the intellect (*budhhi*) which is an "inner sense".

So it can safely and fairly be concluded that his understanding about achieving "imperishable peace" or permanent peace through an inner sense (reason) is a **confusion**. The imperishable, as he puts it, is permanent peace which is a "transcendental state;" the transcendent of the knowing mind, or an *a priori* realm while the reasonable is an *a posteriori* or imperial or sensual realm.

A question can be asked, how will a sensual mind from the imperial side attain the transcendental state of beyond the mind?

Furthermore, giving up ego or individuality not by spoken words, but in and through serious meditation and *Kriya* practice, provide one to be in the desirelessness state [*nirvasana*]; at that time there is no individuality or ego any more – who then will create an organization?

The *Ajna* Center at the Medulla:

According to the teaching of pure *Kriya* tradition, the *Ajna* Center at the medulla, reflection of which is in between the eyebrows, is the center of *Kutastha*, the Inner Self. This is the place where the pure *Kriya* practitioners offer their desires or abandon the expectations of the results of practice **to attain the state of "Desirelessness [*Nirvasana*]".**

The Will Center (The Center of Desire):

On the contrary, Yogananda taught the *Ajna* center at the medulla as being **just the opposite (reverse), as the "Will Center" or the center for Desire:**

"The Will Center becomes the positive pole and the coccygeal plexus becomes the negative pole." *Art of Super-Realization Initiation* by Swami Yogananda, page 7, published by Yogoda Sat Sanga Society [of America, not registered].

This characterization of the *Ajna* Center as the "Will Center" suits very well with his teaching the philosophy of prosperity to his American followers.

It seems that Yogananda's thoughts and understanding were confusing and self-contradictory.

This is a general tendency of the people who get involved in organizations to twist things and make their own history (as suited to their vested interests and the survival for their livelihood).

From an Eyewitness - the Event of his *Paramhansa* Title

"On another day, Ananda-da - Ananda Mohan Lahiri [Only bachelor grandson of Lahiri Mahasay out of eight grandsons] - was with us. It was almost nightfall. Maharaj ji [Sriyukteswar at his Serampore House] was standing on the upstairs veranda and someone was standing next to him. Ananda-da and the writer [Sailendra Bejoy Dasgupta, disciple of Sriyukteswar and private secretary of Yogananda] were downstairs. Before going upstairs, Yoganandaji went to a drainage spot, a bit apart from the area, and began to urinate into the drainage passage. This caught Gurudev's attention and he cryptically joked, "Yogananda has become a 'paramhansa' [great swan, or great soul]!" After urinating, Yoganandaji saw Ananada-da standing at the front door and quietly said, "Ananda-da! Did you hear? Swamiji [Sriyukteshvarji] called me a 'paramhansa'". Later, Ananda-da laughed and said to the writer, "You'll see, Yogananda will one day use this title!" *Paramhansa Swami Yogananda - Life portrait and Reminiscences* by Sailendra Bejoy Dasgupta, disciple of Sriyukteswar, Private secretary of Yogananda, the eyewitness of the event, Chapter 5, page 95.

This paragraph needs an explanation. A Westerner may think that observing Yogananda urinating standing up like a swan which men usually do not do in India, Sriyukteswar jokingly commented that Yogananda has become *Paramhansa* (a great swan). However, the reason was different.

It was a gross violation of Vedic culture. In Vedic culture, there are rules (*bidhi*) and don'ts (*nisedh*) based on the scientific principles. Generally, people eat thrice - breakfast, lunch, and dinner in fixed and specific times. Before taking their meals, with an empty stomach, they are supposed to practice at least twelve *Pranayams* with *Gayatri mantra*. After eating, when they have food in their stomach, they are not supposed to practice *Pranayam* for at least three hours, since breathing is the vehicle of *Pranayam*. All people wash their hands and feet before taking their meals. In India, people being poor, some walk bare foot; as a result, they might have dirty feet. Since they eat sitting with folded legs on a piece of mat or a seat made of wood or of the other materials on the floor the feet are close to the plate. Also they eat without a fork and spoon, only by the right hand (and not by the left hand as it is used, cleaning toilet; hence, considered dirty. Thus offering something to a senior with the left hand by a junior is considered disrespectful). The Lord has given the five fingers to act as a fork. Since eating is an act of worship, the rules are to be clean in body and mind.

In fact, spiritually speaking, in the Vedic society, people do not eat; they simply offer food to the five *devatas* (gods) represented by the five states of *Prana* (*Prana*, *Apana*, *Samana*, *Byana*, and *Udana*). There is a ritual to offer; first put food in five places near the plate; then taking water in the right palm to offer, chanting *mantras,* pouring water around the plate (*gandus*). They are not supposed to talk while eating; or to take a second serving as it has not been offered and it cannot be offered during eating; also one is not allowed to drink water or any liquid substance since that will hamper the already started digestive process, separating the saliva from the food; or to get up or move, as it will hamper the process of digestion also. Since this worshiping is at a fixed time, the organs usually are waiting for this moment to work; if they are disturbed, food will not be properly digested. According to the Vedic culture all these considerations are involved in eating. Practice of *Kriya Pranayam* or Yoga is the backbone of the Vedic culture

Thus, standing up urinating is not simply strange, it is against the Vedic culture and unscientific too. There is another subtle point involved in it. Urinating standing up into the drain water is a matter of disrespecting the water god (Varundev). Taking off clothes the women are not supposed to take bath in water according to the Vedic culture since the water god is present in the water. Once, this statement was uttered by Lord Krisna himself to the gopis when they were in the water of Yamuna River just to free them from timidity or shyness. Observing rules (*bidhi*) and *nisedh* (don'ts) are very important.

Thus the gross violation by Yogananda was joked about by his *Guru* calling him *Paramhansa* (in this case meaning "worthless one" what is, he is not).

His Past Incarnations Described by Yogananda Himself

"The many supernatural experiences that occurred in his life firmly convinced him that he was a maker of history in his previous incarnations, as well as having been persons of formidable power. He came to know these things in transcendental states. He had said that he was in fact the historical British figure 'William the Conqueror.'

"[This paragraph needs an explanation: If Yogananda came to know these things in the transcendental state when the mind merges into oneness with the pure Consciousness of the supreme Self, and the individual self is to be lost, then how did he come to know these things in that state where his individual self already is dissolved? Or was he imagining that he was in the transcendental state, since his individual self was to still exist to remember and to tell his private secretary these things? In that case, it is fair from the common sense point of view as well as from the simple logical and rational standpoint to say that he could not be in the transcendental state. It has to be the product of imagination. He was imaginative. It also gave clear indication of having the seed of a *Dharana* Yogi (will be discussed later). His private secretary, Dasgupta, himself admitted as follows]:

"When examined with an investigative eye, many of the accounts [narrated stories of the *Autobiography of a Yogi*] could have been caused by ordinary means." *Paramhansa Swami Yogananda Life-portrait and Reminiscences* by S. B. Dasgupta, Private Secretary of Yogananda, p. 115

In this connection, something else could be mentioned here. Yogananda was always in the habit of exhibiting powers since he considered himself to have formidable power.

Once, Yogananda said to Satyananda, "Why don't you exhibit some miracles and powers, when people will be attracted, then you serve them."

In reply, Satyananda said, "Anything is possible by the Lord. Who am I to do this? Please don't request me to do such things."

The text book reference of a realized person is for him to not exhibit miracle and power, rather to remain natural in peaceful state.

Lahiri Mahasay himself mentioned dozens of times: "I am nothing and I have nothing." This is the actual description of a realized person.

S. B. Dasgupta continued, "The well-known historical account of William the Conqueror landing on the shores of England and prostrating and kissing the ground – Yoganandaji experienced this within him in a spiritually absorbed state.

"In 1935, when he [Yogananda] and Richard Wright were at that palace at Westminster, Yoganandaji said to Wright, 'You walk behind me. Immediately after I enter the palace, I will tell you which room is where before we ever get there; you'll see, everything will match up.' Wright said later that Swamiji was right every time about the location of the different rooms. Swamiji himself was there at the telling of this event, and Wright was bearing witness to Swamiji's description of the incident. There was no sense of any kind of 'but' [hesitation] in Swamiji's behavior at all!

"[A yogi who has a bit of yogic power easily predicts these kinds of things; although a real Yogi would not use yogic power and be involved in such an insignificant event.]

"Apparently, in yet another life, he [Yogananda] was a vicious and murderous desert marauder. While describing this, Swamiji shivered with horror from time to time, although he maintained a slight smile on the outside.

"Swami Satyanandaji had said that before Yoganandaji went to America and was living at the Ranchi Brahmacharya Vidyalay, one night, he screamed out from his room. He said that a cot penetrated through his closed door and a horrific being was seated upon that cot. From that time on, a student would sleep in a separate cot in his room. Yoganandaji said that if he slept alone, he saw many different beings, and some of the times woke up in fear." *Paramhansa Swami Yogananda – Life-portrait and Reminiscences (paramhansa swami Yogananda - Jivanalekhya o smriticharan- the original in Bengali)* by Sailendra Bejoy Dasgupta, private secretary of Yogananda in 1935-36], page 128- 129, Chapter 7 Epilogue.

In the United States, not explaining to anyone his personal problem of not being able to sleep alone, Swami Yogananda allowed many pretty young Mormon girls to go in and out of his bedroom at night the rest of his life as a defense against those horrific beings who were haunting him, knowing well that there would be someone in his room the whole night while he would sleep at ease.

There were many eyewitnesses in the center about this fact. For example: in this context, it must be mentioned that in the environment of a legal discussion [in a lawsuit, Case No. 445, 883, in the Superior Court of California, in and for the County of Los Angeles, filed October 23, 1939], in which it was alleged by Yogananda's colleague, Nirodh Ranjan Choudhuri, that many beautiful young ladies were coming in and out the whole night, every night, from Yogananda's suite in the center. (Nirod Babu was six years older than Yogananda and he came to the United States from Chittagong, currently Bangladesh, in 1919, that is, one year earlier than Yogananda. He was a Harvard graduate, who joined him later and was in charge of managing his main center Mt. Washington at Los Angeles.

From the viewpoint of the Vedic Culture, it looks odd and unbecoming of a Swami, and the allegations were quite unbefitting with the Vedic Culture in the eyes of average Hindus.

However, personally, the present author thought that there had to be some other valid reasons for these events. Now we know from the statement of Swami Satyananda concerning the eventful night at Ranchi asram set out in S.B. Dasgupta's book quoted above.

From these stories several things can be observed which are very important and somewhat troubling as well. Here are some consequences.

1) Common sense tells us that perhaps those souls whom Yogananda murdered in previous lives were out to get him in his subsequent life and that is why disembodied souls appeared to him as horrible beings and perhaps they would continue to haunt him in revenge. What a predicament and nightmare!

2) In this connection, it should be remembered that a realized person does not dream or see such things. It puts a question mark on Yogananda's achievement of realization.

3) A realized person is always fearless day and night, even during his sleep; he is always in tune with the state of *sahaja samadhi*, spontaneous state of the supreme Self where there is no fear at all and no such ghosts could appear. Again, it raises a question about Yogananda.

In the *Bhagavad Gita* Chapter Sixteen - *Daibasur Sampad Bibhag Yoga* (The qualities of the gods and the anti-gods are described.)

Abhayang *sattwasuddhijnanyogabyabasthiti. Bhagavad Gita* 16:1

The very first word is *Abhayang* which means "absolute fearlessness". The realized yogi is fearless. They do not have anything to fear since they are in oneness with the pure Consciousness of the Self.

In this case, since Yogananda is not free of fear, which means "in the text book sense" Yogananda's position of Self Realization can be in question.

So in his previous incarnation, admittedly, Yogananda was "William the Conqueror", and in addition he was a murderous desert marauder; as a result, he had killed many people as a ruler and as a murderer; the souls of those people were haunting him to take revenge in the subsequent incarnations and would continue in their efforts to get him. Those are the consequences and rules of life.

The Law of Providence

Thus what was supposed to happen had happened; Yogananda could not stop it. That usually happens in everybody's life because most activities of life happen to be dominated by the person's previous life's residual providence, "the resultant force" of activities of previous life.

As per the rules of Providence, it is created out of the person's performed activities in one's previous lives which did not have the chance to give results because in the meantime, the person's body died. So the actions (*Karmas*) performed in life not having a chance to give results, accompanied with the spirit or the individual self of the performer in the last breath remained with the self. This is how the providences are formulated. If we take into account several lives, then the providences are stored like a Himalayan Mountain to an individual self, or to a *jiva.*

At the time of reincarnation, a portion of it is packaged for the forthcoming current life to give results. They stay in the reservoir at the base of the spine in the *Kundalini* Power and look for opportunity (time-wise) to give results. They send out the propensities to act by the person so the providence can find favorable circumstances. When a particular providence gets a favorable situation it becomes a very dominant force to give result pushing and dashing the other factors around; after all, it had waited a long time, even many incarnations. Thus it became destined to happen and no power on earth could prevent it from happening.

Once it gives the result (good or bad) as per the nature of action performed in previous life, it frees the person's self. It does not last longer than its destined tenure. This is how the providence works. The Law of Providence is part of the "Law of *Karma.*"

There is something more to point out here in this regard. If a person of strong personality senses that something bad is going to happen to him and tries to resist it, he may not succeed; but if he does, then the providence goes back to its reservoir and stays there, and waits for another opportunity. So resisting the happening and being able to stop it does not free the person, instead, it grows in magnitude with accrued interest. It never goes away till it gives result, either in the current incarnation or in some subsequent incarnations. The following is a relevant story of providence.

A Story from Lahiri Mahasay's life: On Providence

Lahiri Mahasay used to take a bath in the Ganges every day at the Chousatti Yogini *Ghat* (Chousatti – 64, Yogini – female Yogi, *Ghat* - concrete steps at the bank of the Ganges) since he lived at Benares.

One day, like any other day, his disciple, Krisnaram, who lived nearby accompanied him to the Ganges. They were walking on the narrow lane of Chausatti Yogini *Ghat*; all of a sudden, Lahiri Mahasay said, "Krisna! Tear the cloth." Krisna did not understand why his Baba was asking him to tear his cloth. After they walked a few steps a brick fell from the second floor of a house on the foot of Lahiri Mahasay and it started bleeding. Krisna immediately tore his cloth and bound it. Then he asked, "Baba! Since you knew it why did you not avoid it?" Lahiri Mahasay replied, "That can't be, Krisnaram. If I did, then it could create accrued 'interest' on it."

So the bold and courageous person, who happens to sense a bad thing is going to happen, neither resists nor invites (in that case, he might show the selfish interest to be freed), rather, simply exposes himself to let it happen in its own course and thereafter it would set him free.

These descriptions of the past lives by Yogananda himself bring the inevitable question.

Is Yogananda a *Dharana* Yogi?

What is *Dharana* and who is a *Dharana* Yogi?

The Sanskrit word *Dharana* literally means "concept" or "thought". The state *dharana* falls on the sixth step of the Patanjali's eight-fold Yoga discipline. It is in between the *pratyahara* (interiorizing the senses) and *dhyana* (meditation).

One who contemplates on *dharana* is a *dharana* Yogi. Generally, who contemplates on *dharana*, gains lots of powers. *Dharana* Yogi is an extremely powerful Yogi.

Very interestingly, *Dharana* Yogi has signs of both: *mukti* (liberation) and *bandha* (bondage – ignorance).

Because the signs of both liberation and bondage are present in him, the ordinary people cannot figure out his ignorance aspect. In fact, his status is **intermediate**, in between the ordinary Yogi and a realized Yogi.

Dharana Yogi, being a very powerful yogi, can demonstrate his powers on the manifested external world. He is not a completely realized yogi; his ignorance has not been completely wiped out. As a result, he has attachment to the worldly things. He has tendencies to see the world, travels in the universe extensively, and starts organization after organization with obsession.

It must be mentioned here that before achieving his complete liberation, in the meantime, he has to incarnate several times again and again including even on the lower species depending on the circumstances (deer, swan, *sarava* – eight-legged creature, plant like *haritaki*, vine like *bitapi* and a Bidyadhar or Bidyadhari).

We find reference of *Dharana* Yogi in the *Yoga Vasistha Ramayan.* He is King Bipaschit.

Scriptural Reference: *The Ultimate Book - Yoga Vasistha: In the Light of Yoga Vedanta* by Swami Satyeswarananda Maharaj - *Yoga Vasistha* 6:125:26 *Uttarardha,* Page 1819, Volume II, the Sanskrit text is as follows:

Nityadharma prabuddhanang tayabhutatayataya.
Bipaschito ***Dharana*** *Yogino na parang gatah.*
Yoga Vasistha 6:125:26 *Uttarardha*

The verse says, "Yogi who has received lots of powers by virtue of the blessing of his desired deity [in the case of King Bipaschit, the fire god (Agnidev)]; **but is not completely realized.**

"He lacks the Self-Knowledge, *Atmajnan*; **his ignorance is not completely wiped out. As a result, he has attachment to the worldly things.**"

Dharana Yogi is not liberated.

It fits well and seems the soul of Yogananda is the soul of a *Dharana* Yogi.

The Brief Story of King Bipaschit From the Yoga Vasistha

King Bipaschit, a *Dharana* Yogi, engaged his four powerful generals in four sides to protect his kingdom from the enemies. After a long time his kingdom was attacked by a powerful enemy with a very well planned strategy. They attacked simultaneously on the four sides. After a grim battle, King Bipaschit's generals of east, west and south fell to the enemy. Then the attackers brought their armies to the north and added their force against the northern general of king Bipaschit who realized the situation and not finding any chance to prevail, he felt responsibility to inform his king about the status of the war. Accordingly, he retreated and left the battlefield. Arriving to the king he informed him that the three generals fell to the enemy and the enemy was about to prevail on him too, so he felt the responsibility to come to inform him. Actually, the enemy was chasing him; perhaps they might be near the capital. He asked the king to join the battlefield quickly. A lady from the inner apartment happened to be present. Overhearing the general's report, she also requested the king to protect them and proceed to join the battlefield as soon as possible.

King Bipaschit silently listened to the report and said he would join the battle. Slowly he got up and calmly went to take a bath. Thereafter, he worshiped his desired deity, Agnidev, the fire god. He prayed to him mentioning stories where in the past that he had worshiped him and had his blessings. This time too he would offer him everything and hoped he would have his blessings.

Having said that, he chopped off his own head with his sword and offered it into the fire. Thereafter, four golden hued Bipaschit appeared from the fire and they went to the four sides to battle with the enemy.

Fighting vigorously, the four Bipaschits defeated the enemies. The four Bipaschits continued their lives. After death they were born again; thus they underwent several incarnations after incarnations. The eastern Bipaschit became Yaksha, lion, and so on. The western Bipaschit, at the curse of a Sage, became a *Haritaki* tree and dew, and so on. Once, he became Bidyadhar by the enchanting illusion of a Bidyadhar. Thus their intermediate incarnations continued.

Finally, one Bipaschit got liberation; one became a deer and two, having worldly attachment still were in the universe. Thus is the plight of a *Dharana* Yogi.

As mentioned earlier, *Dharana* Yogis have both signs of liberation and bondage, yet they are not liberated. They have not been able to wipe out their subtle ignorance.

The British and the Indian people had a long history of relationship. Some *Dharana* Yogi from India was incarnated in England as the British king like William the Conqueror. The soul was incarnated back and forth in India and in England. Admittedly Yogananda said he was the King William the Conqueror, which sounds like a *Dharana* Yogi.

Those who were not able to attain their liberation for different reasons, some are like the powerful king Bipaschit who became a *Dharana* Yogi, some are derailed Yogis (*Bhrasta* Yogi) for their undignified and non-spiritual behavior. They have to wander in the world and travel many incarnations before they can attain their liberation. (Reference of a *bhrasta* Yogi):

Prapta punyakrittang lokanusitwa saswati samah.
Suchinang srimatang gehe ***yogabharsto*** *yabhijayate.*
The Bhagavad Gita 6:41

The verse says, "He who is derailed [from Yoga is a Yoga *bhrasta* person] from the path of Yoga and fails to achieve liberation, gets to a higher state like heaven [heaven is not the place of liberated yogis; their place is even higher than heaven], after living there for innumerable years, takes the birth in the house of a Yogi [which is very rare] and wealthy family, which is normal."

Thus Yoga *bhrasta* Yogi, King William, Conqueror, was born in the wealthy family.

Yogananda did not teach *Kriya*. Judge for yourself.

As we mentioned before, Yogananda taught his disciples in the United States prosperity instead of renunciation, forgetting the valuable teaching of Sankaracharya for the Swamis or the renunciates and violating Mahamuni **Babaji's injunction** and Lahiri Mahasay's **prohibition to start organization**.

Once again, let us remember here what is the true and fundamental spirit of the ancient original pure *Kriya*. In the original *Kriya* discipline, there are several fundamental points which represent the true spirit of *Kriya*. We are referring to only two here:

1) To practice *Kriya* strictly according to the instructions one receives from the living lips of the *Guru* (*Guruvrakta-gamya* – learning directly from the mouth of a *Guru*).

2) Abandoning all the expectations in general and the results of the practice in particular.
(As mentioned before, in Bengali, Lahiri Mahasay used just one word in Bengali, *Phalakankharahit*, "Abandoning the expectations of the results of the practice".

In violation, Yogananda taught the philosophy of prosperity; he opened a prosperity bank to get rich and establish name and fame. The example is given below. His teaching totally destroyed the very **SPIRIT** of Pure *Kriya* and altered the teaching entirely in the diametrically opposite direction (spiritually speaking) to a negative one which develops attachment to the worldly things.

This particular violation, for the material prosperity, reduces the spiritual discipline to NOTHING.

Furthermore, the scriptural reference is found from the *Bhagavad Gita* for practicing *Kriya* with attachment to have results.

Karmana sukritasyahu sattvikang nirmalang phalang.
Rajasa phalang dukhamajnanang tamasa phalam.
The Bhagavad Gita 14:16

[This verse explains that the threefold qualities inspire three different types of *Karmas*, or *Kriyas*, and bring the results according to the nature of *Karmas,* or *Kriyas*.]

"The *Sattva guna*, inspires one to act through *Sattvika* (righteousness or Tranquility) *Karma*, or *Kriyas* - for example, to abandon the expectations for results of *Kriya* practice. Those *Kriyas* which are received from the *Guru* personally are *Sattvika Kriyas*, or *Karmas*.

"The *Raja guna*, or active quality, brings the inspiration to work or practice *Kriya* **to receive results, and thus ends in sorrows;** while the *Tama guna* increases ignorance.

"[Thus, Yogananda's followers practicing *Kriya* with the philosophy of prosperity having the attachment to get results, end up in sorrows]". *The Bhagavad Gita* 14:16 Interpretation by Lahiri Mahasay.

Yogananda's followers believed in a God who would help them but not Yogananda who believed in exerting "the laws of prosperity" rather than depending on God. As we have seen in his own handwriting earlier.

By **teaching the philosophy of prosperity** Yogananda accumulated wealth and so the proverb worked: If winter comes can spring be far behind? The lawsuits followed Yogananda.

Another proverb in Bengali: *Bisay bis,* which means "the properties are poisonous". Therefore the lawsuits followed.

The List of Lawsuits

Yogananda himself and his organizations were involved in the following lawsuits. Some of the case references are as follows:

1. Swami Dhirananda vs. Swami Yogananda, Case No. 387 391, in the Superior Court of the State of California, in and for the County of Los Angeles, filed May 3, 1935.

In the above case No. 387 391, Swami Yogananda sued Swami Dhirananda back by filing a cross complaint through his attorney, Willedd Andrews. Cross-Complaint: Breach of contract, fraud and damages on May 10, 1935.

Again, in the above case No. 387 391, Yogananda filed his First Amended Cross-Complaint on May 31, 1935.

One more time, in the above case, Yogananda filed a Second Amended Cross-Complaint on June 28, 1935.

2. Nirod Ranjan Choudhuri, also known as Sri Nerode, vs. Swami Yogananda, also known as Mukunda Lal Ghosh: Swami Yogananda doing business as the Self Realization Fellowship Church: Self Realization Fellowship Church, Inc., Case No. 445, 883, in the Superior Court of California, in and for the County of Los Angeles, filed October 23, 1939.

3. C.W. Eley and Ella Eley vs. Paramhansa Yogananda, also known as Swami Yogananda, Self Realization Fellowship Church, in the Superior Court of the State of California, Case No. 504155 390, in and for the County of Los Angeles, filed July 26, 1945.

This was a case of breach of contract for buying some flowers (worth $80,000.00). SRF reneged on the order after paying for the first batch. The broker Mr. C.W. Eley and his wife, Mrs. Ella Eley, sued the defendants for breach of contract, fraud and damage.

4. Yogananda and SRF sued the Eley's back by filing a cross-complaint in this case.

Again, after three years, the above mentioned case was dismissed. The settlement was signed by the both parties, which meant they mutually agreed on some proposal.

5. Yogoda Sat Sanga Society of India vs. Swami Hariharananda Giri of Puri, India, 1974-75.

6. Coastal Commission vs. Self Realization Fellowship in 1981.

Self Realization Fellowship vs. Coastal Commission (counter suit) in 1981.

7. Self Realization Fellowship Church (SRFC), a California corporation, plaintiff, vs. Church of Self Realization, a California corporation; Fellowship of Inner Communion, a California corporation, and James Donald Walters (also known as Sri Kriyananda), an individual, defendants, in the United States District Court for the Eastern District of California, Case No. CIV-S-90-0846 EJG EM, filed on July 2, 1990.

8. Kriyananda (J. Donald Walters) and Ananda Church of Self Realization, vs. Self Realization Fellowship Church and others in 1992.

9. In re Estate of Vernon Cary vs. Self Realization Fellowship Church, Kern County California, Superior Court, Case No. 43035, Settled in 1994

10. In re Estate of Paulina B. Rima; Prado, etc. v. Self Realization Fellowship Church, New York County Supreme Court, Case No. 94 Civ. 9057 (MBM), Dismissal on July 13, 1994 pursuant to settlement.

11. Ms. Anne-Marie Bertolucci, Plaintiff vs. Ananda Church of Self Realization and Kriyananda (J. Donald Walters) and others, defendants, in 1996, in the Superior Court of the State of California for the County of San Mateo, Case No. 390 230, date January 9, 1996.

In the same suit, on September 26, 1997, Ananda filed 13 "motions" in a bid to knock out plaintiff's case which they lost. They also filed a "cross-complaint" for defamation against the plaintiff and Yogananda's organization, Self Realization Fellowship Church, alleging "conspiracy;" but later on, they dropped it.

The Plaintiff sued the defendant for filing a frivolous claim (the cross-complaint), alleging conspiracy and slander when the defendant, Ananda Church of Self Realization and Kriyananda (J. Donald Walters) and others, dropped the "cross-complaint."

12. Patricia Lyons vs. Self Realization Fellowship Church, Los Angeles County Superior Court, Case No. BC 184382, filed January 16,1998, Complaint

for Negligent Infliction of Emotional Distress, (Plaintiff was ex-employee of SRF).

13. Sunset Palisades, etc. vs. Self Realization Fellowship Church, et al. Los Angeles County Superior Court, Case No. BC212613, filed June 25, 1999

14. Anne-Marie Bertolucci, an individual, plaintiff, vs. Ananda Church of Self Realization, A California religious corporation, James Donald Walters (also known as J. Donald Walters), an individual, defendants, in the United States District Court for the Eastern District of California, Case No. CIV-S-99-1439 LKK JFM, filed on June 27, 1999. Demand for Jury trial.

Anne-Marie Bertolucci, an individual, plaintiff, vs. Ananda Church of Self Realization, A California religious corporation, James Donald Walters (also known as J. Donald Walters), an individual, defendants, in the United States District Court for the Eastern District of California, Case No. CIV-S-99-1439 LKK JFM, filed on August 10 1999, Dismissal of Complaint (FRCP 41 (a) (1).

15. John F. Perry, Executor of the Estate of Richard C. Perry, Vs. Self Realization Fellowship Church, Estate No. 169476, filed on Aug. 4, file No. 2000-CV-29008, District Court.

16. Self Realization Fellowship Church, a California Corporation, Plaintiff-Appellant, Vs Ananda Church of Self Realization, a California Corporation, Fellowship of Inner Communion, No 97-17407, at the United States Court of Appeals for the Ninth Circuit, filed March 23, 2000.

In addition, between 1990 and 2000, Self Realization Fellowship has three personal injury/workers compensation cases and two labor actions.

No wonder Mahamuni Babaji and Lahiri Mahasay prohibited developing organizations around the teaching of *Kriya*.

No wonder Paramhansa Sri Ramakrisna said: *Ami dal pakate asini*, "I have not come to form a group."

The Actual *Kriya* Modifications

Circumstances that led to modifications :

1. Sriyukteswar, disciple of Lahiri Mahasay, had a rational, progressive, and scientific bent of mind and temperament. As a result, he was a giant astrologer. His teaching was influenced by astrology. Sriyukteswar emphasized the astrological meanings of *yuga* in his book *Kaibalya Darsan* ("*The Holy Science*") which may be appropriate in the light of astrology and science, but certainly not in the light of *Kriya.*

In contrast, Lahiri Mahasay defined *yugas* in the light of *Kriya* as follows:

"*Satya yuga* is to hold onto the *Kutastha*, or the inner Self.
"*Treta yuga* is to see the *Kutastha*.
"*Dwapara yuga* is to generate Happiness through *Kriya* practice, and
"*Kali yuga* is to initiate into *Kriya*." 1:86 *Manusanghita*, Commentaries by Lahiri Mahasay (pages 366, and 367, The *Gitas and Sanghitas* Volume 1, Complete Works of Lahiri Mahasay by the Present author).

2. The message of *Kaibalya Darsan* ("*The Holy Science*") is the message of *Kriya*. But it also included a big introduction about astrology which is irrelevant to the message. His preoccupation with astrology caused him to accommodate it regardless of its irrelevancy to the message of the book.

Truth is Eternity beyond space and time. The message of *Kriya* is the message of Eternity, while Time in manifestation is the concern of astrology, to determine the accuracy of happenings.

Kriya is the science of *Avyakta*, inexplicable, unmanifested, ultimate Self; where astrology is the science of manifestation in Time. Eternity achieved through *Kriya* is the destroyer of manifestation and Time.

3. Sriyukteswar's scientific mind failed to grasp the commentaries of the *Bhagavad Gita* by his *Guru*, Lahiri Mahasay. Sriyukteswar had admitted this to Satyananda.

স্বামীজি মহারাজ বলিতেন
"কাশীতে গুরুদেবের পদপ্রান্তে বসিয়া তাঁহার অপূর্ব অনুভূতিপ্রসূত গীতার আলোচনা শুনিতাম; তাঁহার সংক্ষিপ্ত প্রকাশভঙ্গীর ভাষা কখনও বা জটিল বোধ হইত। তাঁহার নিকট উপস্থিত হইয়া ব্যক্তিগত প্রশ্ন দ্বারা এবং সময় সময় পত্র ব্যবহারে বহু বিষয়ের মীমাংসা করিয়া লইতাম। নিজ বোধাবলম্বনে কালোপযোগী বৈজ্ঞানিক ও দার্শনিক দৃষ্টিভঙ্গিতে যেমন সমর্থ হইয়াছি তেমন লিখিয়াছি এবং প্রত্যেক খণ্ড প্রকাশ করিয়া তাঁহার সাক্ষাৎ আশীর্বাদ ও অনুমোদনও লাভ করিয়াছি। তবে এই কার্যে যে গুরুদেবের সম্পূর্ণ ভাব গ্রহণ করিতে সমর্থ হইয়াছি এমন ধৃষ্টতা প্রকাশ করিতে পারি না; তাঁহার সান্নিধ্য-লাভে নিজে যেমন বুঝিয়াছি তাহাই লিখিয়াছি, ত্রুটি বা অসম্পূর্ণতা থাকিলে তাহার জন্য আমিই দায়ী।"

"Arriving at Benares at the holy feet of my *Gurudev* [Lahiri Mahasay], I would listen to his interpretations [of the *Bhagavad Gita*], but his style and precise manner of explanation were difficult for me to follow. Occasionally, I would receive clarification from him through correspondence.

"As far as I was able to understand, I have reinterpreted the *Bhagavad Gita* in accordance with the scientific and philosophic attitude of our modern times [in other words, in the perspective of astrology]." Pp. 1-2, Satyananda's introduction to Sriyukteswar's *Gita.*

4. Sriyukteswar was aware of his limitations. As a result, he tried to preserve the spirit of original *Kriya* and passed it to Satyananda who had been initiated by Sastri Mahasay (Swami Kebalananda). Satyananda had been closely associated with Sastri Mahasay since his young days. Also they had lived together for a long time while both were teaching in Ranchi School, so they had twenty-seven years of association.

That is why Sriyukteswar chose disciplinarian and rational Satyananda to be the leader of the East.

5. Sriyukteswar chose Yogananda as his emissary to the West. He thought liberal and devotional Yogananda could easily modify and adjust

according to time and situation. Time is essence in astrology, especially in determining the course of happenings in manifestations.

6. Sriyukteswar did not receive *Navi Kriya* from Lahiri Mahasay. This *Kriya* primarily balances the subtle energy from *Prana* and *Apana* to direct to *Samana* (the tranquil and equilibrium state).

7. So Yogananda did not know *Navi Kriya.*

8. In the original *Kriya* tradition, initiation is given personally, and *Kriyas* are also taught personally, that is, the disciple learns from the *Guru,* or Master, in person. It is called the *Guru-param-para* way. The scriptures call it the righteous way.

In other words, the disciple learns from the *Guru* in person, having a personal relationship, and not from an institution or lessons. Sriyukteswar neither institutionalized *Kriya*, nor did he introduce written lessons or correspondence courses in *Kriya* teaching. He taught through personal relationship, that which is required according to original tradition.

9. The spirit of modification started with the scientific attitude and astrological spirit of Sriyukteswar. He simply passed it on to Yogananda.

10. Thus Yogananda happened to be the tool of modifications, and he then became eager to introduce some kind of liberalism into the teachings of *Kriya* to popularize it for the masses.

Let us see in the words of Yogananda: "According to the law of change and progress, man's views regarding his institutions undergo constant modifications." "In a word, the minister should get away from the past and perform his duties with a rational point of view, and he should attempt to make the Church adjust itself to the new advanced thought. So as to be more Spiritual." *Inner Culture*, September 1934, Page Twenty-three.

In fact, the case is the reverse. Thought and reason leave us at a certain stage and cannot take us further. It is by dissolving thoughts (regardless of their nature, *tamasika*, *rajasika*, and *sattvika*), and not by adjusting thoughts, that one can be spiritual.

Differences between the Original Pure *Kriya* and the Modified *Kriya*

11. Let us again focus on the fundamental characteristics of the teachings of *Yoga* discipline. For this we will see what is said by Lahiri Mahasay, who is considered to be the polestar of the *Kriya* discipline, as well as the holy Scripture's prescription on the point.

"The seeker receives the true *Kriya* of that state directly from the **mouth** of the *Guru,* or the Master." 2:18 *Manusanghita*, Commentaries by Lahiri Mahasay (pages 385, The *Gitas and Sanghitas* Volume 1, Complete Works of Lahiri Mahasay by the Present author).

Once Babaji said, "Those who are getting *Kriya* from unpermitted and unauthorized persons are not getting *true Kriya*, but rather they are receiving only information on *Kriya*."

Therefore, according to Babaji, Lahiri Mahasay and the holy Scripture, until a person is initiated personally by the permitted master and has received *Kriya* from the mouth of his *Guru,* he has not in reality received initiation and *Kriya*.

Without initiation in a righteous way, nothing becomes operative.

The *Guru-param-para*, that is, learning through personal relationship, provides the vital points, such as *Guru-sparsa,* "touch of the *Guru,*" which provides the life (*Prana*) of the disciple during the initiation. *Gurusakti*, "the energy of the *Guru,*" gives birth to the disciple. In reality, the life of the disciple begins that day; it is the birthday of the disciple.

"The first birth is *Kriya* initiation. The second birth is to pass the air at the waist. The third birth is to receive *Pranayam*, or *Omkar Kriyas*. All these take place in the body." 2:169 *Manusanghita*, Commentaries by Lahiri Mahasay (pages 419, The *Gitas and Sanghitas* Volume 1, Complete Works of Lahiri Mahasay by the Present author).

That is why to receive *Kriya* from the mouth of the *Guru* and the personal relationship with the *Guru* is the life of the *Kriya* teachings.

Thus the modified *Kriya* trend lacks the very life of *Kriya*, and it reduces the teachings to learning information about *Kriya* teachings as if in some academic institution.

Yogananda modified, rather *deviated*, from the tradition on this point and introduced correspondence lesson courses for mass education.

12. Yogananda introduced thirty seven (37) energizing techniques and made them part of *Kriya* discipline, rather part of the modified *Kriya* discipline. These are not at all a part of original *Kriya* tradition.

He found these techniques useful to inspire and motivate his Western devotees who love exercises.

In the original *Kriya* tradition, the *Mahamudra* is practiced in the beginning and serves as an energizing *Kriya* to shake the body. *Mahamudra* is based on the composition of *Paschimuthasana* of *Hatha Yoga*.

13. He changed the composition of *Mahamudra* from the original *Kriya* tradition.

14. He advised that *Kriya* be practiced while sitting on an armless chair, legs hanging and set on the ground.

This is a fundamental modification and deviation from the original pure *Kriya* tradition.

Yoga in general, and *Kriya*, in particular, require a sitting posture with legs folded. The prescribed posture is called *Padmasana* (lotus). All the ancient Yogis prescribed this *Asana* for practicing *Raja* or *Kriya Yoga*.

"In his method of initiation into *Kriya* also, Swami Yogananda added innovations. Perceiving that the average American found it difficult to sit in lotus posture, he taught that he could sit erect on a straight-back armless chair, legs hanging, and practise *Kriya*; initiation was also a mass affair; instead of direct contact between the teacher and the taught - the *Guru* and the novice - the whole affair was reduced to something like an indoor class." p. 168, *Kriya Yoga* written and published by Sailendra Bejoy Dasgupta, Calcutta, 1979. (Dasgupta was Sriyukteswar's disciple and Yogananda's private secretary during 1935-1936).

In the higher stage, the body levitates. At that time the lotus posture serves to lock the body in position. What will happen to the legs which are in hanging position?

Perhaps, Yogananda knew what he was doing. Being compassionate, with much motherly love, he instructed his followers to begin the practice, at least to achieve a step in this life. Customarily, like the other liberal yogis, he offered his work to the Lord that He should take care of it.

The original *Kriya* discipline being the Science of all sciences demands practice very strictly adhering to the rules lest everything be in vain.

Lahiri Mahasay wrote in his letter to his disciple as follows:

অনুগ্রহপূর্ব্বক

বিধিপূর্ব্বক উপদেশমত কার্য্য করিবেন নচেৎ বিড়ম্বনা মাত্র ॥

"Please practice according to the instructions; otherwise all will be a farce. [That is, the *Kriyanwit* will not get results]." p. 66, *Lahiri Mahasay's Personal Letters to Kriya Disciples* by the author.

15. Yogananda introduced *Hang Sa* technique and *OM* technique which he preferred to call *Baby Kriya*, and these are not at all original *Kriya*. These are his introduction to modified *Kriyas*.

In the First *Kriya* (which Yogananda would prefer to call *Kriya Proper*) he brought three modifications:

16. He changed the numbers for the beginners.

17. He changed the instructions of the original *Kriya* and introduced the counting at the end of inhaling. In Original Pure *Kriya* there are specific instructions at the end of both inhaling and exhaling.

18. He advised the practitioner to bring attention from behind to the front underneath the head which is NOT possible for definite physiological reasons according to Swami Pranabananda, disciple of Lahiri Mahasay. The Scripture supports the original Pure *Kriya* tradition and in that respect the comment of Pranabananda.

There is a story which may be appropriate to mention here in this connection.

In the early 70's, the author was visiting Yogananda's hermitage boys' school. Also Panchkori De, disciple of Swami Kebalananda, principal, Postgraduate Teachers' Training College of Sevayatan was visiting Swami Bidyananda (disciple of Yogananda).

Hiralal Chanda, a householder and advanced disciple of Swami Satyananda, was the principal and Abanindra Narayan Lahiri (popularly known as Abani Babu), a bachelor, disciple of Swami Satchidananda (disciple of Yogananda) was the vice principal of YSS boys' school.

Both Hiralal Chanda and Abanindra Lahiri had been the author's teachers in the hermitage school in high school days when he was a resident student. They reserved special affection, as well as regard for the author. Abanindra Lahiri was the host of the author, while Bidyananda was the host of Mr. De.

One afternoon, in the front yard, in front of Abanindra Lahiri's quarters, Hiralal Babu, Mr. De, Abanindra Lahiri, and the author were having *satsanga*, spiritual discussion.

An assistant teacher (a devotee) of the school who happened to be an ex-student of the school, was plucking flowers from the front yard garden in preparation for evening prayer, of which he was in charge.

Meanwhile, Mr. De was taking a break and was looking at some flowers in the garden. When he was near the devotee, he asked him if he was a *Kriya* practitioner?

The devotee replied, "Yes sir, I am."

Mr. De: "Why is it that your health looks so weak? How do you practice *Kriya*?

The devotee brought his hands near his mouth, folded the fingers, touched the tip of the thumb on the tip of the first finger and showed him how he practiced *Kriya* to feel cool current during inhaling and warm current during exhaling.

Mr. De: "From whom were you initiated into *Kriya*?"

The devotee: "By the joint secretary of YSS. [An American]."

Mr. De: "Did he tell you to practice like this?"

The devotee: "He showed me this during initiation."

Mr. De: "How long have you been practicing like this?"

The devotee: "About three years."

Mr. De: "No wonder your health is so weak. You are not supposed to practice like this. Perhaps the secretary wanted you to understand this clearly and that was why he showed you this way. You are bringing the hands from behind to the front to bring attention. Did the secretary instruct this, too?"

"Yes sir," said the devotee.

At this, Mr. De laughed loudly. Everybody's attention was drawn to them. The devotee was eager to know why Mr. De was laughing, but he had no time. He had to leave or he might be late for conducting the evening prayer with the students.

Upon Mr. De's returning to *satsanga*, Abanindra Lahiri asked him for the reason of such loud laughter. It may be mentioned here that both Mr. De and Abanindra Lahiri had been classmates during their one year course of Bachelor of Teachers' training (B.T.) and had been good friends.

Mr. De narrated the story of the assistant teacher to Abanindra Lahiri, the vice principal. Mr. De said that bringing attention from behind to the front underneath the head is incorrect.

Abanindra Lahiri: "To show the bringing of the hands near the mouth to inhale and exhale to feel cool and warm currents was a misunderstanding on the part of the devotee. But what is wrong with the practice of bringing attention from behind to the front side?"

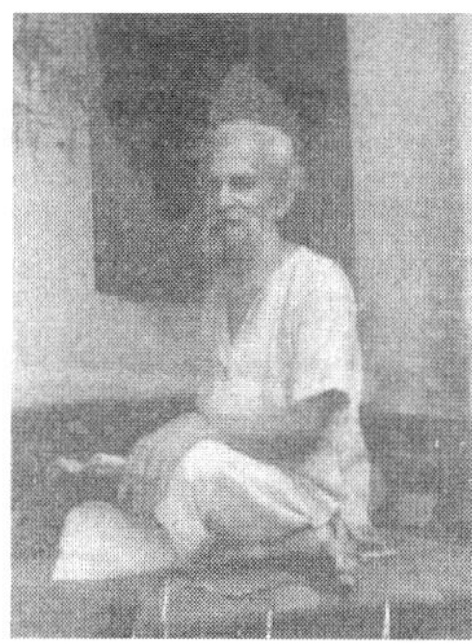

Panchkori De,
Disciple of Kebalananda

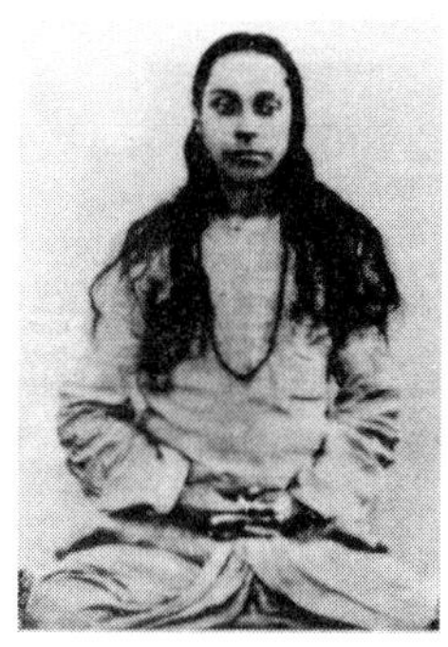

Swami Satchidananda,
Disciple of Yogananda.

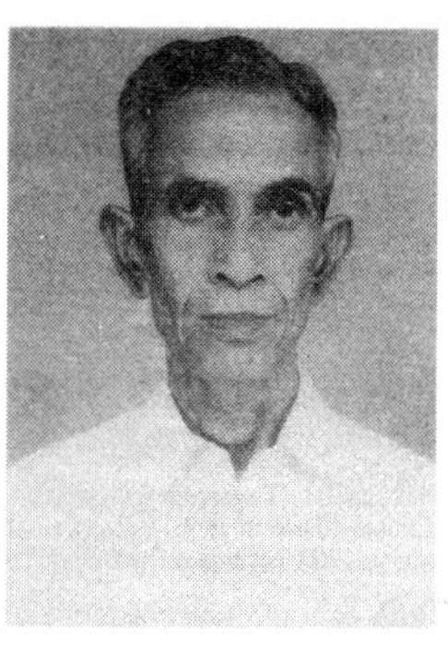

Hiralal Chand,
Disciple of Satyananda

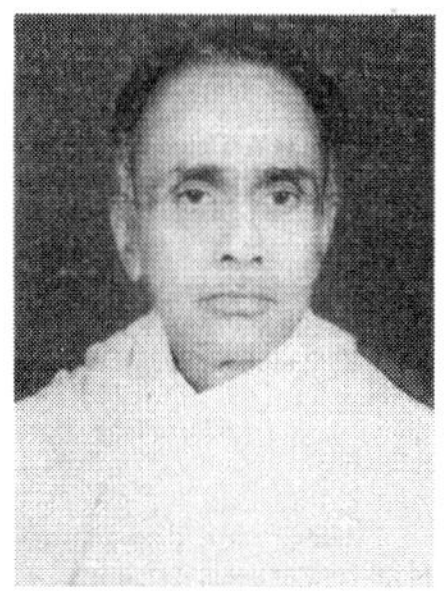

Abanindra Narayan Lahiri,
Vice Principal, Vidyapith

Mr. De said that bringing attention from behind to the front underneath the head is incorrect.

Abanindra Lahiri: "Why is it incorrect?"

Mr. De remained silent.

Abanindra Lahiri looked to his colleague, the principal, Hiralal Chanda, hoping for an answer. He too remained silent.

Abanindra Lahiri, then turned to the author, who too preferred to remain silent.

At this point, Abanindra Lahiri went to his room and brought a big note-book. In fact, it was one of the several volumes Lahiri had bound for his personal use of "the *Preceptom* - the magazine on *Yoga* literature," published fortnightly. Later, these were converted to "Yogoda Lessons" on *Kriya*. In the West, Yogananda's organization has introduced lessons which are not exactly the same. He opened the relevant portion quickly, as important places were underlined. He showed them to Mr. De.

(**NOTE** - After visiting *Kumbha Mela* at Haridwar in 1974, a French lady devotee and a young journalist, an African French, of Paris, who met the author at *Kumbha Mela*, later visited the author, at Dunagiri, Hill, Himalayas. Both wanted clarifications on some of their confusions. At that time, she showed her lessons. Thus the author happened to notice the differences.

(In fact there is a little more to this story. The author, the lover of solitude and silence, never intended to visit *Kumbha Mela* due to the big crowd. But he had to visit Haridwar in 1974, just for three days towards the end of seven weeks duration of the fair because Mahamuni Babaji wanted the author to be there. Babaji had three reasons:

(1. to have the experience of the *Kumbha Mela*, at least once,

(2. to have the author know the differences of the lessons; it indicated that silently Babaji was preparing the grounds by educating the author to commission him later for reestablishing the original *Kriya* tradition and

(3. to respond to the intensive prayers of some devotees.

(Both the devotees, the French lady and the young journalist, had a letter of introduction from Swami Sradhhananda [a Bengali Swami living in Paris, who had received Swami order from Bhola Giri *Sanyas* asram, Haridwar] to Swami Sevananda, a disciple of Yogananda, who was living at that time in Bhola Giri *Asram*.

(The young journalist said, "I have the letter of introduction from Sradhha-nanda to Sevananda. I walked many times in front of Bhola Giri *Asram's* gate, I could walk in and use the letter to see Sevananda, but I did not want to meet an Indian *Kriya* Yogi in this manner. My friend agreed. We prayed to Babaji to bless us so that we could meet an Indian *Kriya* Yogi without formal letter of introduction. And surely, we are glad to meet you Swamiji. We have come, on behalf of two hundred French devotees of Paris, who themselves have been praying to Babaji for this meeting. We want to have clarifications of our doubts regarding our practice in higher techniques according to the teaching through the lessons; and to know the correct pronunciation of the *Mantra* in Sanskrit."

(The author asked, "What about Sradhhananda?)

The journalist replied, "He is very good for the beginners. Whenever he performed *Homa*, the Vedic rituals, many devotees attended."

(Later, both devotees proposed that the author come to Europe. They promised to bear the expenses and do all the necessary arrangements, but the proposal was turned down. Then again, the lady devotee stated that one of her lady friends of Paris wanted to build an *asram* in India, so that she could live six months there and six months in Paris. Her question was, whether the author would be willing to accept and consent to live six months in the proposed asram when her friend would be in Paris.

(The author gently smiled within, observing the tricks of the negative forces to tempt him, and said, "Sorry, this body is not that caretaker person."

(They left Dunagiri Hill after three days.)

Back to the story. Mr. De maintained his silence, and did not comment.

Abanindra Lahiri looked to the author to intervene.

Reluctantly, the author told Lahiri, "The one to whom you are showing these materials was himself in charge of these *Preceptoms* while he was in Ranchi, in addition to his other responsibilities [such as being in charge of Finance, serving as teacher at the *Brahmacharya Vidyalaya* (school), and being assistant general secretary of Yogoda Sat Sanga Society (YSS) from 1936-42. He was even made *Brahmachari* Santananda by Yogananda in 1936. Once, I was told by Satyananda, 'Yogananda wanted to bring him to the U.S.A. in 1936. But in those days, his eyes were focused somewhere else.' In other words, he was focusing inward and everything else was insignificant to him]."

Abanindra Lahiri: "Is this true?" Mr. De nodded his head.

Abanindra Lahiri was shocked by this disclosure. However, he wanted to know the comments of all on this particular point. He looked to Mr. De who maintained his silence. So did the principal, Hiralal Chanda. Then he turned to the author demanding that he say something.

(**NOTE** - Once, Hiralal Chanda was considered to be brought to U.S.A., but it did not materialize. They were highly interested to bring him to the U.S.A. because he was a *Khechari sidhha* Yogi, disciple of Satyananda. He was a householder and had a large family; but they did not like to take responsibility of his family and that became the obstruction).

Again, reluctantly the author said, "As you know, *Kriya* practice is very personal; it is a matter of *Guru-Param-Para* - Master and disciple relationship; that is why no one would answer."

Privately the author told Abanindra Lahiri, "You had better direct your question to Satchidananda (disciple of Yogananda) from whom you are receiving instructions. In this connection, you may look into the comments of Swami Pranabananda (disciple of Lahiri Mahasay) in his *Gita* interpretations - there he said on this particular point that trying to bring attention to the front from behind the head is impossible because the internal tissues in that part of the Spinal Cord are so constituted that if one tries to come from that side it gets tighter and tighter, and blocks it automatically. One could not reach the center this way not to speak of bringing attention to the front side."

By then, it became dark. It was time for evening prayer. Abanindra Lahiri looked very worried, nervous, and saddened. He had been practicing *Kriya* according to the lessons seriously and sincerely for twenty-two years with no results. He complained to the author several times. Now, he began to doubt.

Abanindra Lahiri did not lose time. The following week he made a trip to visit Satchidananda. He told the author, later, on some other occasion, that arriving at Dhanyasol where Satchidananda was staying, "I was so upset, I did not make any introduction, rather, straightforwardly asked Swamiji (Satchidananda), 'Please do not give me a bluff, and answer my questions honestly.' "

Satchidananda: "Let me check your practice."

Abanindra Lahiri said, "When I practiced, he said, 'It is okay.' I tried again to explain to him what had happened and what caused me to direct this question to him, but he said, 'Do not worry; Go on practicing.' "

Abanindra Lahiri asked the author on some other occasion, "Could you comment on Swamiji's (Satchidananda's) treating me like this? What could be the possible reasons?"

Again, the author was reluctant to comment, but Lahiri insisted. He knew that he could count on the author, since the former had known the latter from grade four in the hermitage.

The author said, "I could only imagine two reasons: 1) Satchidananda himself was a disciple of Yogananda and he had no choice but to respect *Preceptom*; 2) he has experienced the Lord's sudden blessing in his *Khecharimudra* practice and, as a result, he understood that unless the right moment comes, things do not reveal. That is why he advised you to continue to practice."

Abanindra Lahiri was not happy with the situation. He knew that Satchidananda, although a disciple of Yogananda, had received instructions from Swami Satyananda. So he decided to seek clarification directly from Satyananda. Accordingly, he contacted the author to make an appointment with Satyananda for three days during the next month.

The principal, Hiralal Chanda and Abanindra N. Lahiri, the vice principal arrived at Sevayatan, Satyananda's hermitage.

On the second day, in the evening, Abanindra Lahiri asked Satyananda an important question in the presence of the author. Satyananda, apparently, said, "Go on practicing. It is okay."

Abanindra Lahiri was shocked. He looked at the author and pressed the author's body hard in such a way that Satyananda could not see. He wanted the author to interfere and help him.

The author said, "It is between you both. It is not the area for another to comment."

Abanindra Lahiri felt helpless and became desperate; he touched the author again and pressed hard by which he meant that he wanted the author to intervene and help him.

At this the author directed a request to Satyananda, "You could throw some light on Abani Babu's question."

Satyananda simply looked at the author and remained silent.

The next day, Lahiri asked the author, during evening walk, "Swamiji! What is your comment about Satyananda's answer?"

The author said, "I have observed on many occasions, whenever one of Yogananda's disciples would come and seek Satyananda's advice, he would not disturb the structure of Yogananda's *Kriya* teachings when giving advice to the devotee. Rather, Satyananda thought this matter to be Yogananda's own responsibility to his disciple.

"Satyananda also knew that he is not supposed to answer until the right moment arrives. Furthermore, looking at the questioner's providential background, advice is given for his benefit. What else can I say? I wish I could be of help, but my hands are also tied; I cannot say any more because the righteous spirit must be maintained. That is, eternal Realization is eternally secret. The Lord Himself kept It secret by means of Silence. I can chant simply:

"*Twamabyaya saswata dharma gopta*, 'You are the custodian of eternal Realization [*dharma*] by means of Silence.' *Gita* 11:18.

"In other words, everything points to the right moment for the fortunate one to receive the right advice in the right time.

"Kabir says, 'The true path is rarely found.' "

The following day both left for Yogananda's hermitage. After a couple of years, Hiralal Chanda, the principal of the Vidyapith (school) retired and Abanindra N. Lahiri became the principal. Then in 1971 Satyananda left body and entered into *Mahasamadhi*. Hiralal Chanda also left body in 1976.

During Abanindra Lahiri's tenure, the author visited him a couple of times. He used to introduce the author to his present students in the evening prayer, advising them to take advantage of author's visit.

Abanindra N. Lahiri left body in November 1983 in Calcutta.

Lahiri Mahasay knew that many initiated *Kriyanwits* might not be able to make progress in *Kriya*, and that is why he emphasized that the first *Kriya* be practiced strictly according to the instruction with all sincerity.

In one letter he wrote to a devotee, "All [complete Realization] can be attained by the first *Kriya*; only sincerity is needed. The After-effect-poise of *Kriya* and blissful addiction are there at the very first *Kriya*. Go on practicing *Kriya*." p. 22 *Lahiri Mahasay's Personal Letters to Kriya Disciples* by the author.

Now to return to the discussion of *Kriya* modification:

19. Sriyukteswar did not teach *Khecharimudra* to Yogananda because he observed that Yogananda had already learned it from Sastri Mahasay (Kebalananda).

Although, in fact, Yogananda was initiated by Sastri Mahasay whom he used to address as *Guru Maharaj-ji* prior to coming to the U.S.A., for some reason afterwards, Yogananda preferred to be identified as the disciple of Sriyukteswar whom he used to call *Jnana Guru Maharaj*.

At that time, Sastri Mahasay was a householder disciple of Lahiri Mahasay, and Yogananda had been made Swami by Sriyukteswar. Perhaps, being a Swami, he preferred to mention Swami Sriyukteswar as his *Jnana Gurudev* over Sastri Mahasay. It may be pointed out here that in spite of his friends' criticisms in India for his apparent changing of *Gurus*, Yogananda never showed disrespect to Sastri Mahasay. Rather he treated him with respect.

Since Yogananda did not learn *Khecharimudra* from Sriyukteswar, he did not teach *Khecharimudra* to his disciples.

Talabya Kriya, or *Khecharimudra*, Its far reaching implications and Yogananda

It will be appropriate to recapitulate once again what we have mentioned before about *Talabya Kriya* and its implications

In the Original *Kriya*, successful *Talabya Kriya* or *Khecharimudra* qualifies a *Kriyanwit* to receive higher *Kriyas*, that is the *Kriyas* of the Tranquil Breath (the *Omkar Kriyas*). *Talabya Kriya* helps to achieve the state of Tranquil breath while practiced in conjunction with *Pranayam*. That is why it becomes a milestone or essential precondition before a *Kriyanwit* is introduced to the *Omkar Kriyas* which require a special procedure to adopt and only successful *Talabya Kriya* or *Khecharimudra* can easily provide it.

In the words of Lahiri Mahasay, "Putting the tongue into the head or to the area between the eyebrows" provides one to be able to connect the individual self of the seeker to the cosmic Consciousness or inner Consciousness of the inner Self, the *Kutastha*.

" ... donation of *Kriya*, that which can be given after the tongue is raised [subject to Master's permission with blessings], ... " 1:89 *Manusanghita*, Lahiri Mahasay's Commentaries (p. 29, *Hidden Wisdom,* Com. Vol. III by the author].

It will be helpful to put things in sequence and in proper perspective. As mentioned before Satyananda and Yogananda first learned *Kriya* in 1906 from Bhagavati Charan Ghosh and then from Kebalananda in 1907 and 1908 before they met Sriyukteswar in 1909.

Let us see what Satyananda, the best friend, colleague, and brother disciple of Yogananda has to say regarding their teenage days.

> শাস্ত্রীমহাশয়ের সান্নিধ্যে মুকুন্দলাল সাধনজীবনে নবজীবন লাভ করে অগ্রসর হতে লাগলেন। অল্প-দিনের মধ্যে ক্রিয়াযোগের প্রাথমিক স্তর অতিক্রম করলেন, তাঁর জিহ্বা-গ্রন্থিভেদ হল।

It says, "Under Sastri Mahasay's [Kebalananda's] teaching Mukundalal [Yogananda] received a new life in his *Sadhana*, pursuit of meditation. Within a short period of time he crossed the first step; his *jiohagranthi*, knot of his tongue, was crossed." *Yogananda Sanga* by Satyananda p. 33

> শাস্ত্রীমহাশয়ের সঙ্গসময়ে যে রকম কঠোরভাবে সাধনানুষ্ঠান করেছেন তাঁর জীবনে আর কখনো সে রকম তপস্বীর ভাব দেখেছি বলে মনে হয় না।

The above quote says, "I [Satyananda] never saw him [Yogananda] so intensely practice his *Sadhana* any time in his life except in those teen years of ours when we were associated with Sastri Mahasay [Kebalananda]." *Yogananda Sanga* by Satyananda p. 30

The successful *Talabya* or *Khechari* has its positive impact; it increases inwardness in the seeker's pursuit of Truth. The outwardness of mind from all the three planes: physical, mental, and cosmic begin to transform into inwardness. The seeker generates greater strength to restrain his senses particularly touch (skin or sensual attachment), smell (nose), and taste (tongue). See discussion of Chapter 4 "The *Kriya* Science."

> এই সময় হতেই মুকুন্দ গৃহ, পাড়া প্রতিবেশী, স্কুল প্রভৃতি সর্বত্র এক বিশিষ্ট চিহ্নিত ব্যক্তি হয়ে উঠলেন। সহপাঠী, সমবয়সী প্রভৃতি অনেকে বন্ধুভাবে এসে তাঁর প্রভাবে আধ্যাত্মিক জীবনের সন্ধান নিলেন। অনেকে শাস্ত্রী মহাশয়ের নিকট ক্রিয়াযোগে দীক্ষা গ্রহণ করলেন।

It says, "During this period Mukunda started drawing attention of others at home, neighborhood, and at the school from friends, classmates, and the boys from his age-group. Many came his way and received spiritual life. Many were initiated into *Kriya* by Sastri Mahasay [Kebalananda]." *Yogananda Sanga* by Satyananda, p. 31

Successful *Talabya* or *Khechari* at a young age has its down side also; it brings some yogic powers: It ignites inner visions, tempts one to see in the future, and tempts one to tell future happenings, etc. (It may be mentioned here that being able to see and tell future happening is not an advanced state of inner Realization, rather a preliminary state.) It creates greater temptations to use these powers in practical life for personal success. One has to handle the situation and to channel this inspiration into a positive direction, or else it causes an impact in a negative way in the entire life of the person. The application of yogic powers for drawing attraction upon oneself, generating name and fame, and gaining comforts, builds obstructions, and that is why Yogi Patanjali condemned it in his *Yoga Sutras*.

ते समाधावुपसर्गा व्युत्थाने सिद्धयः ॥ ३७ ॥

Te samadhabupasarga byuthane siddhaya. Yoga Sutras 3:37

The verse says, "The sixfold yogic powers are the obstruction in achieving success [Liberation]."

The successful *Talabya* or *Khechari* in the young age also brings frequent failure of memory in practical life. As the tongue intends to go upwards always to be in touch with the inner Self within, the individual's material aspect of life automatically is being ignored. It happened to Dukori Lahiri, the youngest son of Lahiri Mahasay. (Lahiri Mahasay watched his youngest son, Dukori Lahiri, and once he said, "Keep yourself secret. Do not worry about what the people say about you." Once, some devotee drew Lahiri Mahasay's attention requesting him to do something to cure Dukori Lahiri. Lahiri Mahasay replied, "Do you think that he is my only son? What about all these people?" He pointed to the attending *Kriyanwits*.)

In Yogananda's case, successful *Khechari* in youth brought excessive enthusiasm in his life to help others. He started initiating his friends in those days as a young boy's play, though he was not permitted either by his father or by Sastri Mahasay (Kebalananda). The question of permission from Sriyukteswar did not arise, because he was yet to meet Sriyukteswar. He assumed the role of a *Guru* by himself in his teens, and the style continued. In his young days, he developed interest in hypnotism, etc,. For details, the reader may look at "*Biography of a Yogi*" by the author.

The following year, after graduating from high school, in October 1909, Mukunda left for Benares to stay at Sri Bharat Dharma Mahamandal hermitage. Coincidentally, Sriyukteswar was visiting his old mother at Benares, where Mukunda first met him. (Discussed in Chapter 7 in the title "*The Original Kriya*" by the author).

Later, observing Yogananda's ability for publicity and the spirit of liberalism, Sriyukteswar chose him as his emissary to the West.

Sangjam, or Restraint of the Senses

The characteristic of a realized person is to be restrained. *Sangjam*, the restraint of the senses is the primary ingredient of inner Realization. Yogi Patanjali mentioned *Sangjam* in his *Yoga Sutras*:

> त्रयमेकत्र संयमः ॥ ४ ॥
>
> *Trayamekatra Sangjam. Yoga Sutras* 3:4

The verse says, "Three [*Dharana* - glimpse of Tranquility, or concept, *Dhyana* - meditation and *Samadhi* - attunement in Oneness] being united into One constitutes the state of *Sangjam*, or the state of restraint."

There is a nice story on this point: Gargya, son of Valaka, one day, visited King Ajatsatru of Benares. Gargya was proud of his *Brahmana* heritage. He wanted to teach the king who was a *Khatriya*. So their conversation began:

Gargya (G) said, "He who is in the wind and who is also as breath within, I meditate upon as *Brahma*."

Ajatsatru (A) said, "You should not say like that about *Brahma*. I worship Him as invincible and unconquerable."

G: "He who is in the fire and who is in the heart, I meditate upon as *Brahma*."

A: "No. You should not speak thus of *Brahma*. He is the embodiment of forgiving; I meditate upon Him as forgiveness."

G: "He who is in the water and in the heart, I meditate upon as *Brahma*."

A: "No. Do not speak thus of *Brahma*. I meditate upon him as harmony."

[Thus both continued back and forth for a while. Finally Gargya said the following; and Ajatsatru replied appropriately.]

G: "He who lives in the heart as Intelligence, I meditate upon him as *Brahma*."

A: "Please do not speak of *Brahma* in that manner. He who meditates upon *Brahma*, achieves *atma sangjam*, self-control. I meditate upon *Brahma* [the supreme Self] as *Sangjam*, or self-control."

Gargya reflected on what the king has said and became silent for a while. Then he approached the king, "Please accept me as your disciple."

The king said, "You are a *Brahmana*; your profession is to teach spiritual discipline. I am a *Khatriya* and my duties are to rule, make gifts and to support the *Brahmanas*."

Gargya again approached the king with folded hands to accept him as his disciple. This time, the king said, "Well then, I will teach you."

Gargya was advanced but not a realized *Brahmana*. So quickly he understood that he needed to learn the discipline directly and personally from the King who was a realized yogi and was established in self-control.

In fact, it is *atma-sangjam*, self-control, or restraintment, that provides *Sthirattva*, eternal Tranquility, or eternal Realization. Lack of *Sangjam*, or the state of restraint of the senses, induces one to obsession to save souls.

Before leaving India, and after returning to India in 1935-36, Yogananda did not teach *Khecharimudra* to his disciples, but rather he asked them to learn and check *Kriyas* with Satyananda, who never disturbed Yogananda's structure of *Kriya* teaching and never initiated any disciple of Yogananda into *Khecharimudra*. Rather Satyananda considered Yogananda to be primarily responsible for them.

For example, as mentioned before, in spite of the repeated insistence of Swami Satchidananda (then *Brahmachari* Animananda), disciple of Yogananda, Satyananda did not teach Satchidananda *Khecharimudra*. He had to learn it from Sriyukteswar's household disciple, Bijoya K. Chatterjee of Howrah.

In the original *Kriya* tradition, *Khecharimudra* is very essential. One must be initiated into it directly from the permitted teacher. It is so important that in the original *Kriya* tradition, nobody is initiated without it into the second *Kriya* and all the remaining higher *Thokar* and *Omkar Kriyas*.

Khecharimudra provides a special capacity (resulting in the second birth into the *Kriya* path), which is required to function in the special procedure which is adopted in the higher *Kriyas*, and without this capacity, or second birth, *Omkar Kriyas* simply do not become operative, no matter how perfect one is practicing them.

The life of the practice of higher *Kriyas* is gone if the blessings of *Khecharimudra* are missing. It should be mentioned here that it is fatal to practice those *Omkar Kriyas* without *Khecharimudra*.

Successful *Khecharimudra,* or *Talabya Kriya*, as Lahiri Mahasay mentioned, provided a capacity to connect the seeker to the *Kutastha*, the inner Self, the eternal Master. At this stage the seeker becomes *Dwija*, "the twice born."

When a *Kriyanwit* seeker in original *Kriya* tradition succeeds in *Talabya Kriya*, he is initiated into higher *Omkar Kriyas*. This is the *Kriyanwit* seeker's third birth.

Practicing higher *Kriyas*, that is, *Omkar Kriyas*, without *Talabya Kriya,* brings a qualitative change in the approach of *Kriya* Science. With this significant modification, whether the approach or practice remain a *Kriya* approach is very much questionable.

Yogananda, Sriyukteswar's emissary to the West, who did not learn *Talabya Kriya* from him, reduced the importance of *Talabya Kriya* from "must" to "may." At least, that is what the author was told by Yogananda's dear and close Western disciple, president of SRF and YSS, in their second meeting, one to one, at Calcutta in November, 1972.

Liberal Yogananda was trying to respect the original *Kriya* tradition by indicating that he was the last *Guru,* or Master, of his line of teachings since he dropped the teaching of *Talabya Kriya,* or *Khecharimudra*.

As mentioned before, in the original *Kriya* tradition, nobody is initiated in the second *Omkar Kriya,* or higher *Kriyas,* without *Talabya Kriya*. Yogananda modified the teaching and taught *Omkar Kriyas* without introducing *Talabya Kriya* at all.

"Another startling innovation introduced [by Yogananda] was that [the] Second or the Third *Kriya* was allowed to be practised without having to do *Khechari Mudra*. All these innovations or rather deviations from the regular methods [Original *Kriya* Tradition] could not find favour with devotees and lovers of *Kriya Yoga*.

"It is pertinent to note that an American intellectual, Dr. Wendel Thomas, an American professor, - in his book *Hinduism Invades America* (New York, 1930) while eulogising the broadness of outlook of Swami Yogananda and comparing him as the best among all the Hindu Missionaries that ever came to America, pinpointing adoption of American methods by him remarked, 'He has plunged headlong into American life ... who knows if the message itself is not changed in the long run.' " p. 168, *Kriya Yoga* written and published by Sailendra Bejoy Dasgupta, Calcutta, 1979.

Recently, on August 8, 1991, a devotee had an appointment with the author to have *Satsanga*, spiritual meeting. Being asked by the devotee in that *Satsanga*, the author explained something on *Jnana Yoga*, the path of Knowledge, and then explained the same in the light of *Kriya Yoga*. The following day, the devotee called the author to have some clarifications. He had developed some questions from yesterday's *Satsanga*.

The devotee said, "Baba (the author)! Yesterday, you were explaining the path of Knowledge to me. Were you suggesting to me that my path is the path of Knowledge?"

The author said, "No. It was a general discussion. It does not necessarily apply to you. That is why the point was explained to you again in the light of *Kriya*".

The devotee said, "Another question: I heard from a friend that he knew one gentleman who received *Khecharimudra* from Yogananda. Would you please comment on this?"

The author said, "In India, Yogananda did not teach *Khecharimudra*. At least, that is my observation. In the West, people have a tendency to assume things personally. Yogananda might have discussed it with some devotees during *Satsanga* and the devotees assumed that they were taught *Khechari*. It may be of that nature. Think about yourself M; you thought that you were taught the path of Knowledge just yesterday. This is an example of how average American people take things or relate to themselves personally. They think that there must be some reason and connection, otherwise, why would Baba say this? In *Satsanga* things are discussed in general. If there is personal instruction then it is told personally with a special emphasis."

The devotee said, "Now I understand and see your point. Thank you Baba for your kind answer."

Observing the average American's physical construction, in his time, Yogananda instructed his students to sit on a chair instead of on the floor with folded legs or lotus posture for their *Kriya* practice. Perhaps, for the same reason he dropped advising *Khecharimudra* to his students. He may have thought that the practice of *Khecharimudra* might horrify them.

The author feels embarrassed to point this out, but remembering Babaji's instruction, and considering that someone has to tell the hard Truth, he must mention that this is a very significant change, or modification. The implications are so far-reaching that the entire practice would lose the credibility of being called the *Kriya* approach.

In his teaching of *Omkar Kriyas,* Yogananda made three changes:

1. He modified the nature of the head movement.

2. He changed the place for *Viksha* (begging).

3. Also, his teaching instructs that the last three *aksaras* of the *Mantra* be put in places which are different than in original *Kriya* tradition.

If the *Mantra* is chanted in the wrong places, bad results are produced. Lahiri Mahasay clearly wrote in two of his *Letters to the Disciples* that one should practice strictly according to the instructions.

"Many put attention in each center and do not make *Japa* in each center. In this case, the practice becomes negative. Therefore, during the practice of *Pranayam,* or *Kriya*, *Japa* should be made properly at the six centers in the Spine." p. 58, *Lahiri Mahasay's Personal Letters to Kriya Disciples* by the author.

"Making oneself interiorized during inhaling and exhaling, *Japa* should be proper at each center. If such *Japa* is not practiced strictly according to the instructions, then the *Kriya* practice becomes negative." p. 58, *Lahiri Mahasay's Personal Letters to Kriya Disciples* by the author.

In his teaching, Yogananda made no mention of the Fifth *Omkar Kriya* and all the remaining higher *Kriyas* simply because he was not taught by Sriyukteswar who himself did not receive these from Lahiri Mahasay.

It would be appropriate to mention some references here on this point. The references of Sixth and Seventh *Kriyas* are found in the letters of Lahiri Mahasay's disciples.

"I practice in the evening as follows: *Pranayam* 108, the second *Pranayam* 28, the third *Pranayam* with *thokar* 175, the fourth 200, the fifth 200 and the sixth 175, *Mahamudra* 9." p. 44, *Lahiri Mahasay's Personal Letters to Kriya Disciples* by the author. I practice according to the instructions of Dukori *Dada* [*Dada* means elder brother, while the word *Bhai/Vai* is an affectionate Bengali term for younger brother], 144 the first, 144 the second, 144 the third, 288 the work of meditation, staying inside, 336 the fifth [*Kriya*], with *Mantras*, and in tranquility 12 X 14 the sixth [*Kriya*] with *Mantras*, and later the seventh [*Kriya*]." p, 68, *Lahiri Mahasay's Personal Letters to Kriya Disciples* by the author.

The reference of the fifth *Kriya* is found in the Lahiri Mahasay's reply.

"When some *Kriyanwits* receive higher [*Uccha*] *Kriya*, then they think they shall not have to practice *Pranayam*. For this reason sometimes among the advanced *Kriyanwits* there is confusion. You should practice six hundred *Pranayam*, fifty/sixty *Mahamudra*, *Navi Kriya* and the fourth and fifth *Kriya*." Pp. 38 & 40, *Lahiri Mahasay's Personal Letters to Kriya Disciples* by the author.

In fact, there are 108 steps of *Kriyas* in the original *Kriya* discipline.

Yogananda, during his young days, learned meditation from the Radha Swami group. They emphasized meditation on *Jyoti* (Light) and *Nada* (Sound). He was benefited by the Light in his life on many occasions. He was so influenced by the Light that he even named a *mudra* for it, called *Jyotimudra*. There is no reference in the Vedic Scripture of *Jyotimudra*.

In fact, there is *Yonimudra* in the original *Kriya* tradition. As a matter of fact, Yogananda took some part of *Yonimudra*, especially the Light aspect of it, and called it *Jyotimudra*, since the word *Jyoti* in Sanskrit means "Light."

(NOTE – *Yoni* literally means, sex organ, birth place. In *Kriya*, it means the place of creation of the individual self, that is, *Kutastha*, in between the eyebrows.)

In teaching his *Jyotimudra*, Yogananda changed the positions of the index fingers from the original *Kriya* tradition, so that the practitioner could easily have a glimpse of the flash of light between the eyebrows due to the pressure on points of meridian lines.

Thus, one assumes the flash of light generated in this way to be inner Light. In fact, inner Light, as well as inner Sound, are produced and generated from the tranquil Breath.

The flash of light produced from the pressures on the nerves is not inner Light, not to speak of tranquil inner Light; since it is not produced from the tranquil Breath generated through the practice of *Pranayam*.

In reality, *Talabya Kriya,* or *Khecharimudra,* helps transcend three sensations (smelling, tasting and touching). *Yonimudra* helps transcend two sensations (seeing and hearing - that is, light and sound).

In the original *Kriya* tradition, one is advised to practice by integrating both the *mudras* and simultaneously to dissolve the operation of the five sensations.

The question arises: Since *Kriya* is a positive science, if the integrative aspect of the approach to *Kriyas* is disturbed, how could the practice dissolve five sensations simultaneously, when major parts which deal with four sensations are dropped from the practice? The obvious answer is that it is doubtful.

To put it in plain English, can anyone fill up a pot with water, pouring from the top, when there are four big holes at the bottom? You know the answer.

A devotee commented the other day, that perhaps, observing his Western followers' difficulties, Yogananda, being kind, simplified the *Kriya* approach for them.

Towards the end of dissolution of the individual self, according to the original *Kriya* tradition, integration of *Talabya Kriya*, *Yonimudra* and *Omkar Kriyas* is very much necessary.

On the contrary, in the modified *Kriya* trend *Talabya Kriya* or *Khecharimudra* is dropped, *Yonimudra* is partly practiced in the form of *Jyotimudra*, and *Omkar Kriyas* are practiced with several modifications without first doing anything with *Talabya Kriya.*

So the question remains to be answered as to whether the modified *Kriya* trend would work for the practitioner? Is it possible to conduct an experiment in the laboratory of physics (physical body of the seeker) when all the equipment is assembled on the table and the electricity, that is, the power line (in this case, the *Talabya Kriya,* or *Khecharimudra*) is not connected?

During the author's stay at Ranchi (when they tried to recruit the author) in October, 1972, he wanted to test the spirit of the joint secretary YSS (American) as to whether the joint secretary could digest the author's outspoken character.

The author asked him, "Perhaps, you have heard by now, that there is a controversy in India about Yogananda's teachings of *Kriya* in a liberal way, what are your comments about the modifications of the integrated aspect of *Kriya* by Yogananda?"

He said, "*Guruji* [he meant Yogananda; the author is not aware if he had met Yogananda.] experimented, then taught."

Then the author asked him, "What can you tell me about your president? She came first time to India known as sister. Now the printed papers here say *Mata* (means mother). She was then president, the head of your organization, so who made her Mata?"

The joint secretary did not reply to the question. He prepared to leave abruptly. Then the author asked him, "If nobody made her such, then was it self styled?" He then left speedily and entered the office, leaving the author in the verandah of Ranchi asram. His actions were understood. The author then left to go to the garden on the campus.

The joint secretary's comment brings another question. A realized person's experimental techniques have every chance of being influenced by his own realized state, but whether or not this would be workable and beneficial to the ignorant and ordinary seeker is questionable.

Conclusion on Modifications in General

In conclusion it can be pointed out that in the Vedic culture there are many spiritual disciplines; for example, *Jnana Yoga, Raja Yoga, Kriya Yoga, Karma Yoga, Bhakti Yoga, Tantra Yoga, Mantra Yoga* and *Laya Yoga,* etc.

These ancient oriental spiritual disciplines propagated by the ancient yogis have no inadequacy in themselves. These are the paths to Eternity. All these paths are there to cover the various sentiments of the whole human spectrum, so that everyone should have a path of his own.

In the words of Paramhansa Sri Ramakrisna, "*Jata mat tata path* - As many as there are sentiments, opinions, or convictions, among men, that number of paths there are."

In other words, each individual self must find his enrichment, contentment, and fuller life in the state of inner Realization of the ultimate Self.

Each path has its own rules and regulations; each path is complete in itself, a proven path. Some ancient yogis among the realized have revealed the message, or the discipline.

It will be in the fitness of righteous spirit to accept the discipline in entirety with all its implications.

No one, Indian or Western yogi, has any right to amend, modify, or adjust anything of an ancient Indian spiritual discipline. In fact, there is no room for it, as the disciplines are all proven paths to Eternity.

Western devotees visit India and study in some hermitage for a time to learn some spiritual discipline and return to the West. Some study in the West under an Indian Yogi. Then they start their own schools and teach in Europe and in the U.S.A.. They add more techniques, developed by themselves, to the discipline that they have studied. In the name of making the discipline more powerful and effective, they add techniques of their own.

(NOTE - In the light of *Kriya*, 'Studying' does not mean learning the discipline in the conventional way; rather 'Studying' means 'dissolving the intellect and holding onto the supreme Self.')

In fact, they are in a confused frame of mind wherein it never occurs to them that the discipline they learned is complete in itself and there is no room for improving it. All they are doing is showing their egotistic and imaginary experiments. They are trying to accommodate their own weaknesses in the name of making a spiritual discipline more effective. They want to add their contributions, rather confusions, to the discipline.

Neither do these novices understand the path of Eternity, nor do they realize anything. Had they realized, they would have developed the spirit of tranquility, contentment, and found eternal Silence and Peace.

Instead, they developed eagerness to show their ego, trying to help others in the name of God's work. It is the same old game of displaying ego; and starting a school or organization is a good way to display it.

In society, in the average person's mind, the common psychology to measure realization of a yogi or sage is to see how big his organization is. It never occurs to them that organizations, groups, buildings, and numbers of centers, are not the true vehicle to measure the state of inner Realization of a Yogi. The whole world is his reflection and for that matter all are in him.

In India, the spiritual teachings are handed down through Master to disciple which is called *Guru-param-para.* It is the righteous way (discussed in the tenth chapter of the book, *the Original Kriya* by the author). It is a tradition; it has its own value and place.

In the Vedic society, it is inconceivable to amend a spiritual discipline or the tradition since there is no space of inadequacy in the established and proven disciplines.

A Westerner, growing up in the Christian culture, which basically has one discipline, the path of Love, cannot even conceive of the seriousness of amending a proven spiritual path of the Vedic culture. They simply fail to understand it because they are so conditioned in their minds with their 'ego trip' and ignorance.

The Conclusion on the Modified *Kriya*

It seems the original pure *Kriya* tradition is a proven discipline while the modified *Kriya* trend is an experimental discipline based on Yogananda's liberal method of teachings.

On the face of all these substantial changes and modifications, it can be pointed out that one should keep one's mind open and check it out for oneself and do not allow oneself to be deceived.

If one concentrates on Babaji and Lahiri Mahasay and reads their message and lifestyle between the lines, one will understand that Babaji and Lahiri Mahasay are the role models for the renunciates and householders respectively.

Mahamuni Babaji and Lahiri Mahasay both specifically advised not to develop organizations around the teachings of *Kriya*.

Now, we know why both Babaji and Lahiri Mahasay specifically advised their disciples to remain free from being involved in organizations. Yet many could not help themselves, in terms of *karma,* because of their particular providential debris.

It can be safely said that the *Guru-param-para* is the righteous way of learning any spiritual discipline: that is, the seeker has to learn directly from the mouth of the *Guru*, in a personal relationship.

On the contrary, the learning of any spiritual discipline through easily available materials, such as, lessons, books, literature, lectures, seminars, and through organizations, is not the righteous way. Learning through these means could never solve the subtle problems of the seeker.

In fact, the *Guru-Sakti*, "the power of the *Guru*" is not there, because there is no *Guru-Sparsa*, "touch of the *Guru*," which is required to ignite or invoke the blessings of the *Guru*. The inner Realization of the ultimate Self is beyond the scope of comprehension even by the sharp and subtle intellect of the seeker.

The negative forces find an easy time to target and to tempt the residents of the hermitage and the people involved in the spiritual organization around the teaching of spiritual disciplines through their traditional weapons, such as name and fame, post and positions, the use of the occult powers to attract more people as followers, and the development of bigger organizations in the name of God's works.

In fact, the style of the negative forces to attack the seeker is very sophisticated and subtle. Sometimes they camouflage themselves to the seeker in the name of positive forces; for example, the seeker may think, "I shall be the honest seeker of truth, I will love God, with all my heart I will serve God, I will be the honest servant of God, I will be the humble servant of God, I will be the best teacher, etc." The seeker is not aware of what is happening here. He or she thinks these are positive thoughts and that he or she is in the right direction; but the seeker is not aware that he or she is individualizing himself or herself, and is looking forward to his or her own enrichment and development or progress.

In doing so, the seekers are developing a strong and subtle ego and a strong base to maintain the state of dualism, instead of dissolving the ego or the individual self to merge in Oneness with the supreme Self to achieve eternal Tranquility, or *Sthirattva*. Achieving *Sthirattva* is the ultimate aim of *Kriya*, as well as of many spiritual disciplines that are aimed at providing permanent Peace through liberation from attachment and dualism.

Until the *Kriyanwit* seeker is in Oneness with the ultimate Self at the After-effect-poise of *Kriya*, he or she is not in the position to say: "I and my Father are one." And until one has achieved that state while one is living in the body here on earth, one has not achieved anything.

Brahmabit Brahmaiba bhabati, One who knows *Brahma*, the ultimate Self, becomes *Brahma*.

Atmabit Atmaiba bhabati, One who knows *Atma*, the ultimate Self, becomes *Atma*; One who knows the Father, becomes the Father.

Yogananda introduces Lessons of Correspondence Courses

It is common practice to advise seekers to read some books to prepare their minds to be aware of the discipline they are about to practice.

Characteristically, Lahiri Mahasay used to advise the seekers to read twelve verses from the *Bhagavad Gita* every day.

The Yoga path is suited to those who are calm in nature and have a body that is exceptionally good anatomically; while *bhakti* is suited to those who are emotional, devotional and affectionate in nature. Yogananda belonged to the second. His nature was observed by many people, for example:

On November 29, 1935, an excerpt from the following conversation took place. It was recorded in the book: *Talk with Sri Ramana Maharshi*.

Yogananda: How is the spiritual uplift of the people to be effected? What are the instruction to be given them?

Maharshi: They differ according to the individuals and according to the ripeness of their minds. **There cannot be any instruction *en masse.***

Finally the Yogi rose up, prayed for Sri Bhagavan's blessings for his own work and expressed great regret for his hasty return. He looked very sincere and **devoted,** even **emotional**.

Being questioned, Maharshi pointed out to Yogananda the righteous way and how instruction is to be given. The advice echoes a Bengali proverb: *Adhar vede upadesh*, "Spiritual advice or instructions must be given according to ripeness of the seeker."

It seemed Yogananda did not learn anything from Maharshi's advice.

Devotional people adore the Lord naturally. In doing so, they do not know where and when to stop; usually they are carried away; and so they fail to hold the balance, equilibrium, or tranquility.

A student of mathematics may not do well in literature and vice versa. Similarly, it is the same in the Vedic spiritual disciplines; one has to find the right discipline first; then a teacher from the same discipline.

Most Westerners do not understand this point at all because they are exposed only to one discipline, the devotional path of the love of Jesus. They think, when they are to practice a spiritual discipline, they can qualify and practice any discipline, and with this thought they fall into the trap of their ego.

Thus the introduction of written lessons through a correspondence course or mass education and to impart *Kriya* discipline through mass initiation is wrong for the following reasons:

1. There is no room for generalized instructions or advice in a spiritual discipline.
2. Each seeker has different providential background and ripeness for which he must be evaluated personally and individually by his *Guru*.
3. The purpose of meditation, or practicing *Kriya*, is to go beyond thoughts while the lessons burden the seeker with thoughts.
4. No lessons of the correspondence course can replace advice from the "Living lips of the *Guru* [the state of *Guruvaktragamya*]."
5. A *Guru* has a tremendous responsibility to advise at the right time and not before.

We are going to elaborate on these points.

1. There is no room for generalized instructions or advice in a spiritual discipline.

As we have seen in Maharshi Ramana's answer to Yogananda, there is no scope for generalized advice or instruction in spiritual disciplines. Generalized **instruction *en masse* for a group will inevitably lead to confusion** and some will be affected mentally and physically. Practicing under the generalized instructions for mass education, the seekers will jeopardize their spiritual lives.

Example: Many of Yogananda's followers, being affected physically and mentally, discontinued their years of modified *Kriya* practice. They formed groups to help each other, and also are seeking help from the health professionals. They are of such a large number that many counselors in the Los Angeles area call it a 'syndrome' after the name of his organization.

2. Because of different providential background and ripeness, each seeker needs to be evaluated, diagnosed and then his spiritual discipline should be chosen. Thereafter, the question of advice arises. Advice should be in such a way so that the disciple will be able to complete his providential debris to be free from such bondage.

His *Guru* must evaluate and diagnose his needs to match his providential background so that the advice is appropriate to his practice or else the seeker will be confused with generalized advice and the practice will not be effective to work through one's providential debris.

For example, after *Kriya* initiation at Dunagiri Hill, Himalayas, Lahiri Mahasay requested Babaji if he could enter into the order of Swami and follow him; but Mahamuni Babaji, considering Lahiri Mahasay's providential, background sent him back to his household life to complete his providences.

In a marketplace, in group initiation, the scope of personal relationship and the chance of having advice from the living lips of the *Guru* is destroyed; as a result, the seeker is in a precarious position from the very first day.

Lahiri Mahasay used to give advice personally and individually. Sometimes, he advised one of the spouses separately, when the situation so required.

3. The purpose of meditation, or practicing *Kriya*, is to go beyond thoughts and to attain the state of *Sthirattva*, eternal Tranquility.

The introduction of written lessons overburden the student with thoughts and feelings; instead of decreasing one's thoughts, the unnecessary and untimely advice through voluminous written lessons increases one's thoughts and feelings. Thus the introduction of written lessons in *Kriya* discipline is **counterproductive**. The seekers get confused regarding their spiritual duties, in the context of *Kriya* discipline.

The fundamental and basic feature of the Original *Kriya* is **to practice *niskam karmas*, that is, practicing *Kriya* without expectations of the results of the practice.**

4. No lessons of the correspondence course can replace the "Living lips of the *Guru*."

The inherent mystic Power in the living lips of a *Guru* generates in the following manner. The *sabda*, or "sound" of the word of speech (*bak*) from the mouth of the *Guru* comes directly from awakened *Kundalini* (mystic Energy) from the coccygeal center to the throat through the spinal cord where it strikes the *swarayantra*, larynx, to vibrate and to create sound; then it travels to the mouth. Thereafter, it comes out from the mouth as *bak* (speech), which is *Bagdevi*, Goddess of Speech, or *Swarasati* (coming from *Swarayantra*, larynx), Goddess of Knowledge. That is why the *Guru Gita* says:

Dhyanangmulang Gurormurti pujamulang guro padam.
Mantramulang Gurorbakyang mokshamulang Guro kripa.

Guru Gita 38

The verse says, "This is the image of *Guru* and root of meditation. Basically, worship is the practicing of *Kriya*. *Kriyas* are the legs (*Charan*) of *Guru*. Verbal Speech (instructions from the "living lips of *Guru*") is the sound of *OM*, that is, the essence of all the *Mantras*. Holding onto the After-effect-poise of *Kriya* is the instrument for attaining eternal Liberation." *Guru Gita* 38, Commentary by Lahiri Mahasay.

According to the verse, the *bakya* or speech from the living lips of the *Guru* is *mantra* for the disciple.

(It must be pointed out here that the speech must be from the living lips of the *Guru* and not from the speech recorded by a mechanical device, either of a living or dead teacher).

This is how sound from awakened *Kundalini* Power through the living lips of the *Guru* becomes *mantra* for the disciple and practicing *Kriya* with *mantra* infuses *Atmajnan*, or Self-Knowledge, to the mind and spirit of the seeker.

The absence of *sabda*, or "sound.," or "words," from the *Guru's* awakened *Kundalini* Power is like conducting an experiment in the physics laboratory with all the equipment without connecting the electrical power. As you can imagine the experiment goes nowhere; in fact, it cannot start at all.

Similarly, learning from lessons and modified *Kriya*, having no words from the living lips of a *Guru,* the practice is ineffective even from the very beginning.

As mentioned before, from the spiritual point of view, the whole practice is nothing but a physical and mechanical exercise.

5. A teacher has a tremendous responsibility to advise at the right time and not before.

In this regard, in the Original *Kriya* Discipline, the teacher may be pressured by his own students (especially by those who are eager and lack understanding of the process). They may request to have more *Kriyas*.

A Story from Lahiri Mahasay's life:

Example: Once, a disciple requested Lahiri Mahasay in the midst of many attending devotees in his Benares house at Garureswar to have more *Kriyas*. Lahiri Mahasay heard the disciple's request and waited a while to answer. In the meantime, another disciple, Brinda Bhakat, a postal peon [mailman] entered the house.

Lahiri Mahasay said, "Brinda! come here. I want to give you more *Kriyas*."

Brinda said, "Baba! I have come here just to request you to please not give me any more *Kriyas*. I am sinking in joy; and I am afraid that I might be run over by a vehicle on the street while I am delivering letters."

(Actually, in Benares the houses are not separated on one side by odd numbers and the other side by even numbers (like in the U. S. A.), as a result, Brinda had to cross the street back and forth to deliver letters. It should be mentioned here that house numbers in most cities in India are in the same manner).

The disciple who pressed for more *Kriyas*, hearing Brinda's request got his answer and kept his head bent down.

Another example of advising at the **right time and not before** can be cited here from the Kurukshetra War of *Dwapara Yuga*.

(One has to understand that there is a **right-combination** between the positive and the negative, which positive force would kill which negative and **when** [at the **right moment**] according to providence. Then again, it varies according to the individual.

(The inner War of positive and negative forces through meditation or *Kriya* practice, is a very subtle and complicated one; and hence, without the direct, personalized advice from the living lips of the *Guru* is not possible to win.)

The war between the cousins, the *Kauravas* and the *Pandavas* to regain the empire, lasted for eighteen days. The example is taken from the battlefield of fourteenth day.

(We are going to reproduce it here briefly. For a detailed description of the fourteenth day battle of the *Kurukhestra* war the reader may see the present author's title: The *Mahabhrata*, Commentaries Volume 2, pages 262- 274.)

On the thirteenth day the negative side killed Arjuna's son, Abhimanyu: ACTIVELY BEING CONSCIOUSNESS, violating all rules of war.

In the evening, returning from the battlefield, Arjuna learned of the terrible event. After inquiring from King Yudhisthira, Arjuna became aware that at the gate Jayadratha (who had blessings from Lord Siva to prevail over four *Panvdavas*) obstructed reinforcement and assistance to his son. So he held Jayadratha responsible for his son's death.

So Arjuna, ENERGY OF THE SEEKER'S BODY, vowed to kill Jayadratha, COURAGE TO DO NEGATIVE THINGS; failing to perform his vow before the sun set, Arjuna would kill himself in the fire.

At the beginning of the fourteenth day, when the *Pandava* armies came to the battlefield, they observed that on the *Kaurava* side, Dronacharya made several *vhuhas*, military strategies arrayed one behind the other:

In the front, *Chakravyuha* (circular formation), then *Sakatavyuha* (wedge formation), then *Padmavyuha* (lotus formation) and finally *Suchya-vyuha*, or the needle formation). Then at the end of the needle formation, Jayadratha was stationed and protected by able generals. The purpose was that Arjuna might not have time to pass through all of these during the entire day and would fail to reach Jayadratha and thereby not be able to kill Jayadratha and, therefore, have to kill himself being true to his vow.

Krisna and Arjuna stationed Satyaki (disciple of Arjuna in weapons) to protect King Yudhisthira from Dronacharya. They said until they returned from killing Jayadratha, Satyaki must under no circumstances leave King Yudhisthira. It was very important. They could not trust what Dronacharya, the old

Brahmana, then the commander-in-chief of the *Kauravas*, might do. Krisna and Arjuna did not see anybody who would be a good match for Dronacharya except Satyaki.

Both Krisna and Arjuna took off to find Jayadratha.

After fighting the whole day, finally, ENERGY OF THE SEEKER'S BODY (Arjuna) found Jayadratha and approached COURAGE TO DO NEGATIVE THINGS (Jayadratha), but only a very short time was left. COURAGE TO DO NEGATIVE THINGS (Jayadratha) was surrounded by six divisions of chariots led by six prominent generals.

Lord Krisna then advised Arjuna, "The sun is about to set, but there is still time for you to keep your vow. I will create clouds on the western horizon so that the *Kauravas* will think that the sun has set. Take this opportunity to kill Jayadratha." So through yogic powers, Lord Krisna created a volley of dark clouds to hide the sun.

King Jayadratha, observing the darkened sky thought to himself, "I am safe now. Evening has approached." Lord Krisna then said to Arjuna, "**Now is the time** [**right time**] to kill Jayadratha. He is off guard. Quickly cut off his head and fulfill your vow."

Arjuna released a large crescent-shaped *anjalika* arrow which flew through the air like Indra's fiery thunderbolt aimed at Jayadratha's neck, whereupon Jayadratha's head was chopped off. Lord Krisna then commanded Arjuna, "Quickly send the severed head through the air guided by arrows straight to the lap of Jayadratha's father who is sitting in his evening meditation outside the battlefield (*Samantapanchaka*). Place it down very gently."

(Arjuna did not know even for a moment before the right time that he had to send the severed head of Jayadratha outside the battlefield on his father's lap.

(Krisna was waiting for the event to take place; when Arjuna accomplished this feat, only then did he consider that it was the right time to advise to send the severed head outside the battlefield where Jayadratha's father was meditating.

(Thus the teacher or the *Guru* has tremendous responsibility not to impart the disciple with advice in advance which could confuse or overburden the disciple's mind and prevent him from concentrating properly. Thus Yogananda's lessons can be counterproductive.)

In the absence of *Guruvaktragamya*, learning from the living lips of the *Guru*, the seeker is deprived of the right doses of advice to eliminate vibrations and to get rid of his providences in the right time. How can he make an effective spiritual life? How can he win the battle in meditation?

An organization cannot contribute to enhancing one's spirituality, and those who are involved, rendering social service in the name of God's work, simply support themselves by the donations they collect and confuse others regarding the performance of their spiritual practice without attachment to results.

These so-called renunciates, themselves, are not clear about the true path of *Niskam Karma* (practice without attachment to the results therefrom), which is the fundamental basis of achieving eternal Tranquility, or Liberation.

How can they help others when they are themselves involved with organizational debris?

As the proverb goes: It is like the blind leading the blind.

The Traditional Way of Disposing the Body According to the Hindu Rite

After Sriyukteswar left body (1936), Yogananda brought a former Ranchi student, his disciple, Sudhir Choudhuri, made him Swami Sevananda Giri and put him in charge of Puri Karar Ashram. It was he who removed the sign board of Puri Karar Ashram and put up a new one reading Yogoda Ashram.

After about nine years, in 1945, he left the asram and joined his beloved Principal of Ranchi Brahmacharya Vidyalay (high school), Swami Satyananda, who left Ranchi in early 1941. At that time, Satyananda being the Asram Swami of Puri and the third president of Sadhu Sova, sent his disciple Swami Ushananda (Later, Swami Hariharananda, not to be confused with Swami Hariharananda of Puri who was there after Ushananda left Puri) to Puri Asram to take charge.

After some years, Sevananda wanted to live at Haridwar. So Swami Satyananda requested his good friend, Swami Mahadevananda, the president of Bholananda Giri Sannyas Ashram of Haridwar, to accommodate Sevananda.

Accordingly, he moved to Haridwar. Swami Mahadevananda asked Sevananda, if "*Viraja Hom*" part of *sannyas* vow was observed during his *sannyas*. Sevananda said he did not think so. Then Mahadevananda said, "it has to be done again, technically and strictly, without *Viraja Hom* the vow of *sannyan* is not completed.". So *Viraja Hom* had to be performed before he was taken to their ashram.

When Yogananda took *sannyas* from Sriyukteswar in 1915, he was young, only twenty two years old; perhaps he was not aware of it. Even if he was aware, being liberal and not being able to follow rules, he had a tendency to violate the Vedic Culture, Vedic tradition and the rules.

Whenever he violated the rules, Satyananda reminded him once, and then left it to his decision. Examples, when he planned to found Yogoda Sat Sanga, Satyananda said, *Yogoda* is incorrect in Sanskrit; it should be *Yogad*. Yogananda said, "For us, everything is fine." Again, Yogananda informed Satyananda that he was thinking to make his American disciple, James J. Lynn, President of Yogoda. Satyananda wrote, "I will be the first person to come out from your organization [since, in Vedic Tradition, Swami does not serve under the householders], but if he entered some sort of renunciate order, then I will not have any problem". Yogananda wrote, "Then forget it".

When Satyananda met Sister Daya, he also reminded her in front of this writer thinking the American lady may not be aware of the Vedic Tradition that there were some Swamis in the organization. She appointed an outsider and a householder, Mr. Binay Narayan Dube as general secretary. Swamis do not serve under the householder in the Vedic Tradition. She replied, "I need this man to revive Guruji's ashram".

In Vedic Culture, most people are cremated, and are hardly ever buried; when they are buried it is not in a casket like in the Christian tradition, but the body is put in the ground with four/five hundred pounds of salt to decompose the body.

As mentioned, the average Hindu used the process of cremation. Lahiri Mahasay was cremated at Manikarnika *ghat* at Benares. There was a note found in Lahiri Mahasay's diary that when he dies, at that time, he wanted his body to be buried, that he may rise again; when he wrote that note he did not complete his realization and when the note was found it was too late

Regarding the Swamis, there are two different ways. First, to bury in the ground like Sriyukteswar and Satyananda were; second, put in the current of a river or in the water (this process is called *Salil Samadhi*: *salil* means water);

like Trailanga Swami was put in the Ganges at Benares. He was a good friend of Lahiri Mahasay.

For the violator of Vedic Tradition, in liberal Yoganada's case, none of these happened; his body is still lying in some park at Los Angeles. Daya wanted to bring it to their center, but the city did not allow it.

The Conclusion

The Modified *Kriya* followers, Yogananda's disciples Kriyananda and Roy Eugene Davis were highly interested in the Lahiri Mahasay's materials (manuscripts), especially the *Bhagavad Gita* and *Yoga Sutras* of Patanjali. Swamiji Maharaj knew that they would not be able to understand at all the original *Kriya* interpretations.

Since they were taught the philosophy of prosperity, and not renunciation (*phalakankharahit*), how could they understand the ancient pure original *Kriya*?

Being highly motivational (attached with the results), they only knew how to compete with their organizational skills.

It seems Yogananda showed to his followers how to be prosperous and successful in material life (in the garb of proud spiritual beings) and if necessary to protect their interests and engage in the path of litigation instead of liberation.

In the next chapter, we will discuss them and present their letters.

Chapter 7

The Interested Publishers

Hereunder, there is a list of very enthusiastic, tempted, presumptuous, and aggressive publishers for the highly sensitive information about the original pure form of *Kriya* discipline. Since *Kriya Yoga* is internationally known, some had a vested interest in this information and some saw a potential goldmine. They are as follows:

1) Kriyananda, disciple of Yogananda,
2) Roy Eugene Davis, disciple of Yogananda,
3) Motilal Banarsidass, Publisher, New Delhi, India,
4) Arurverlag, Germany,
5) Mrs. Michele Champy, French lady (Atmananda Mission),
6) Ranjit Ganguly, West Bengal, India.

And Others from the following countries:

7) Bulgaria (formerly a Communist country) could not resist the temptation and already translated a book without valid permission and so was advised to destroy the translation.
8) One gentleman (Marcel Jullion) from Lyon, France translated a few chapters and sought permission, later which was denied.
9) One from Portugal was seeking permission to translate into Portuguese.
10) One from Slovakia (one of the oldest publishing houses in the country) requested twice. Permission was denied.
11) One from Russia, the permission was denied.

The scriptures of the vast Vedic culture are not like the one holy book of the Jews (Written Torah), of the Christians (the Old and New Testaments of the Bible), or of the Islamic people (the Holy Quran).

There are so far as many as one hundred twelve (112) *Upanisads*, innumerable *Puranas*, *Smriti Sastras, Yoga and Tantras Sastras* (scriptures) in the Vedic culture.

However, the message of all these vast and voluminous scriptures can be summarized in one book which has all the essential elements, that is, *The Bhagavad Gita*. It has eighteen chapters (18) comprising seven hundred (700) verses.

Again, out of these seven hundred verses only one verse can explicitly express the spirit of the teachings of the entire *Bhagavad Gita.*

Karmanyebadhikaraste ma phalesu kadachana.
Ma karmaphalaheturbhurma te sangayastwakarmani.
The Bhagavad Gita 2:47

The verse says, "You have the right to work only, but never to expect the results from your actions. You should not be the cause of making the results from your actions, nor should you have attachment to inaction either."

Once again, we have to remember the explanation of the "Law of *Karmas*", the results are in the hands of the Lord of Providence (*Daiba*).

If the actions performed in the previous lives by the individual *jiva* (*jivatma*) had no chance to give results to the performer in that life and in the meantime, the body dies, the results of those actions formulate the providence (*prarabddha Karma*), and so the balance of the results of the past lives carry forward to the current life.

When the individual being (*jiva*) performs actions in the current life, often the results are given from the previous life's balance carried forward by the deity in-charge of the providence, *Niyati* or *Bidhatri*, the one who awards the results. She is very hard (*kathin*) and tough (*kathor*).

That is why one has no way of knowing whether one will get the results at all.

Usually the man expects high, though destiny might have decreed against him, and he receives happiness or sorrow as it might chance. Binding himself into the results through expectation [*vasana*], he attracts bondage into the cycle of birth and death and cannot release himself.

The above paragraph needs explanation. According to the Yoga systems (whether one believes it or not, yet, it is the science, happens to every individual regardless of one's belief system) life is construed mainly with the results of providence (*prarabddha karmas*).

Because of the many lives one is living, one after another, the accumulation of the providence becomes a Himalayan height. They stay in the individual's continuous life system.

During the formation of the next life some of them eagerly stand in a line to be packaged, as they are waiting for a long time being impatient. Sometimes, they already had missed a chance in the previous incarnation. That is why they start pushing and dashing in line impatiently. That is one reason why most portions of the next life are filled in with these providential results or debris. That is the reason why some people do not understand certain things when these happen in due course. In a guessing game, one can say that 90% of the current life is filled with providence and only 10% left with things to do with free will.

The current life is a big battle between the providence (destiny) and the person's free will (will power).

It must be pointed out that Providence has to be enjoyed or suffered according to the nature of the actions performed and by the performer only. There is no escape from it, as the works had been done in the past life and it had no chance to give results.

Most importantly, providence has no law of limitation. It stays in the system of the individual. Also, in the meantime, it increases like interest owed.

The only comforting thing of providence is, when it gives results, it releases the person and it does not last longer than it has its tenure.

On the practical plane, the reason nowadays man and woman are changing their life partners is because when one of the partners in the relationship, or even marriage, sees the destined man or woman partner, as per providence, the parties make their move faster as both attract each other; the tremendous powers start working with the force of providence and the party deserts the living partner immediately, who becomes totally stunned and devastated and begins to search for reasons as to what he or she has done wrong in the relationship. No reason can be found as it was rooted in the previous life's activities. What a nightmare for the losing partner! But wait, he or she will be fine. After a while the losing partner will find the destined other partner and life will go on. Since they had messed up their lives even in the previous life how can they expect to finish with one partner the rest of their life in the current one?

As mentioned, the most important thing in spiritual life in adopting any spiritual discipline is one needs to abandon the expectation of the results of practice. That is why Lahiri Mahasay, the polestar of *Kriya*, put two fundamental conditions in the *Kriya* discipline.

1) Practice every day strictly according to the instruction one receives from his *Guru's* mouth (*Guruvraktagamya*).

2) Abandoning the expectation of the results of the practice of *Kriya* (*Phalakangkharahit*).

It seems Yogananda had completely forgotten the second fundamental condition when he was teaching the philosophy of prosperity to the American devotees.

James Donald Walters (Kriyananda), disciple of Yogananda

Naturally the question arises, how can the disciple of Yogananda be able to understand the true spirit of *Kriya*?

Both Kriyananda and Roy Eugene Davis, disciples of Yogananda although were not highly educated, met Yogananda in 1949 just after their high school graduation. How can they understand, at such young age and such a short period of association (only 3 or 4 years), with a teacher who was teaching just the opposite philosophy of *Kriya* (the philosophy of prosperity). Whereas the true spirit of *Kriya* is the spirit of Renunciation of the material world as well as the reward of merits of the practice?

One has to remember where Swamiji (Swami Satyeswarananda) was coming from. On the academic side, Swamiji has an M. A. degree in philosophy, specializing in Vedanta philosophy, and a law degree, both from the Calcutta University, and *Vidyaratna,* a special degree in Sanskrit. He was an attorney and a law professor. On the spiritual side, since the age of eleven he was associated twenty years with Swami Satyananda who was the boyhood best friend of Yogananda, and who became Sriyukteswar's chief disciple in India, the leader of the East appointed by Sriyukteswar himself. Thereafter, leaving the law practice as an attorney and law professor, spending the next twelve years in the Dunagiri Hills, Himalayas, for a secluded meditative life, and under the instruction of Mahamuni Babaji having been commissioned by him to present the *Kriya* interpretation of Lahiri Mahasay to re-establish the original *Kriya*, Swamiji landed in the United States.

Swamiji was eight years a residential student in the YSS Vidyapith (high school). As a result, he was fully aware of the situation of Yogananda's modified *Kriya* teaching and practice in India as well as in the United States.

On their part, the disciples of Yogananda were thinking that they were quite capable and confident to edit and publish the books. All they needed to do was to look at the manuscripts (or just have the manuscripts). Since they had written books and published them, they considered themselves experienced.

Ordinarily speaking, there would be justification of their claim; but not with Lahiri Mahasay's *Kriya* interpretations of twenty six classical Indian scriptural texts with the technicalities of Yoga and Sanskrit, when even their *Guru*, Yogananda, did not venture into any Indian scripture (which are all in Sanskrit, the language of God) except the *Bhagavad Gita* which is much of Sriyukteswar's *Gita* interpretation (in Bengali). Sriyukteswar published only the first nine chapters. He admitted there were mistakes (admitted to Satyananda) on those, and it needed corrections if it was published again. Swamiji has translated it into English and published it. (The *Bhaagvad Gita* interpretations of Swami Sriyukteswar, ISBN No. 1877854123). One can see that Yogananda had copied the features of Sriyukteswar's presentations without giving him credit.

(In this respect, one should see in the Sanskrit Classics section what Swamiji had laid down about the vibrations of the letter - *akshara* in the Sanskrit literature in which all the Indian scriptures of *Vedic* disciplines are written.

(Some relevant paragraphs are mentioned from the section of the Sanskrit Classics here as follows:

(Each odd letter (*Aksara*) of the alphabet contains a smaller degree and number of atoms of inner Light and atoms of inner Sound; while each even letter contains a greater degree and number of atoms of inner Light and atoms of inner Sound. The word, therefore, expresses the composite vibrations of inner Light and inner Sound depending on how many odd letters and even letters there are in the word.

(Similarly, a sentence carries the composite degree of vibrations of inner Light and inner Sound depending on how many words are there in a sentence.

(For example, "Sanskrit" is an English word, its equivalent is *Samaskrita*. If the word *Samaskrita* is scanned it will be two words: *Sama* means "Tranquility," and *krita* means "done." Therefore, *Samaskrita* means "the state of Tranquility;" it happens when the restless breath is made tranquil.

(So the word *Samaskrita* for a Yogi and spiritual person is the "state of tranquility of the breath;" while for a linguist it is the name of an ancient language and for an intellectual it is merely a word, indicative of an ancient language. From all the words and sentences they want to make a meaningful concept which makes SENSE.

(Unfortunately, Spirituality or the Self is beyond all senses including reason and thoughts. That is why the intellectuals call "Spirituality," the world of mystics. Therefore, as far as the intellectuals are concerned, they are BARRED to the spiritual world; until they get *mantras* and till they make the *mantra* conscious (*mantra chaitanya* – making the *mantra* alive by constant practice), they will remain blind and will live in the world of intellectual fools.

(Swamiji had to transfer the atoms of inner Light and the atoms of inner Sound from the verses of the Sanskrit texts and from the Bengali interpretations of Lahiri Mahasay, making an appropriate "Interface" of the accumulated vibrations of the message into English language.

(How can only an English knowing person or an intellectual editor have penetration into the world of vibrations when their primary concern and focus would be only to express the well meaning concepts with flowery words with their assumption that the materials are perfection?

(Here is an example; in the beginning, once, an American devotee mentioned, "Baba! this sentence is missing the verb". Swamiji looked at the sentence and said, "You have your problem, and I have mine."

(The devotee was looking at the grammar of the sentence and he was right in his place; while Swamiji was looking at the accumulative vibrations of inner Light and inner Sound, and from the point of view of denotation and connotation to present the pure Consciousness of the Self in the message; again, keeping in the mind the "Interface" from Sanskrit and Bengali. If he used a verb it will disturb the total vibrations and so Swamiji changed some word of the sentence to accommodate the verb not suggested by the devotee but Swamiji selected his own verb which in devotee's opinion was not exactly an appropriate verb but could make "sense." This is what Swamiji meant - "it is all they want to see that it makes sense from their grammatical and intellectual point of view;" which is the world of the intellectuals and linguists. Just the opposite of the spirituality where vibration of the pure Consciousness is the primary concern and Swamiji was concerned to see that it remain intact in the presentation.

(To Swamiji, it was ridiculous to give the books for editing and publishing to Kriyananda or Roy Eugene Davis, or to the other publishers as well, for this reason).

May 7, 1982

Swami Satyeswarananda
P.O. Box 9823
Santee, CA 92071

Dear Swamiji,

Thank you for your recent letter, and welcome to America.

I think I may be able to help you with publishers, and my great interest is in the manuscripts by Lahiri Mahasaya and Sri Yukteswar. If there is any way that we might be able to publish any of them, or arrange for their publication, that would certainly be our first choice, and so, of course, I would like this to be my first offer to you, before suggesting other publishers. The greatest blessing would be to see these writings shared in English, and I would like to encourage this, however it might be possible. To be able to help, I will need to see the manuscripts, and to see what I could help directly on, and what I would refer to other publishers I am in contact with. Keshava tells me that the manuscripts are still in a rough form. That is really quite all right. Being a writer myself, I think I will still be able to get a good feeling for the manuscripts, and I would like to help you get started now toward their publication so that as much of the arrangements as possible can be made while you are still in this country. I have, as yet, no plans of going to southern California soon, and I am committed to being here during July and August. For this reason, would you be kind enough to arrange to xerox and mail to me a copy of Lahiri Mahasaya's Gita and Patanjali interpretations in both English and Bengali? I would be happy to cover all of your expenses. These would be just as samples, and I would keep them in my possession and do nothing with them until a formal agreement is reached with you. Please let me know if this arrangement is agreeable to you, and let me know what the expenses will be. I am looking forward to hearing from you very soon.

Swami Kriyananda
14618 Tyler Foote Road
Nevada City, CA 95959
(916) 265-5877

In divine friendship,

Swami Kriyananda

kr/ke

May 7, 1982

Swami Satyeswarananda
P.O. Box 9823
Santee, CA 92071

Dear Swamiji,
Thank you for your recent letter, and welcome to America.

I think I may be able to help you with publishers, and my great interest is in the manuscripts by Lahiri Mahasaya and Sri Yukteswar. If there is any way that we might be able to publish any of them, or arrange for their publication, that I would like this to be my first offer to you, before suggesting other publishers. The greatest blessing would be to see these writings shared in English, and I would like to encourage this, however it might be possible. To be able to help, I will need to see the manuscripts, and to see what I could help directly on, and what I would refer to other publishers I am in contact with. Keshava tells me that the manuscripts are still in a rough form. [This sentence needs a note see below*].]That is really quite all right. Being a writer myself, I think I will still be able to get a good feeling for the manuscripts, and I would like to help you get started now towards their publication so that as much as of the arrangements as possible can be made while you are still in this country. I have, as yet, no plans of going to southern California soon, and I am committed to being here during July and August. For this reason, would you be kind enough to arrange to xerox and mail to me a copy of Lahiri Mahasaya's Gita and Patanjali interpretations in both English and Bengali? I would be happy to cover all of your expenses. These would be just as samples, and I would keep them in my possession and do nothing with them until a formal agreement is reached with you. Please let me know if this arrangement is agreeable to you, and let me know what the expenses will be. I am looking forward to hearing from you very soon.

In divine friendship

Swami Kriyananda

kr/ke

* This is a very strange comment from out of the blue. Keshava is the Indian name of an American secretary to Kriyananda who had no way of knowing anything about the status of the manuscripts. They simply assumed that since it is prepared by an Indian man it has to be in a rough state.

(In this connection, Swamiji remembered Kriyananda's comment that Swami Satyananda's knowledge of English was poor. The attitude of these people is very strange. Swami Satyananda having secured a higher position in merit in his B.A. (Honours) in philosophy wrote the answer scripts in English more than his classmate Rash Behari Das who later became the Dr. Rash Behari Das, Prof. of philosophy at the University of Calcutta who was the guide for Swamiji in his Ph. D. program.

(On the other hand, Kriyananda was born to an America couple in Romania, Europe, and he went to school there in his childhood, then moved to America. Thus his English grammar in the school stage got confused and somehow became high school graduate).

The sentence was projected intentionally and diplomatically to create the ground for future editing, in case he was involved in the book publishing project.

(Once, Bholananda, an American living in Ranchi in YSS many years, made a trip to the Himalayas to see the place where Lahiri Mahasay was initiated before returning to the United States. A hill boy brought him to Swamiji in the evening at Dunagiri Hill, so Swamiji had to give him shelter for the night. He could not resist asking where Swamiji had learned English. In the United States too, once a lady visitor asked where Swamiji has learned English? American people are so naive, majority of them simply do not want to learn anything other than English for themselves. Many of them do not know that even before America was discovered or born, India was ruled by the British and Calcutta had dozens of English Medium Schools and several English Medium Colleges where Indian people were educated in English. The tradition is still maintained today, even more English Medium Schools and Colleges are opened in all parts of the country and are producing millions of English knowing graduates.

(Indian people, about 60%, that is, now six hundred (600) million people, are English educated; they know English very well (reading and writing) but are poor in 'fluency in spoken English' as they do not speak daily but only when it is absolutely necessary. That does not mean they are poor in English knowledge. It can be said that India today is the largest English knowing country in the world; the population of the five English speaking countries: England,

America, Canada, Australia, and New Zealand combined cannot match the number of English knowing people in India.

July 1, 1982

Swami Satyeswarananda

Dear Swamiji,

I just got back from Europe and received your letter of May 16th. I certainly respect your wishes for not wanting to share the manuscripts.

Perhaps you will find the enclosed helpful.

Swami Kriyananda
14618 Tyler Foote Road
Nevada City, CA 95959
(916) 265-5877

In divine friendship,

Swami Kriyananda

kr/ke
enclosures

July, 1, 1982

Swami Satyeswarananda
P.O. Box 9823
Santee, CA 92071

Dear Swamiji,
I just got back from Europe and received your letter of May 16th. I certainly respect your wishes for not wanting to share the manuscripts.

Perhaps you will find the enclosed helpful.

In divine friendship

Swami Kriyananda

kr/ke
enclosures

NOTE - The enclosures were four printed and four typed pages, explanations of his marriage with a young Italian lady (he called her Parameshwari). There was also a two page letter from an American lady devotee (Shibani), a founder member of Ananda Village, explaining the situation.

What a Deal!

There was a direct instruction from Yogananda to his inner circle of devotees, particularly to those who were dedicated workers with him, that they have to sacrifice and to set aside their salvation in this life to bring the teaching of Yogananda to the world. They will achieve their salvation in the next life through devotion to him.

The most devotional energetic young boys and girls, many of them fresh from the high school, some who did not finish the school, joined him. Among the girls, many were from the Mormon community (a Christian group, some of whom still believed in polygamy and living in a community set up).

The reflection of this inner circle ordinance was found in the letter of a former *brahmachari* in a ten page handwritten letter to Swamiji.

A Portion from the ten pages handwritten letter of *Brahmachari* Kebali (David Braner) to the author

BRAHMACHARI KEBALI
c/o DAVID BRANER
1951 W. Cullom Ave., #1
CHICAGO, ILL. 60613

November 14, 1985

Swami Satyeswarananda Giri

Dear Swamiji,

Thank you very much for "Biography of a Yogi," and also for the tape of Vedic Chants and, particularly, Kriya Master's songs.

"Biography of a Yogi" is a wonderful book which you have given, containing much valuable knowledge and inspiration. And I have long desired to hear the vibrations of your voice, and speaking the names of Lahiri Mahasay, Sriyukteswarji, and OM Mantra (or "twelve-accent" mantra, Lord Krishna (Basudeva) Mantra) used in

over→

2)

Omkar Kriyas. Thru the cassette tape my desire has been fulfilled.

I was first made aware of the divine sage Yogiraj Sri Sri Shyama Charan Lahiri Mahasay many, many years ago through reading "Autobiography of a Yogi" when I was a young boy of about 12 yrs. I was not much interested in school but rather in the holy science of yoga. I was inwardly praying for, and outwardly seeking, my Gurudev. I was very much attracted to Lahiri Mahasay. I often prayed intensely to him that I might somehow receive his holy Kriya techniques.

I also felt great reverence for the divine Himalayan yogi Babaji, and for Sriyukteswar. Paramhansa Yogananda, I had deep respect for— as the bringer of this higher knowledge to me thru his autobiography. I could also feel that he, himself, was a great soul, and highly advanced in yoga. In fact, I eagerly studied his books and "Praecepta" teachings.

3)

The shining jewel of my heart, however, continued to be Lahiri Mahasay.

Later, about the age of 17 years, I entered the monastic Order of Self-Realization Fellowship in California, where I eagerly hoped to receive personal guidance in the practice of Kriya Yoga. Instead, I found that this desire for deep Kriya practice was discouraged, and that service and devotion was greatly stressed as being most important. I was often told that: ...."we have already received everything that we need for Self-realization in the Praecepta teachings of Yogananda....." Further inquiry was considered wrong. A high official of the Order once told me that probably none of us (in SRF) would achieve Self-realization in this life — that we are pioneers, meant to sacrifice our salvation or set it aside in this life, in order to devote ourselves to bringing the Master's teachings — missionary-like — to the world. We would find realization, then, thru devotion to the Master, service to the

over→

4)

Cause, and divine grace. He very often quoted saints such as St. Francis, St. Theresa, & Brother Lawrence. He had known Yogananda personally and did possess much devotion, faith, and an almost fanatical attitude of dedication. He was my personal counselor.

I remained in the Order for 8 years, keeping much to myself. For this, I was criticized, but left alone. I felt great progress in the practice of Kriya, often experiencing joy and bliss in the feeling of current in the spine, and experiencing divine Light and expansion beyond body-consciousness in higher Kriya's. I also received ordination as a "Brahmachari" which I have kept all my life. I attended Kriya initiations given by the President of the Order, with reference to the First Kriya, or Pranayam, and the Second, Third, & Fourth Kriya's (as taught by Yogananda). However, I constantly felt a growing gap between my own desire for Self-realization, and what was expected of me as one w would be asked to become a touring minister of SRF (or similar position). I also

From Page 3

Later, about the age of 17 years, I entered the monastic Order of Self Realization Fellowship in California, where I eagerly hoped to receive personal guidance in the practice of *Kriya Yoga* instead, I found that this desire for deep Kriya practice was discouraged, and that service and devotion was greatly stressed as being most important. I was often told that :

"We have already received everything that we need for in the Precepta teaching of Yogananda ...

"Further inquiring was considered wrong. A high official of the Order once told me that probably none of us (in SRF) would achieve Self-Realization in this life - that we are pioneers, meant to sacrifice our salvation or set it aside in this life, in order to devote ourselves to bringing the Master's teaching - missionary like - to the world. We find realization, then, thru devotion to the Master, service to the cause, and divine grace. He very often quoted saints such as St. Francis, St. Theresa, and Brother Lawrence. He had known Yogananda personally and did possess much devotion, faith, and an almost fanatical attitude of dedication. He was my personal counselor.

"I remained in the order for 8 years, keeping much to myself. For this, I was criticized, but left alone. I felt great progress in the practice of Kriya, often experiencing joy and bliss in the feeling of current in the spine, and experiencing divine Light and expansion beyond body-consciousness in higher Kriya's . I also received ordination as a 'Brahmachari' which I have kept all my life. I attended Kriya initiation given by the President of the order, with reference to the first Kriya, or Pranayam, and the second, third, and fourth Kriya's (as taught by Yogananda)."

[The following is a comment by S. B. Dasgupta, about four higher *Kriyas* taught by Yogananda without *Khecharimundra*,

("The central or fundamental Kriya is the 'Hangsa' mantra manifesting in the form of pranayam [mystic yogic breathing]. Because of Yoganandaji's method of initiating many people at once, or because of having to learn the teaching from the Precepta Lessons, quite a few misunderstandings can come about. This has been seen in many of the practitioners in both India and America. It is imperative to correct these errors through the direct company of one's guru. Going further, one is only fit to practice the higher Kriyas after one accomplishes Khechari Mudra. This absolutely essential technique is also not very easy to attain. For this reason, Yogananda gave instructions for higher Kriyas even without Khechari. In the perspective of pure Kriya practice, this is not proper; and furthermore, the purpose of practicing higher Kriyas cannot be brought to fruition without Khechari. It seems that because of perceiving this fruitless possibility, 'mental Kriya' [mental practice] was given the emphasis in the Precepta Lessons. Mental practice is also a practice of scriptural injunction; however, the second, third, fourth and such higher Kriyas cannot ever be varied by methods such as that [mental kriya]. From the second Kriya onward, all of the higher Kriyas must be performed with Khechari Mudra. Without Khechari, neither 'Thokar' Kriya nor 'Omkar' Kriya can be performed; if anyone says otherwise, then he is not speaking about Kriya Yoga. Mental practices are proper for many other paths. But it is impossible to ever accomplish the distinctive aspects of Kriya Yoga via that method [mental kriya]." *Paramhansa Swami Yogananda Life-portrait and Reminiscences* by S. B. Dasgupta, disciple of Sriyukteswar and the private secretary of Yogananda during 1935-1936, Page 126).

The reflection of the great deal of the inner circle of Yogananda which was also found in Kriyananda's enclosures with the letter to Swamiji which were printed (October 15, 1981) for mass distribution as an explanatory measure for understanding of his recent marriage with Rosanna Golia, a young Italian lady; he called her Parameswari; follows:

"My [Kriyananda] whole life has been offered to Master for his work. Long ago I decided [Kriyananda did not decide, it was a deal from Yogananda himself for his inner circle devotees] it didn't even matter if my salvation was deferred, so long as I might serve him."

This great deal of Yogananda with his inner circle disciples, to set aside their salvations or self-realization was possible only because of their background of being young, having blind devotion, and being naive. They were innocent, and spiritually hungry.

The tradition in the Vedic culture was closely to observe a man at least twelve years before he could be given a *brahmachari* initiation; another twelve years of strict observation usually was considered for the Swami order. Yogananda being a very liberal person, quickly after the initiation of someone into *Kriya,* always had a tendency to make healthy young boys a *brahmachari* so that he could have a dedicated worker while simply providing food and shelter. His necessity was the primary consideration for him instead of considering whether the boy would qualify. In India, he practiced this style (examples - *Brahmachari* Kripananda and *Brahmachari* Robi). In the West examples were these two young high school graduates and many others like (*Brahmachari* Nerode and *Brahmachari* Khagen) in the United States. Later, if they wanted to get out of *brahmachari* vow for some reason, then Yogananda would use their own vows against them, pinching into their own conscience. He was such a practical and liberal organizer.

In fact, Kriyananda wrote Swamiji (the author) in the Himalayas having obtained that address from Krispien. He would like to buy one hundred acres of land in the Ranikhet area to start an International English School. Swamiji advised him to try either in Bengal or in other parts of India, but not in northern India.

(The reasons and explanation for not trying an International English school in north India were the following:

(Politically speaking, India never was a country. There were more than six hundred twenty five (625) kings and they had their defined territories as their kingdoms. Sometimes they had fights with the neighboring kings to conquer the other's land or the entire kingdom. It is the British during their rule in India who made India politically a country and defined its boundaries. The English language played a prominent role for unification of the country.

(In 1947, when India got independence from the British, there were fourteen languages which were recognized in the Indian Constitution. The north Indian four or five states were Hindi speaking and made up about 35% of the population of India at that time. Hindi happened to be the largely spoken of the fourteen languages.

(Hindi remained as the proposed to be the national language of the country. The rest of the country, the east, the west and the south opposed it. So a compromised formula found that both English and Hindi would be the official language (not national language - Hindi remained as proposed national language, even today) of the Government of India. The arrangement would continue till the non-Hindi speaking states agree.

(In the early sixties, one day, the people of the state of Madras - currently Tamilnadu, and the city called Chennai, found themselves in a very strange situation. All the English signs and writings were removed by painting over them with black tar and only the Hindi writings were left alone on the trains stationed at Madras. The south Indian people do not know Hindi at all. So they were all surprised and felt very bad and angry. Soon thousands of passengers gathered. They started shouting that the north Indian people made them foreigners in their own home state. Soon the anger grew and about thirteen trains were burnt.

(The language issue is very touchy in India and tension has always remained high for this sensitive issue. A member of the parliament (M.P.) from south India asked a question in the parliament in English to a minister from the north Indian Hindi speaking state who knowing English very well intentionally chose to answer in Hindi so that the south Indian M. P. would not understand. Immediately, all the members of the south went to the well of the house and the speaker of the house could not control them. A pandemonium took place and the house adjourned for the day. This kind of thing happened in Indian parliament dozens of times on the language issue.

(That was the reason Kriyananda was advised to change his plan to either Bengal or any other parts of the country except north India to avoid trouble. His plan never got off the ground).

When Swamiji arrived in the United States, he was staying with a family who were his host. Swamiji wrote to Edith Krispien in Germany that he was visiting the United States. She replied that she would visit the United States to see him. In her letter she mentioned that Kriyananda got married. (Edith did visit Swamiji in America). So Swamiji wrote a letter to Kriyananda also (as both were in contact by letters) informing him that Swamiji arrived in the United States and mentioned that he learned about his marriage from Edith Krispien.

The understanding of the word "playboy" in India is simply a school age boy who goes on dates with many different girls, even innocently. This is very different from the American concept of a "playboy" as someone who pursues a life of pleasure and is irresponsible or sexually promiscuous.

With this understanding and not knowing what the word meant in the United States, Swamiji wrote to Kriyananda that his action was "like a playboy."

When Swamiji told the hostess, her reaction was kind of horrified. Swamiji did not understand at that time why it was such a big deal; later, he understood her reaction. Then it was too late for cultural counseling.

In reply, through his secretary, Keshava, in one of his letters wrote that he was glad that Swamiji addressed him as "A spiritual boy". When Swamiji received his letter, he was stunned. This is a man who once was the vice president of the Self Realization Fellowship (SRF) who losing all his senses twisted the word "playboy" to "a spiritual boy" and sent it through his secretary making the secretary think that Swamiji greeted him with honor as "a spiritual boy."

Another example of the twisting-master Kriyananda, when Sister Daya as president of SRF and YSS first went to India, he was in the party as he was the vice President. He was planning to stay in India for a long time and so he was working hard in New Delhi. As the vice president of SRF at that young age of thirty, the active,energetic, young *brahmachari* Kriyananda trying to prove his organizational skill, quickly rented seven houses in New Delhi in different parts of the nation's capital and started meditation centers with the local devotees of Yogoda. They started working very well with the enthusiastic devotees.

Prior to arriving at Delhi, Kriyananda in West Bengal quickly learned a few songs in Bengali and sang with the harmonium (a very common musical instrument used in India), with a devotional overtone beautifully, and won the hearts of the Bengali *Kriyanwits* of YSS group. Most people know that from Lahiri Mahasay down to Kriyananda's *Guru*, Yogananda, till the present day almost 90% of *Kriya* teachers happened to be Bengali. Thus, winning the hearts of the Bengali was very important to Kriyananda. With a definite personal plan, he was trying to make ground work for staying in India for an indefinite period. Swamiji heard him singing in an asram the following music, the first line of which was as follows:

Satya mangala premamaya tumi,
Dhrubajyoti tumi andhakare.

It meant "You are truly the embodiment of well being and the embodiment of love. You are the true Light in darkness."

Sister Daya was a simple hearted nice lady. Swamiji met her in 1957/58 on her first visit at YSS asram. He met her in her second visit in 1963 at Serampore accompanying Swami Satyananda who was chief guest at Chatra, Serampore asram (at the place of Motilal Mukhopadhtaya, the chief household disciple of Sriyukteswar) when Sister Daya was to preside at the function, because that branch was affiliated with YSS.

Swamiji met her on a one on one basis again at Calcutta in 1972. Their Joint General Secretary, Shantananda, arranged the meeting. Before meeting her, Shantananda sent a note of caution and Swamiji happened to notice it: "He could be a stalwart". In that meeting they wanted to recruit Swamiji to work with them. Swamiji took the opportunity to ask Sister Daya directly if Yogananda taught them *Khecharimudra*. She mumbled at first to answer as she was not expecting such a direct question. Later, she managed and said, "*Guruji* told us both ways; we may or may not practice *Khecharimudra*."

Sister Daya happened to be so simple she even did not like to be president, although she was Yogananda's private secretary and served him well, as well as was loved by him. She realized that if she would become president, then her meditative life would be ruined. That was the primary reason for her unwillingness to accept the post. In the meantime, they found out startling information about Swami Premananda of Washington D.C. He happened to be Yogananda's student at Ranchi, a disciple of Yogananda who made him Swami in the United States in 1941 and appointed him in 1942 as the International Secretary of the organization to avert a crisis facing the organization at that time when Satyananda left Ranchi and Premananda at that time; separating from Yogananda started working in co-operation with Swami Satyananda who was his beloved principal at Ranchi school, as well as the *Guru* of *brahmacharya* initiation.

Under these circumstances, it was her sister, Ananda Mata, who found a note which once Yogananda wrote to Daya, and a sentence was found in the note: "Only Love can take my place". She brought that letter and disclosed the information that Premananda was coming to Los Angeles from Washington D.C. to claim to be the president of SRF. There was no reason to hesitate and to waste time. Thus her sister Ananda Mata practically forced Daya to be SRF president. They put out a sign board that "Sister Daya becomes the president of SRF." That is why she wrote a book the title "*The Only Love*". Again, it was intelligent Ananda Mata who told Daya that she must bring back the dashing boy (meaning Kriyananda), or else he could kick her out of the post of President.

(As far as Premananda was concerned, Sister Daya already had direction about him from Yogananda himself.

("When Daya was asked [by S. B. Dasgupta] about Premananda's separation from the organization, she said, 'One day, a letter addressed to Swamiji (Yoganandaji) came from Washington, D.C. As his personal secretary, I used to open most of his letters and read them first if Swamiji was not present. Because Swamiji was not there that day, I opened the letter and saw that it was written by Swami Premananda. There was an improper statement about Swami Sriyukteswarji in the letter. As soon as I read that, I became very worried about the kind of effect that comment would have on Swamiji (Yoganandaji), and I closed the letter without going further. I placed it under Swamiji's pillow as was the usual practice. Swamiji arrived, opened the letter and immediately became extremely somber. He asked me, 'Did you read this letter?' With great trepidation, I said, 'Yes. I opened it and read it.' He replied, 'I'm extremely sad that you read this letter!' After remaining quiet for a while, Swamiji said, 'When I am not here, you all should cut off all association with all of these people!' *Paramhansa Swami Yogananda Life-portrait and Reminiscences* by S. B.

Dasgupta, disciple of Sriyukteswar and the private secretary of Yogananda during 1935-1936, Page 123.

(Comments like "cut off all association with all of these people!" reveals Yogananda was not only assertive, but on occasion, dictatorial too like a king).

Sister Daya did not have to bring back Kriyananda, it happened as per natural course. He was caught red handed taking a photograph of a prohibited area of a military place in New Delhi. The sign board was displayed there: "This is restricted area. Taking photograph is prohibited". Still he took the photos. His camera was snatched and he was arrested. Subsequently, the first prime minister, Mr. Nehru, ordered the Home Department to deport him and not to allow him to enter India for four years.

After the sexual harassment case, with Ms. Anne-Marie Bertolucci, Kriyananda resigned as director of his Ananda Village, founded by him, and left for Italy. Going back and forth between Europe and America, he ended up in India to fulfill his dream, and made some centers in big cities in India. In Delhi, he used Mr. Nehru'a photo in the web site for Delhi center "twisting" the word mentioning that Mr. Nehru was very helpful to him.

Kriyananda enclosed some printed papers, four pages in one (date October 15, 1981) and four pages typed in another (date May 13, 1982) also two pages written by Shibani, a female founder member of Ananda Village.

He sent a letter (date July 1, 1982) with a comment: "Perhaps you will find the enclosed helpful." At one place, Kriyananda wrote in those enclosures the following :

May 13, 1982

Dear Friends:

As many of you know, last year was an important year for me personally. I took a step I'd never believed I would ever take: I got married.

Actually, it was not marriage in the usual sense, but rather a soul commitment -- a spiritual, not a physical union. Though I confess to having felt terrified of the risk I was taking, I didn't feel that this step meant the breaking of my monastic vows. Rather, what I felt was the strongest inner guidance to broaden my commitment to God's service, by showing people the ideal of renunciation as the basis of true spiritual marriage.

For Parmeshwari, my spiritual partner, and me it was a union of souls -- inward to the point where the essence of our relationship became, for each of us, an experience of joy rising up through the spine, drawing us into a state of meditation.

I had never experienced a magnetic exchange of this kind with anyone before -- except, indeed, in the company of saints. Nor had I realized that anything remotely like such an exchange was even possible. For me, Parmeshwari was a channel through whom the Divine Mother Herself magnetized me, changing me in ways that were, I knew, vitally important for my spiritual growth, but that were too subtle for me to grasp on my own.

Parmeshwari, too, grew immeasurably through our association.

The change in both of us had also a positive effect on others. As one friend put it, "I love seeing the two of you together, because of what it does for me!" Another friend, after accompanying us on a tour of Egypt and meditating with us in the ancient shrines, remarked later to the group, "What I got most out of this trip was just seeing Swami and Parmeshwari together." And many people remarked to us, "I don't know what it is, but there is something magic in the combination of the two of you."

For myself, all I can understand clearly of our relationship is that it brought more of a divine flow into my consciousness, where before I had been too much inclined to analyze everything -- to look too carefully (if I may put it this way) for the caterpillar in the salad.

As I say, the basis of our relationship was almost wholly spiritual. If anything, indeed, it was almost <u>too</u> spiritual -- in the sense that it failed to take into account the molasses-like quality of reality on this material plane.

My tendency always has been to view the spiritual potential

of a situation as though it were an already-existing fact. One of the hardest lessons I've had to learn, indeed -- and one I've yet to learn well -- is that matter obstructs change.

Despite the obvious gains from Parmeshwari's and my relationship, it took all my courage to enter into a commitment that seemed to me (though actually it wasn't) so much in conflict with my monastic calling. It was the intensity of the guidance I felt that determined me -- this, and the positive reassurance everyone gave me to whom I turned for external guidance.

But how strange: Having summoned up all my courage and embraced this new direction, I had it thrown back in my face!

What happened was that Parmeshwari, lacking the years of experience with inner guidance that I've had, and the many opportunities to test it and see it working in the laboratory of daily life, panicked and fled.

Consider it from her point of view: The relationship to which we both felt called placed her in a position of unprecedented prominence -- a position for which nothing in her past had prepared her. Suddenly the whole situation seemed to her unreal -- as indeed it was, when viewed in the light of all that had been familiar to her in her life so far. Her panic is very understandable.

But I am now left with several very big questions, and with few answers -- both for my own life, and for my life's work.

Was my guidance, after all, wrong? Say, rather, did I merely imagine it all?

Was it wrong for me to follow this inner experience, as opposed to my objective belief system?

Was I more foolhardy than courageous, to risk so much on a single venture?

Sounding a more positive note: Was God merely testing me -- as He did Abraham -- to see if I would do whatever He asked of me?

I had never had a desire for marriage. Nor did I enter this commitment out of desire, except to do God's will. Indeed, shortly before Parmeshwari decided to withdraw from the commitment, I prayed earnestly to Divine Mother: "If in any way I've misunderstood Your will, and You haven't wanted this relationship, please take Parmeshwari away from me!"

So, then, another possibility: Was her leaving me an answer to that prayer? But if so, why not sooner? Certainly I'd prayed as sincerely before. Nor for a moment before or since her departure have I wanted anything but God's will in this matter.

Shortly after she left, I felt a strong pull at the spiritual eye -- a sensation that I have learned to associate with new guidance, and new directions. "What is it you want, Master?" I prayed, keeping my heart open with all the sincerity of which I was capable to any new direction in which he might want me to go. Immediately I felt pushed right back to Parmeshwari -- the one direction over which I had absolutely no control!

Since then I have received much new guidance for Ananda, but, until lately, none for myself. It is almost as if Divine Mother were saying to me, "I have given you many reasons over the years to have faith in Me. If now I give you none, will you still have faith?" Yes, I have faith! Nor for an instant has my faith wavered. And though I have known much pain through this whole experience, not for a moment have I regretted the pain, nor sought anything for myself but Divine Mother's will. For I know that Her will is true, and that it is never anything but benign. What She wills must in the end prove perfect for me, for Parmeshwari, and for everyone else concerned. Thus, along with the pain, I have known great inner freedom, and great joy.

I no longer live in a monastery as I did in Self-Realization Fellowship, with the comfort and security of people around me whose experience on the path was greater than my own. There are risks involved in following my own inner guidance. I must bear them bravely, knowing that the gains will be greater if I follow the guidance truly, but that the dangers also are greater. Until this experience, my track record, fortunately, has been very good. But is it possible that in this test, involving as it does the most crucial decision I have ever had to face in my own spiritual life, I have erred?

Of this much I am certain: If we do anything sincerely, with a continuing desire to please God alone, He cannot let us down! I have not allowed myself to be influenced by the possibility of public criticism, even ridicule, for having made a wrong, and therefore a foolish, choice. I am concerned only with pleasing God. Whether people shower me with praise or with blame is to me the same.

As far as I am concerned, the issue is entirely this: What does God want of me? My test, then, is that He has chosen to make me wait for His answer. But never mind: I am certain His will is going to be made clear to me, in His time -- and His is the only time that matters to me, also. If, moreover, He wills that I look like a fool, then I embrace that, too. In no corner of my heart is there the smallest plea: "I want Thy will, Lord, but please let it be this -- and please also, that!" Even if He wants to destroy my life work, it is His work, not mine -- His to do with entirely as He wills.

Will Parmeshwari come back? If I was right last year, and her destiny lies here, she will have no other choice. But it is not for me now to probe this question further. For myself, I have committed myself to her -- or say, rather, to Divine Mother through her. This is, indeed, a commitment to Divine Mother alone, and one therefore in which there is no bondage. But as long as my guidance continues to flow, as it does, in the direction of this commitment, I have no choice but to hold it in my heart despite the impossibility, objectively, of bringing that guidance to fruition. Should Divine Mother and Guru point me in another way, I will walk that way equally readily, and with the same freedom in my heart.

Meanwhile, I feel that Divine Mother was the true source of all the blessings I received through Parmeshwari. To Her I bow. To Her I look now for the same blessings, seeing her in my heart as encased in the form She chose to take for me, as my spiritual partner.

With love and joy,

S. Kriyananda

Swami Kriyananda

While meditating lately on this question of new direction [getting married] I've **felt** his [Yogananda's] answer: "It has been good until now, for the work that you've done, for you to be a monk. You may continue happily as you are, and certainly with my blessings. But if you do so, you will not be serving the present needs of my works. The world is not now in need of examples of withdrawal. People are suffering and confused. They need relevant guidance in their day-to-day lives."

"What then," I asked, "is needed? Where can I serve best?"

"Isn't the greatest need, as you yourself have seen it, in the area of marriage and male-female relationship? You have wanted Ananda Village to set an example in this area. Is it doing so yet? Will it ever do so, without your leader ship and guidance?"

"But Master, I'm a monk! I've vowed my life to God."

"And what are your vows, ultimately, if not to serve Him as *He* wants?"

"But I've never felt the slightest desire to be a husband!"

"[That's right as it closes the door to date other girls].

"What if you were to live as one time only - to set an example for others? Your motive is pure: It is to God's will, and to serve Him in your fellow man. With such complete dedication your attunement with Him can only grow. Later, you and your divine partner could graduate to the higher more impersonal level of union together in God, as was commonly practiced in ancient India."

The printed enclosures were distributed to people by Kriyananda as an explanatory measure about his marriage at the age of fifty two (52) with the Italian young lady (he called Parameshawri). He was trying to fool his fellow Americans with his predicament. Similarly, he sent them to Swamiji too when he knew that Swamiji had heard about his marriage.

The whole thing he was trying to thrust upon Yogananda as if it was Yogananda's direction putting words into the imaginative mouth of imaginative presence of Yogananda; in the name of direction, he was so consumed with these thoughts, he was indulging his own imagination and feeling like a naive school boy at the age fifty two (52). He continued in another paragraph as follows:

"And I did feel it, repeatedly, every time I prayed:"

This word "feel" or "feeling" is extremely tricky. It is a sense and it works in the field of sensation. Whatever is in the field of sensation is not spiritual. The spiritual field is beyond the sensation and the intellectual arena, since the intellect too is an inner sense like the mind, the heart and the ego. One's "feeling" never can be trusted as spiritual.

Let us see what happened to Kriyananda when his partner, Parameshwari, left him very soon.

In one of those enclosures (date May 13, 1982) he wrote:

But I am now left with several questions, and with few answers -- both for my own life, and for my life's work.

[Attachment to work (characterizing life's work), is another big problem].

Was my guidance, after all, wrong? Say, rather, did I merely imagine it all?

[Yes, it was just an imagination, and he knew that it was imagination and he knew that he wanted his Guru to be on his side to approve his feeling. There lies the unique play of *maya* (illusion) and *moha* (attachment) to blind one's understanding and reasoning. He failed to recognize her, considered

Parameshwari, a newly found soul-friend, as divine mother, when she was merely a trick of *maya*].

Was it wrong for me to follow this inner experience, as opposed to my objective belief system?

[That was not an inner experience, it was an inner urge to get the girl.]

Was I more foolhardy than courageous, to risk so much on a single venture?

[Yes, losing his reason, he fooled himself and then surrendered to her! From the description and his helplessness, it appears that she could have been his partner or wife in previous life and that is why he could not survive but to marry her].

Sounding a more positive note: Was God merely testing me -- as He did Abraham -- to see if I would do whatever He asked of me?

[This last question is really a desperate one].

In another paragraph he wrote - "This needed direction came as the result of seemingly chance meeting with someone in whom found already highly refined those very qualities which I so much wanted to develop in myself. It was an encounter such as I'd never had before in my life."

[The question is which qualities he was referring to? Qualities of an artist? What a confusion? He did not realize that he had already made up his mind to find a girl outside his organization and then prayed to disembodied Yogananda to grant his desire and put words in the mouth of an imaginative figure.

[The present situation of Kriyananda, reminds the author about his *Guru*, Yogananda. Somehow, after graduating in B. A. from the Serampore College under the Calcutta University, in 1915, Mukundalal Ghosh, renouncing all the worldly interests, entered into the order of Swami, and left for Benares. Just after six months, he came to Calcutta and put up with his father of former ashram, Bhagavati Charan Ghosh, which as a Swami, as per the rules of *sannyas*, he should not do. It violated the vow of *sannyas* (Swami order). The rule says that the newly entered into the order of Swami is not supposed to enter the house of former ashram (the former family). Then the second violation, in 1916, he became again Mr. Mukundalal Ghosh. The third violation, he left for Japan to study agriculture while a renunciate has no business anymore other than spirituality. Then just after one week, he returned to India and became Swami Yogananda again; that was the fourth violation. Then came the fifth violation, he enrolled in the Philosophy, M. A. class in the Calcutta University for just two months and discontinued. All these changes from one thing to another and so soon, are clearly signs of restlessness and lack of maturity. One cannot be so fickle; it shows the unpreparedness before acting and disrespect for established rules, practices and traditions. It seems like *Guru* like *Chela* (disciple).

[When there are many more interests of diversified nature including different spiritual disciplines, the essence of Self Realization (*Atmatattwa* or *Samatattwa*) is never revealed to those seekers. When all those cravings of the heart are destroyed or overcome completely only then a person receives the science of Breath or *Kriya* for attaining the realization of the Self.

[*Abhabe sarbatattwanang samang tattwang prakasate.*
The Siva Sanghita 2:58

[The verse says, "When all *tattwas* (doctrines of essences), in other words, all craving (*trisnas*) of the mind, all desires (*vasanas*) of the heart, are zeroed in the individual *jiva*, **then and then only**, the *sama tattwa* (*Atma Tattwa* – The Science of the Self), that is, the ***Atma Kriya*** is revealed to a seeker."]

Kriyananada continued, "I have met many thousands of people in my life, but no one ever affected me like this [Because Miss Golia sought him by a *sammohan* (mesmerism) *ban* or *Goli* (bullet)]. Even with my *Guru*, I've first visualized his outward appearance, and then felt his spiritual presence. But with my new soul-friend I found that her inner presence was my first reality, on the basis of which I might mentally reconstruct what she looked like. It was as though I were looking at the world *through* her eyes, rather than seeing her from the outside."

So admittedly, she was more powerful than his *Guru* to him. It seemed he was no match for her; with her vibration, she already flattened him internally to his knees. In such a confused situation, this is what usually happens very fast when a person trusts one's sense particularly "Feeling".

Dhayoto bisayanapungsa sangstesupajayate.
Sangatsangjayate kama kamatkrodhayabhijayate. Bhagavad Gita 2:62
Krodhatbhabati sangmoha sangmohatsmritibibhrama.
Smritibhrangsatbuddhinasobuddhinasatpranasyati.Bhagavad Gita 2:63

The verses say, "The man dwelling on the sense-object [feeling] develops attachment for them; from the attachment springs up desire; and from the unfulfilled desire ensues anger.

"From anger arises infatuation; from infatuation, confusion of memory; from confusion of memory, loss of reason; and from loss of reason one goes to complete ruin."

The moment one trusts a sense like "feeling" (which is such a tricky stick) one immediately starts developing step by step and in an orderly fashion as stated in the verses to complete ruin to a measurable state. Being a rational being when a man loses his reason and conscience, he meets a devastating state in life.

In reality, when such a crisis time occurs, one's intellect (*buddhi*) starts working in the "opposite or reverse order", the famous saying is: (*Apatkale biparit buddhi* - During crisis, the reverse reason starts working). As a result, it is really difficult for one who simply cannot help himself or herself.

Being devotional in nature, if one trusts one's heart, one faces the same result. Feeling and the heart are relative terms of the same sense world.

Since with Yogananda's deal "to set aside salvation in the current incarnation" there was left no serious sentiment to practice with modified *Kriya* practice instead plenty of time was left to work on the different fields and directions of setting examples for the fellow man. What a confusion and mess in understanding of life! It seemed his whole life was that of an imaginative, ambitious, manipulative, and demonstrative entertainer without proper understanding of the goal.

To make one life's works so important in this world one goes blindly to such an extent when the world itself is a product of Illusion.

Na biswamasti naibasinna cha nama bhabisyati.
Idamabhasate ***santang chidbyoma paramatmani****.*
Yoga Vasistha Ramayana 6:103:82(*Uttararddha*)

The wise are like mad men (*Pagalbat*); according to them, the world in front of you is void (illusion): It never was, it is not now and it will never be in the future; as it was never created in the first place (simply reflected in illusion).

"Oh Rama! As in a dream one sees one's own death and performance of one's funeral by the relatives and friends, but in fact it is not so, such is this world [illusion like a mirage in the desert, silver in shells, snake on rope – non-existent]."

"*And the earth was without form, and void* [illusion like a child's seeing a goblin – non-entity]." *Genesis* 1:2

For such an illusory world, the man's ego wanders endlessly in the state of illusion.

After the marriage at the age of 52, Kriyananda was again in trouble at the age of 62; he was sued for sexual harassment (stated below). To hide his past in the United States about his marriage and the sexual harassment case, etc.,

Kriyananda resigned as director of Ananda Village which he founded, and moved to Italy and then to India. Thus, Kriyananda's original idea to live in India was fulfilled. He lived in Italy and in India the later part of his life and was acting there as an accomplished Yogi. The ignorant Indian people thinking the American, (rich person), renouncing everything accepted the life of a *sanyasi*, renunciate, accepted him. Unfortunately, the servitude mind to the British in India still continues. In Delhi, he became sick. So he left for Assisi, Italy, where he died April 20, 2013.

Kriyananda was involved in the following lawsuits : Some of the case references are as follows:

1. Self Realization Fellowship Church (SRFC), a California corporation, plaintiff, vs. Church of Self Realization, a California corporation; Fellowship of Inner Communion, a California corporation, and James Donald Walters (also known as Sri Kriyananda), an individual, defendants, in the United States District Court for the Eastern District of California, Case No. CIV-S-90-0846 EJG EM, filed on July 2, 1990.

2. Kriyananda (J. Donald Walters) and Ananda Church of Self Realization, vs. Self Realization Fellowship Church and others in 1992.

3. Ms. Anne-Marie Bertolucci, Plaintiff vs. Ananda Church of Self Realization and Kriyananda (J. Donald Walters) and others, defendants, in 1996, in the Superior Court of the State of California for the County of San Mateo, Case No. 390 230, date January 9, 1996.

4. In the same suit, on September 26, 1997, Ananda filed 13 "motions" in a bid to knock out plaintiff's case which they lost. They also filed a "cross-complaint" for defamation against the plaintiff and Yogananda's organization,

Self Realization Fellowship Church, alleging "conspiracy;" but later on, they dropped it.

The Plaintiff sued the defendant for filing a frivolous claim (the cross-complaint), alleging conspiracy and slander when the defendant, Ananda Church of Self Realization and Kriyananda (J. Donald Walters) and others, dropped the "cross-complaint."

5. Anne-Marie Bertolucci, an individual, plaintiff, vs. Ananda Church of Self Realization, a California religious corporation, James Donald Walters (also known as J. Donald Walters), an individual, defendants, in the United States District Court for the Eastern District of California, Case No. CIV-S-99-1439 LKK JFM, filed on June 27, 1999. Demand for Jury trial.

Anne-Marie Bertolucci, an individual, plaintiff, vs. Ananda Church of Self Realization, A California religious corporation, James Donald Walters (also known as J. Donald Walters), an individual, defendants, in the United States District Court for the Eastern District of California, Case No. CIV-S-99-1439 LKK JFM, filed on August 10 1999, Dismissal of Complaint (FRCP 41 (a) (1).

6. Self Realization Fellowship Church, a California Corporation, Plaintiff-Appelland, Vs Ananda Church of Self Realization, a California Corporation, Fellowship of Inner Communion, No 97-17407, at the United States Court of Appeals for the Ninth Circuit, filed March 23, 2000.

Roy Eugene Davis, disciple of Yogananda :

Like Kriyananda, Roy Eugene Davis, the moment he heard about the release of the biography of Lahiri Mahasay, wanted to see the manuscript. In the meantime Swamiji got it published. He received a copy and had gone through it. He contacted Andrew Ciaramitaro whom Swamiji had earlier asked to contact his literary agent.

Roy E. Davis visited Swamiji in 1985. He introduced a lady who accompanied him as his wife, Molly. Roy said that he once requested Sister Daya to do something about the works of Lahiri Mahasay to make them available in English, but they were not interested.

In fact, in 1935/36, when Yogananda visited India, he appointed Ram Kisore Roy, an attorney of Ranchi to the board of director of YSS. In exchange he collected from him some books of Lahiri Mahasay's works. Those books were with Devendranath Roy, disciple of Lahiri Mahasay, Ram Kisore Roy's uncle. Thus they (SRF) were aware about the original *Kriya's* status; the English presentation could confuse or ruin Yogananda's entire *Kriya* teaching in the United States in their opinion.

Roy Davis did not know that they (SRF) already knew that Lahiri Mahasay's presentation and *Kriya* interpretations could confuse the modified *Kriya* of Yogananda.

Roy added that he went to India looking for Lahiri Mahasay's published books and he did not find them. It was not possible to find them as they were printed by his chief disciple, Sri Panchanan Bhattacharya, at the instruction of Lahiri Mahasay. The limited copies were distributed among the Lahiri Mahasay's disciples and the *Kriyanwits* and not outside *Kriya* people. So those who were his disciples and disciple's disciples had those copies. Today, their descendents possess them and they would not part with them. Usually, those copies were in their altar rooms and were worshiped every day.

Swamiji remembered once Swami Sadananda at Risikesh told him that one of Yogananda's disciples, Roy Eugene Davis, met him and was looking for Lahiri Mahasay's works.

Like Kriyananda, Roy E. Davis was highly interested and confident that he could help in the project.

CENTER FOR SPIRITUAL AWARENESS
POST OFFICE BOX 7
LAKE RABUN ROAD
LAKEMONT, GEORGIA 30552-0007

Roy Eugene Davis
President & Director

(404) 782-4723

June 7, 1983

Dear Andy,

It was a pleasure talking with you and Swamiji last evening. I called him right after I had talked with you.

I am interested in seeing a copy of the manuscript of Lahiri's biography. I will then be in a position to decide whether I can purchase large quantities, when published. And, perhaps even enter into a cooperative publishing arrangement with you.

I am well acquainted with publishing, having written some twenty books, with some of them also published in Japanese, Portuguese and German languages. We use R.R. Donnelly & Sons Co., who usually produce books for us within 4-5 weeks after they receive typeset pages. As a usual procedure, we typeset materials here and prepare everything for the printer. The printer then manufactures and binds to our specifications.

As to our possible distribution potential: we have 7,000 active names on our list. 1000 of these are our supporting members. We publish Truth Journal magazine and send to 7,000 persons ten times a year. We also send book announcements to key metaphysical book dealers and to over 400 book departments of Unity, Science of Mind and Yoga groups. So we have a well established book experience,having been active in this procedure for 20 years.

We also have a branch organization in Europe and I lecture there annually. We also have a branch in Ghana, West Africa.

At our meditation retreat here in north Georgia (photos enclosed) we invite students to come for retreats and seminars. As a disciple of Paramahansa Yogananda (initiated by him in 1950 and ordained by him in 1951) I also give Kriya Yoga instruction.

I met Paramhansaji in 1949, right after highschool, and was resident minister for SRF in Phoenix, Arizona until I left of my own free will in late 1953. There was no philosophical differences, only that I felt the need to be independent. I mention these matters so that you and Swamiji will understand my back-

-2-

ground.

I have long felt that a biography of Lahiri and of Sri Yukteswar should be published for English speaking students. And that Lahiri's commentaries on scripture should likewise be published.

Therefore, I am extremely interested in your present publishing projects and will do what I can to assist in their completion.

As I mentioned to Swamiji, on the telephone, I will be in Phoenix this August (first week) to attend a conference and could then also fly to San Diego for a personal visit. In the meantime, we can communicate by mail and telephone.

All good wishes,

Roy Eugene Davis

P.S. Under separate cover I am sending you sample issues of Truth Journal magazine and gift books to further acquaint you with our work and presentation. Let me explain that we have an outer ministry and an inner one. The outer ministry includes popular and inspirational writings and programs to serve a large number of people. The inner work is with sincere students who are interested in Kriya Yoga practices.

Center For Spiritual Awareness
Post office Box 7
Lake Rabun Road
Lakemont, Georgia 30552-0007

Roy Eugene Davis **(404) 782-4723**
President & Director

Dear Andy,

It was a pleasure talking with you and Swamiji last evening. I called him right after I had talked with you.

I am interested in seeing a copy of the manuscript of Lahiri's biography. I will then be in a position to decide whether I can purchase large quantities, when published. And, perhaps even enter into a cooperative publishing arrangement with you.

I am well acquainted with publishing, having written some twenty books, with some of them also published in Japanese, Portuguese and German languages. We use R.R. Donnelly & Sons Co., who usually produce books for us within 4-5 weeks after they receive typeset pages. As a usual procedure, we typeset materials here and prepare everything for the printer. The printer then manufactures and binds to our specifications.

As to our possible distribution potential: we have 7,000 active names on our list. 1000 of these are our supporting members. We publish Truth Journal magazine and send to 7,000 persons ten times a year. We also send book announcement to key metaphysical book dealers and to over 400 book departments of Unity, Science of Mind and Yoga groups. So we have a well established book experience, having been in this procedure for 20 years,

We also have a branch organization in Europe and I lecture there annually. We also have a branch in Ghana, West Africa.

At our meditation retreat here in north Georgia (photos enclosed) we invite students to come for retreats and seminars. As a disciple of Paramhansa Yogananda (initiated by him in 1950 and ordained by him in 1951) I also give Kriya Yoga instruction.

I met Paramhansaji in 1949, right after high school, and was resident minister for SRF in Phoenix, Arizona until I left of my own free will in late 1953. There was no philosophical differences, only that I felt the need to be independent. I mention these matters so that you and Swamiji will understand my background.

I have long felt that a biography of Lahiri and of Sri Yukteswar should be published for English speaking students. And that Lahiri's commentaries on scriptures should likewise be published.

Therefore, I am extremely interested in your present publishing projects and will do what I can to assist in their completion.

As I mentioned to Swamiji, on the telephone, I will be in Phoenix this August (first week) to attend a conference and could then also fly to San Diego for a personal visit. In the meantime, we can communicate by mail and telephone.

All good wishes

Roy Eugene Davis

P.S. Under separate cover I am sending you sample issues of Truth Journal magazine and gift books to further acquaint you with our work and presentation. Let me explain that we have an outer ministry and an inner one. The outer ministry includes popular and inspirational writings and programs to serve a large number of people. The inner work is with sincere students who are interested in Kriya Yoga practices.

CENTER FOR SPIRITUAL AWARENESS
POST OFFICE BOX 7
LAKE RABUN ROAD
LAKEMONT, GEORGIA 30552-0007

Roy Eugene Davis
President & Director

(404) 782-4723

December 7, 1983

Dear Swamiji,

I recently received your book about Lahiri.

I have read it carefully and am so pleased that you have made this material available in English to a wider reading public.

We will offer this title to our disciples and students and they, too, will very much appreciate it.

Thank you for this service to all of us,

Roy Eugene Davis

P.S. I will arrange to visit you when I next travel to California, in March.

Center For Spiritual Awareness
Post office Box 7
Lake Rabun Road
Lakemont, Georgia 30552-0007

Roy Eugene Davis
President & Director

(404) 782-4723

December 7, 1983

Dear Swamiji,
I recently received your book about Lahiri.

I have read it carefully and am so pleased that you have made this material available in English to a wider reading public.

We will offer this title to our disciples and students and they , too, will very much appreciate it.

Thank you for this service to all of us.

Roy Eugene Davis

P.S. I will arrange to visit you when I next travel to California, in March.

Motilal Banarsidass Publishers (P) Limited
Indological Publishers and Distributors

41 U.A. Bunglow Road, Jawahar Nagar
Delhi 110 007 (India)

As mentioned before, in 1975 Swamiji was in Germany in his world lecture tour under the instruction of Mahamuni Babaji. He took the opportunity to visit the International Book Fair at Frankfurt. It was a huge book fair for ten days. His hostess, a professor at Gothe University, took him in the fair during the time (between 10 A.M. and 2 P.M.) when only the publishers were allowed and the rest of the day was for ordinary people.

As mentioned also, Edith Krispien, the literary agent was authorized to find a possible publisher for Swamiji's new title - *Kriya* in English.

She found one publisher which was interested. It was a very reputed and a big publishing company, Motilal Banarsidass from New Delhi, India. Their proposal was that Edith be a co-publisher with them contributing one thousand U.S. dollars (US $1,000.00) which Edith did not have and so it did not work out.

Swamiji returned to India. Three years later, in 1978, a devotee learned of this contact with Motilal Banarsidass for Swamiji's book *Kriya*. The devotee happened to be a magistrate and a literary professional and asked Swamiji's permission to write to the particular publisher. Swamiji said, "It is of no use. His writing has a special reason and these have to be published under direct supervision of Swamiji properly, otherwise, publishers would alter the presentations for their primary interest to make maximum profit."

The magistrate continued insisting to let him try. Reluctantly, Swamiji permitted him to contact the particular publisher at Delhi. After a long time not having any answer from them, the magistrate informed Swamiji.

Then in 1982 Swamiji moved to the United States and had to start the Sanskrit Classics, the self publishing firm, and managed to write and publish several books. So many years passed by, then came 1995, the year which happened to be the centenary year of Yogiraj Shyama Charan Lahiri Mahasay's leaving the body in *Mahasamadhi*.

All the *Kriya* practitioners (*Kriyanwits/Kriyanwitas*) in India, especially in Bengal, and all the hermitages around the world celebrated for several months. In Delhi SRF/YSS and Kriyananda's group celebrated in such a way that it became a very eventful happening in Delhi. It caught the attention of Motilal Banarsidass Publisher. They suddenly realized the tremendous spiritual influence of Lahiri Mahasay on the entire planet. They wanted to know about Lahiri Mahasay. All they could find in English was a chapter on him in the *Autobiography of a Yogi*.

Then they found Swamiji's comprehensive biography of Lahiri Mahasay and the title Babaji.

When the celebration started in October,1995, they almost immediately wrote to Swamiji on 16th November,1995.

Swamiji did not like to respond for the simple reason: Since it was not possible to give them the book, and books published in the U.S.A. would be expensive for Indian readers. As a result, books could not be given to them for distribution as well. They desperately wanted a response, but to no avail.

On 27, November,1999, after four years, again they wrote. They saw a goldmine in Lahiri Mahasay's complete works of 26 books on the classical Indian scripture in Bengali but their complete English version was translated into English for the first time by Swamiji who published them as well. It is not easy to translate them. One has to be very well versed in at least four languages:

1) Sanskrit,
2) Bengali,
3) Hindi, and
4) English.

5) Besides, one has to be expert in the *Kriya* discipline, and conversant in Indian philosophy and Vedic culture. These do not come by so easily.

Finally, Swamiji sent them an e-mail explaining why he did not respond to their letters all these years. Still they pleaded to have permission and right to bring a cheaper Indian edition for the greater benefit for the people.

Being frustrated they contacted Kriyananda, disciple of Yogananda, there at Delhi and cut a deal publishing his writing on the modified *Kriya*.

In the meantime, Swamiji arranged to print books in Calcutta and Lahiri Mahasay's complete works were published in a four volume hard cover set and were given with other books to Motilal Banarsidass for distribution.

The following were the correspondences with Motilal Banarsidass.

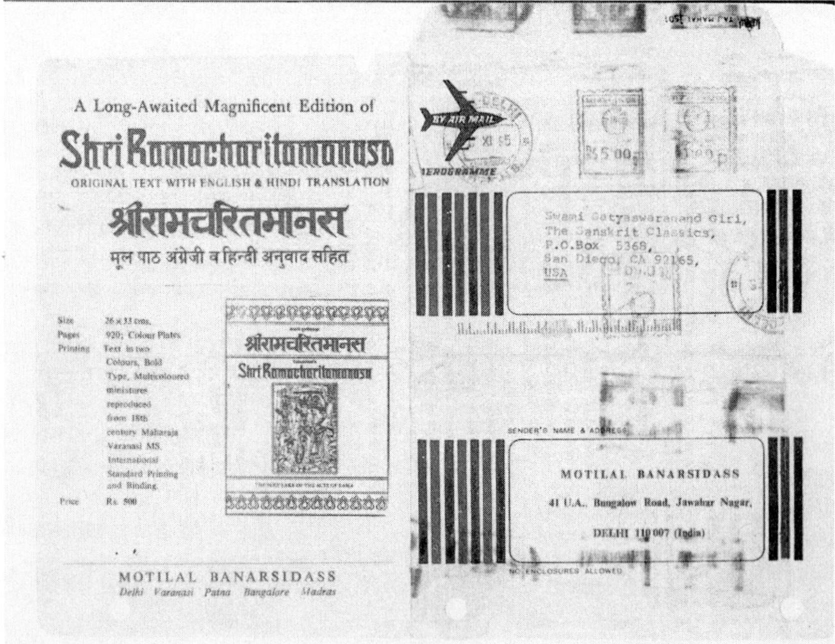

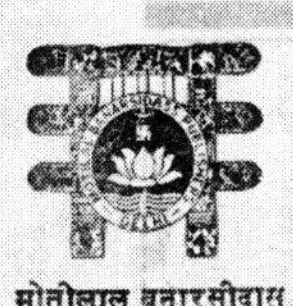

मोतीलाल बनारसीदास
Delhi Varanasi Patna
Bangalore Madras

ESTD. 1903

Tele Gram : GLORYINDIA
Phones: (O) 291-1985
291-8335
(R) 29-17335

MOTILAL BANARSIDASS
INDOLOGICAL PUBLISHERS & DISTRIBUTORS

41 U.A., BUNGALOW ROAD,
JAWAHAR NAGAR,
DELHI 110 007 (INDIA)

Ref. No. JPJ/USA/2957

16th November,95

Respected Swami Satyaswaranand Ji,

You will be pleased to know that we are a renowned publishing house for the last nine decades dealing with all sorts of publications.

I happened to see some of your publications including that of 'Babaji: Lahiri Mahashaya'. We would like to review your publications and would request you to please send two copies each of them by Airmail for our consideration. Moreover, if you want us to distribute your books in India, we can consider this proposal too, after receiving your books for perusal.

With best regards,

Sincerely

(J.P. JAIN)

Swami Satyaswaranand Giri,
The Sanskrit Classics,
P.O.Box 5368,
San Diego, CA 92165,
USA

Motilal Banarsidass
Indological Publishers and Distributor

41 U.A. Bunglow Road
Jawahar Nagar
Delhi 110 007 (India)
16th November, 95

Ref. No. JPJ/USA/295

Respected Swami Satyeswaranandaji,

You will be pleased to know that we are a renowned publishing house for the last nine decades dealing with all sorts of publications.

I happened to see some of your publications including that of "Babaji: Lahiri Mahasay".

We would like to review your publications and would request you to please send two copies each of them by Airmail for our consideration. Moreover, if you want us to distribute your books in India, we can consider this proposal too, after receiving your books for perusal.

With best regards.

Sincerely,

(J. P. JAIN)

Swami Satyeswarananda Giri
The Sanskrit Classics,
P.O. Box 5368
San Diego, CA 92165,
USA

Gram : GLORYINDIA
Tel : 291-8335, 291-1985
252-4826, 293-2747
Faxes : 011-293 0689/579 7221
Emails : mail@mlbd.com
gloryindia@poboxes.com
Web Site : www.mlbd.com

MOTILAL BANARSIDASS PUBLISHERS (P) LIMITED

INDOLOGICAL PUBLISHERS AND DISTRIBUTORS

मोतीलाल बनारसीदास पब्लिशर्स (प्रा०) लिमिटेड, दिल्ली-११०००७

Ref. # JPJ/ 9099

41 U. A. Bungalow Road, Jawahar Nagar,
Delhi 110 007 (INDIA)

November 27, 1999

Swami Satyeswarananda Giri
THE SANSKRIT CLASSICS
P.O.Box 5368
San Diego, CA 92165
USA

Dear Swami Giri,

Hope, you are aware about our Publishing House. We regularly print our monthly Newsletter,circulation of which is about 20,000 all over the world. In our Newsletter, we publish reviews of various books. I am sending herewith a copy of our Newsletter and will appreciate if you kindly send me a copy each of the books by LAHARI MAHASHAYA, published by you so that we can publish their reviews in our Newsletter.

Further, if you wish that the books by Lahari Mahashya should be marketed and their sale is promoted in India, kindly let us know your terms and condition.

With best regards,

Sincerely,

J.P.JAIN

ENCL: Newsletter

Regd. Off. A-44, Naraina Industrial Area, Phase I, New Delhi 110 028, Phones: 5793423, 5795180, 5792734

Motilal Banarsidass Publishers (P) Limited
Indological Publishers and Distributors

41 U.A. Bunglow Road, Jawahar Nagar
Delhi 110 007 (India)
November 27, 1999

Ref. # JPJ/9099

Swami Satyeswarananda Giri
The Sanskrit Classics,
P.O. Box 5368
San Diego, CA 92165
USA

Dear Swami Giri,

Hope, you are aware about our Publishing House. We regularly print our monthly Newsletter, circulation of which is about 20,000 all over the world. In our Newsletter, we publish reviews of various books. I am sending herewith a copy of our Newsletter and will appreciate if you kindly send me a copy each of the books by LAHIRI MAHASAYA, published by you so that we can publish their reviews in our Newsletter.

Further, if you wish that the books by Lahiri Mahasaya should be marketed and their sale is promoted in India, kindly let us know your terms and conditions.

With best regards,

Sincerely,

J.P. JAIN

ENCL: Newsletter

Subject: Ref: JPJ/USA
Date: Sat, 25 Dec 1999 14:01:13 +0530
From: Motilal Banarsidass Publishers <mlbd@vsnl.com>
To: ssg@sanskritc.com

Dear Swami Satyeswarananda Ji,

Thanks for your email of 8th December'99 and noted the contents. I am thankful to you for providing us the information about LAHIRI MAHASHYA's books which people are not much aware in India and moreover, Indian readers are not able to afford foreign editions. I will, therefore, appreciate if you kindly send reading copies of each of the books of LAHIRI MAHASHYA for our considering to publish their Indian edition so as to make the same available to Indian readers within affordable price. We will publish review of these books in our monthly NEWSLETTER also. Send other literature pertaining to LAHIRI MAHASHYA's books so as to popularise the same among readers.

Looking forward to hear from you soon.

With best regards and wishing you a Happy New Year.

Sincerely,
J.P.Jain

--

Motilal Banarsidass Publishers
41, UA Bungalow Road, Jawahar Nagar
Delhi-110007, India
Tel : (011) 3274826; 3911985; 3918335; 3932747
(011) 5795180; 5793423; 5797456
Fax : (011) 3930689; 5797221
Email: mlbd@vsnl.com & gloryindia@poboxes.com
Website: www.mlbdbooks.com

Subject: Ref: JPJ/USA
Motilal Banarsidass Publishers <mlbd@vsnl.com>
To: ssg@sanskritc,com

Dear Swami Satyeswarananda Ji,

Thanks for your email of 8th December 99 and noted the contents. I am thankful to you for providing us the information about LAHIRI MAHASHY's [MAHASAY'S] books which people are not aware in India and moreover, Indian readers are not able to afford foreign editions. I will therefore, appreciate if you kindly send reading copies of each of the books of LAHIRI MAHASHYA [MAHASAY] for our considering to publish their Indian edition so as to make the same available to Indian readers within affordable price. We will publish review of these books in our monthly NEWSLETER also.
Send other literature pertaining to LAHIRI MAHASHY's [MAHASAY's] books so as to popularise [popularize] the same among readers.

Looking forward to hear from you soon.
With best regards and wishing you Happy New Year.
Sincerely,
J.P. JAIN

Swami Atmananda Giri (Prakas Chandra Das), Secretary YSS

In Calcutta (currently Kolkata), near Garpar on the Upper Circular Road (currently Acharya Prafullya Chandra Road) there is Greer Park (currently Ladies' Park). In December, 1911, the meeting of National Congress was held there. The boys and girls of Nava Bidhan Samaj's Sunday school were selected to sing at that meeting. Among the boys, Prakas Chandra Das (Swami Atmananda Giri, now deceased) who had a good voice came to sing. Through the Sunday school connection, Prakas Chandra came to know Tulasi Narayana Bose. Young Prakas easily attracted the affection of Tulasi Narayana. He used to bring the boy frequently to his house. Prakas was at that time a young boy who had lost his father.

Prakas began to live in the house of Tulasi Babu and was treated like a member of the family. So Tulasi Babu, being kind, enrolled young Prakas in the Metropolitan School of Bahubazar branch, where the revered Swami Kebalananda Maharaj was the chief teacher of Sanskrit. When Tulasi Babu came to know Hangsa Swami Kebalananda he was initiated by Kebalananda. Thus he became a *Kriyaban*. Being a very sincere seeker, Tulasi Babu arranged an altar in one part of his house, and there he began to worship in each month on the Day of New Moon the Goddess Kali: and young Prakas Chandra used to sing songs there.

Tulasi Narayana Bose, resident of Pitambar Bhattacharya Lane, became Mukunda's friend who being kind later offered part of his house to start the Asramic school at 17/1 Pitambar Bhattacharya Road so that the three friends, Basu Kumar (Dhirananda), Satyananda, and Yogananda could start their first Asram and *Brahmacharya* school.

Prakas Chandra, being obedient to Tulasi Narayana and being initiated and by virtue of his living in the house of Tulasi Babu became part of the *Kriya* group.

Later, growing up, Prakas became *Brahmachari* Prakas. He began to write to Yogananda in the U.S. against Satyananda to become the secretary of YSS. As mentioned before he succeeded when Binayananda appointed him as secretary. Then in 1955 he went to the U.S. and found out that Yogananda had written in a note that *brahmachari* Prakas would be Swami Atmananda and *brahmachari* Animananda would be Swami Satchidananda. (This information was mentioned before). So when he returned to India he became Swami Atmananda Giri.

In 1958 when Sister Daya visited India for the first time, observing their behavior unbecoming of a Swami, removed both of them (Binayananda and Atmananda) from YSS.

Swami Atmananda had four principal disciples.

1) *Brahmachari* Sraddhananda, a Bengali gentleman,
2) *Brahmachari* Brahmananda, a Bengali gentleman,
3) Swami Jnanananda, a Swiss gentleman. and,
4) Yogamaya, a French lady.

Since Atmananda was removed, these people also were not welcomed in YSS. As a result, Sraddhananda left for France, Brahmanada stayed in Calcutta, Jnanananda, the Swiss gentleman, left to Simla, north India and began to live there, and Yogamaya continued to live in India in different places although her health started deteriorating. Her parents wanted her back in France since she was the only child but she did not respond to them. (This information was told to Swamiji by a French lady, Blanche, when she visited him at Dunagiri Hill. Even her parents approached her to bring back their only daughter but she refused- will be discussed later).

Brahmachari Sraddhananda arriving at Paris, got involved in the timber business. His ritualistic worship making *Arati,* flame works offering to the deity in Vedic tradition, were appreciated by many French people especially the older French ladies.

In the meantime, *brahmachari* returned to India for a brief period and was initiated into the Swami order from Sri Bholananda Giri Sanyas asram and became Swami Sraddhanada Giri.

Swamiji once visited the famous Kumbhamela, the largest gathering of Swamis, Sadhus, and religious people in India at Haridwar. It was just a once in a lifetime experience. He could not go before as there was always duty to stay in the hermitage during that time which was the government financial year ending on the 31st March and April 1st was the beginning of the financial year. So it was necessary to stay at the hermitage which run schools (general and technical) also post graduate teacher's training college; and all were government sponsored. As a result, it was necessary to deal with the government during that time.

Swamiji met unexpectedly, or probably was destined to meet, two French people at the Kumbhamela: one was a French Lady who came for the second time to India and the other was a young black African journalist who was brought to France when he was just three years old and educated in France. They were together.

Meeting with French devotees Blanche and Babu

On the third day at Kumbha, the author was sitting under a tree alone outside the camp of the Guru of the two Americans devotees. At about 10:30 A.M., an African man of late twenties came there. He was staying in the next camp.

After a formal gesture of *pranam* (bowing) according to Indian style which he had learned, he sat on the sand. After observing silence for about thirty minutes, he asked which path the author was following.

Perhaps, he failed in his guess work of observing the outfits and outward sign of renunciates in India, which he had begun to learn, in guessing at the author. The author had no *malas* [garlands of beads] or sign on the forehead. It was difficult for the young foreign visitor to guess.

Not getting any answer, he tried a different approach. Slowly he started to tell his story carefully looking at the author to see if he was disturbing him. He was cautious and made his story short, about why he had come with an old French lady friend to Kumbhamela to look for an Indian *Kriya* Yogi.

After listening to his story and hearing that they were looking for an Indian *Kriya* Yogi, the author smiled gently. The young man happened to be a graduate in journalism and social science. He was born in Africa; while a baby he was brought to France where he was educated and lived.

Observing the author's gentle smile he guessed and said "Maharaj-ji, You are a *Kriya* Yogi."

The author nodded his head.

At this point, he became very excited and continued to tell his story with enthusiasm. He said that his friend had been to India before; this was her second visit and that he came for the first time. Actually their friends in Paris, a couple of hundred year old ladies, requested their friend, Blanche Sibole, who already visited India once, to find an Indian *Kriya* Yogi.

The French devotees felt tired listening to their American counselors from Los Angeles, Yogananda's organization, who could not even pronounce the Sanskrit correctly.

Blanche told them that she was not feeling good those days. That was the reason why the old French lady devotees selected the twenty seven year old African young man who (called himself Babu) to accompany Blanche Sibole in search of an Indian *Kriya* Yogi and they considered Kumbhamela to be the best place to find one.

At this point, the author opened his mouth and said, "I heard that one Swami Sradhhananda Giri, disciple of Swami Atmananda Giri, a Bengali gentleman, is there in Paris."

Babu said, "We know him. Actually, the old ladies consider him to be for beginners and not for advanced people or seekers. In fact, before we left France, he wrote an introductory letter to Swami Sevananda Giri, disciple of Yogananda, who lived at Bholananda Giri Sannyas asram, from where he took *sannyas*, vow of renunciation. We have walked by Bhola Giri Sannyas asram several times, but did not use the introductory letter to Sevananda.

"We are, as well, two hundred year old ladies from Paris, praying to have the blessing of Babaji and to meet an Indian *Kriya* Yogi without anybody's formal introduction. It seems our prayer is granted and is blessed by Babaji.

"My friend stayed at Gujrathi *Dharmasala*. Will you kindly give her *darsan*?"

The author said, "I am leaving Kumbha today, this evening."

Babu, the African journalist devotee, got alarmed. He asked, "Maharaj-ji! When are you leaving? Kindly have some *prasad* from our camp and be kind to give *darsan* to my friend before you leave Kumbha."

The author said that he had eaten and he was staying in the next camp with two American devotees.

Babu said that he knew those two Americans, Barnic and Stephen.

The author said that he would leave by the evening train and possibly could see his friend on the way to the railway station.

After hearing the news that the author was leaving Kumbha, the American devotees said that the author must stay another three days to have the last bath; as the Kumbha mela would end after two days. The author felt it would be very difficult to get out of Haridwar, such a small town, then, especially with such a large gathering at Kumbha to clear. He decided that his leaving was final with no second thought.

Babu informed his friend, Blanche, that he would be coming to see her in the afternoon with an Indian *Kriya* Yogi he met by the grace of Babaji.

When both arrived at Gujrathi Dharmasala (pilgrims residence), the author saw that some other Americans were staying there. Meeting Blanche who was a very nice person, he did not like to lose time. She took her "lessons file" and all three went to the roof and closed the door. She was showing the author the lessons where she was facing problems or confusion. She had marked those places.

The author was familiar with the "Preceptom," lessons, even from his school days from his Vice Principal, Abanindra Narayan Lahiri.

According to Blanche, all of her friends, the old ladies of Paris were having such problems, that was why they were looking for a *Kriya* Yogi in India. She wanted to hear the correct pronunciations of the *mantras* in Sanskrit. She requested the author to repeat them several times so that they could hear several times.

Soon the sun was bending to the west, the sun light began to fade. It was hard to see. Then all stayed for a while in silence. The author prepared to leave. Babu and Blanche wrote down information on how to get to Dunagiri Hill, Himalayas, where the author was going. Then they accompanied the author to the railway station and bid him farewell.

As the train left Haridwar station, Babu and Blanche were looking as long as they could see.

The author arrives at Dunagiri Hill, Himalayas

The author arriving at Dunagiri Hill, Himalayas, stayed at a small hut adjacent to the Temple of Vaisnabi Mata Sri Sri Bhagavati Jagadamba, known as Ram Kuti Baba.

Fifteen days later, Babu and Blanche arrived at Dunagiri Hill. The author arranged for their stay of three days.

They saw Bhagavati Temple and other places in the valley. Babu took many photos with his video camera.

The author rejects Babu's proposal and Blanche's request

One day, Babu said. "Maharaj-ji! Would you consider coming to France? Many people are interested to learn *Kriya* directly from an Indian *Kriya* Yogi."

The author said, "Sorry Babu, it is not necessary to step out of India for anything. The Himalayas is the abode for this body."

Then Babu said, "Someday, I would like to bring this *Kriya* Science to my people in Africa."

One day, Blanche told the author that one couple in France asked her to find their only daughter in India and if possible to bring her back to France; she was living in India almost twenty years practicing *Kriya* Yoga and was not in good health.

The French girl had taken the Indian name Yogamaya. A Swiss gentleman who went by the name Jnanananda was a brother disciple of Yogamaya, and he had met Blanche at Gujrathi Dharmasala.

Through him Blanche found out that the French girl was living in Delhi. She was interested to come to Dunagiri Hill, but her health did not permit her to visit.

Blanche continued, "Maharaj-ji! I have a request to make and hope you will grant this. An old friend of mine in Paris wants to build an asram in India and live here for six months and the other six months she wants to stay in France."

Anticipating Blanche's next sentence, the author interrupted her and said, "This Swami is not that person who would look after her asram the other six months as a caretaker when she would not be in India."

Blanche was surprised to hear that. She commented, "I was hoping that you would agree. Since you do not like to leave the Himalayas, you could stay here. I can suggest to my friend to build the asram here. You do not have to move anywhere. We could easily come and go."

The author said, "Sorry. This body prefers to live alone."

After three days, Babu and Blanche left Dunagiri.

Mrs. Michele Champy, a French woman, disciple of Swami Sraddhananda (disciple of Swami Atmananda Giri)

In 1984, Swamiji wrote the following book and published it.

A) *Babaji: The Divine Himalayan Yogi* and published it through self publishing - The Sanskrit Classics. ISBN Number 1877854344, Copyright Registration number is - TX 1-470-585 Sep 21, 1984.

In 1985, He also translated Lahiri Mahasays' *Kriya* interpretation in Bengali into English of the following books including his personal letters to the *Kriya* disciples:

B) Under the general title *Commentaries Volume 1* (in English) which included the following Books: Copyright registration number is - TX 1-402-082 Aug 6, 1984.

1) *The Guru Gita*,
2) *The Kabir Gita,* and
3) *The Tejbindu Upanisad.*

C) In a separate title:

4) *Personal Letters of Lahiri Mahasay.to Kriya Disciples.*

In addition to getting these books published, Swamiji managed to get these books translated into French language, and considering the materials high in demand registered the manuscripts with the Copyright Office at the Library of Congress. The registered number of the manuscripts were as follows:

D) Babaji: Le Yogui Divin de I' Himalaya (in French)

The Manuscript's Library of Congress Copyright registration number is - TXU 172-902 Sep. 21, 1984.

E) Under the general title - *Commentaries Volume 1* (in French)
The Manuscript's Library of Congress Copyright registration number is - TXU 172-901 Sep. 21, 1984.
The manuscript title included the following books in French.

1) *La Gita du Gourou* (*The Guru Gita*),
2) *La Gita de Kabir* (*The Kabir Gita*), and
3)*L'Upanisad de Teja Bindu* (The Tejbindu Upanisad),

In a separate title:

4) *Les Lettres Personnelles Aus Disciples de Kriya de Lahiri Mahasay* (*Personal Letters of Lahiri Mahasay.to Kriya Disciples.*)

There were copyright registration of the manuscripts in French. As to the title *Babaji: Le Yogui Divin de I' Himalaya*, violating the International Copyright Mrs. Michelle Champy, a French lady, disciple of Swami Sraddhananda, translated the English version of the book into French in 1991, claiming the Copyright.

Then she wrote to Swamiji for permission on August 7, 1992, to translate the book when she already translated and published it one year before in July 1991, without prior written permission. The relevant documents are reproduced here. For obvious reasons, permission was denied since we had our own French translation of the title and the manuscript was copyrighted at the Library of Congress, the registration number - TXU 172-902 Sep. 21, 1984.

In July, 2010, to our utter surprise we found on the internet that our book was translated into French without our written authorization and published. She was also the publisher. Then she sold the books long nineteen (19) years. Having this information from the internet we first procured a copy of the book to see for ourselves. Indeed it was our book published in such a way as gave a false perception as if it was authorized.

When the attorney of the Sanskrit Classics, Stephen Gorey, contacted some bookstores and the distributor in France they said that she became a woman renunciate and her spiritual name was Swami.Amritananda Giri and that she died just two months before. The attorney said to them that they could not sell the book; since it was not authorized to translate the book by the original writer Swami Satyeswarananda Giri. They were interested to know if Swami Satyeswarananda would authorize it as as they had invested some money. The attorney said, he did not think so.

Such is the saga of internationally and highly sensitive materials of the Original *Kriya* information.

Copyright violation
Copyright page of the book

Titre original :

B A B A J I
The Divine Himalayan Yogi

ISBN 2-901.054-15-3

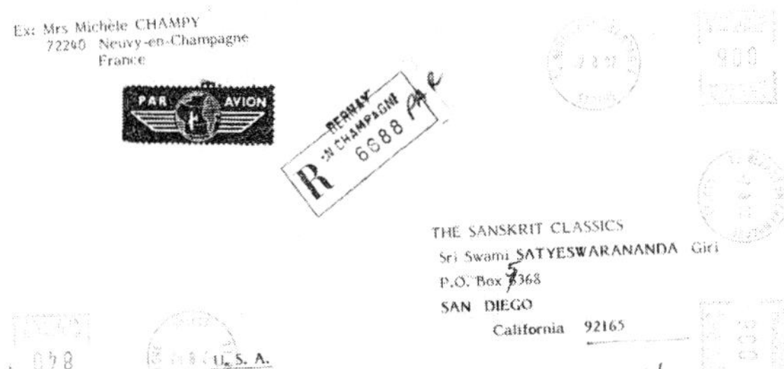

Ex: Mrs Michèle CHAMPY
72240 Neuvy-en-Champagne
France

PAR AVION

R BERNAY EN CHAMPAGNE 6688

THE SANSKRIT CLASSICS
Sri Swami SATYESWARANANDA Giri
P.O. Box 5368
SAN DIEGO
California 92165
U.S.A.

« La Fleur d'Or »
Neuvy-en-Champagne
72480 BERNAY-EN-CHAMPAGNE
(France)

Tél. (43) 20.71.16

Narod Baba Math
108, Suren Sarkar Road
CALCUTTA - 700 010
India

Tél. 35.54.58

MISSION SWAMI ATMANANDA

Association déclarée selon les lois des 1-7-1901 et 9-12-1905
Fondateur et Directeur Spirituel : Swami BRAHMANANDA Giri

La Fleur d'Or, 11th of July, 1991

THE SANSKRIT CLASSICS
SAN DIEGO

Dear One,

I have all the books written by Swami Satyeswarananda Giri, and I am unable to know where he is living. I need to know for some reason.

It is why I write that letter to you. Please can you inform me if you know the adress of Swami Satyeswarananda Giri.

With thanks for your kind reply. In Divine Friendship.

M. Champy

(Mrs M. Champy)

Mission Swami Atmananda

La Fleur d'Or, 11th of July 1991
The Sanskrit Classics
San Diego

Dear one,

I have all the books written by Swami Satyeswarananad Giri, and I am unable to know where he is living, I need to know for some reason.

It is why I write that [this] letter to you . Please can you inform me if you know the adress [address] of Swami Satyeswarananda Giri.

With thanks for your kind reply. In divine Friendship.

(Mrs. M. Champy)

7th of August, 1992

Sri Swami Satyeswarananda Giri Maharaj

Reverend Swami Satyeswarananda Giriji,

Once I called your book shop to search for you and what was my desire I wanted to tell you. But I was so unfortunate that I could not have direct connexion on phone with you.

But by the grace of God I found one of my friend staying in Louisiana (U.S.A.) who is lucky to have you on phone. I told him also my desire about the book "Babaji" what you have writen, to translate in French, just only with that idea that many french people do not know english so much and for which they are in complete darkness to know what the real Babaji is. You know there are many books in European country in English and French about Babaji, where there is nothing reality about our true Babaji.

So if by the grace of God and your permission may allow me to translate in French with the idea to get the light of Babaji what is there in your book, I will be ever grateful to you.

I have no other wish but that.

If you permit me to visit you in San Diego I will try my best to avail that opportunity as early as possible.

My earnest and sincere desire what I have expressed can only be satisfied through your grace.

Awaiting your reply with your convenience, thanks and Pronam to your Feet.

Michèle Champy

P.S. Enclosed 2/3 pages of your book in French what I have done for your inspection.

Mrs Michèle CHAMPY
72240 NEUVY-en-CHAMPAGNE
France

Mrs. Michelle Champy wrote this second letter on August 7, 1992 seeking permission to translate into French the title Babaji: The Divine Himalayan Yogi when she had already translated without permission and had published it as a publisher herself and claimed its copyright. The produced documents prove it.

7th of August, 1992

Mrs. Michele Champy
72240 Neuvy-en-Champagne
France

Sri Swami Satyeswarananda Giri

Reverend Swami Satyeswarananda Giriji,

Once I called your book shop [Publication] to search for you and what was my desire I wanted to tell you. But I was so unfortunate that I could not have direct connexion [connection] on phone with you.

But by the grace of God I found one of my friend staying in Louisiana (U.S.A.) who is lucky to have you on phone. I told him also my desire about the book "Babaji" what you have writen [written], to translate in French, just only with that idea that many french [French] people do not know english [English] so much and for which they are in complete darkness to know what the real Babaji is. You know there are many books in European country in English and French about Babaji, where there is nothing reality about our true Babaji.

So if by the grace of God and your permission may allow me to translate in French with the idea to get the light of Babaji what is your book, I will be ever grateful to you. I have no other wish than that.

If you permit me to visit you in San Diego I will try my best to avail that opportunity as early as possible.

My earnest and sincere desire what I have expressed can only be satisfied through your grace.

Awaiting your reply with your convenience, thanks and Pronam to your Feet.

Michele Champy

P.S. Enclosed 2/3 pages of your book in French what I have done for your inspection.

BABAJI

LE DIVIN YOGI DES HIMALAYAS

CHAPITRE I

APERCU SUR LE LIVRE

Ce livre a deux objectifs : celui d'apporter la lumière sur les principes et les pratiques qui aident le chercheur de Vérité à avancer rapidement et méthodiquement vers l'éveil, et celui de tenter d'expliquer, autant que cela soit possible, le caractère universel de Mahamuni Babaji et son influence dynamique sur cette planète et sur ses habitants. En poursuivant la lecture de ce livre, le chercheur se rendra compte que Babaji, bien que conférant le Kriya comme un puissant moyen de progrès spirituel, n'est nullement limité par cette discipline particulière. Il est au-delà de toutes les disciplines.

Le livre est divisé en trois parties correspondant respectivement aux trois états de compréhension de la Réalisation intérieure. Ces trois états sont : Sravan, Manan et Nididhhasan, soit : "écouter", "analyser" et "s'abandonner".

Cette première partie, "Les réminiscences de Baba", correspond à Sravan, ou écoute d'histoires à propos de l'auteur (populairement connu sous le nom de Baba), et de sa vie avec Babaji, le mystérieux Yogi Himalayen, considéré comme l'Etre Eternel. Cette "écoute" des récits ésotériques inspirera le chercheur pour harmoniser sa vie en vue d'atteindre le bonheur éternel. Dans un sens spirituel plus profond, "écouter" signifie "écouter le Son intérieur, ou Son de OM."

La seconde partie, "Les Disciplines", correspond à Manan, ou analyse de l'écoute. En outre, elle expose des dialogues entre le Maître et le disciple, obligeant le lecteur à observer soigneusement l'attirance de son mental afin de déterminer quelle discipline est la meilleure pour son avancement spirituel. Ferme dans sa détermination, le disciple obtient alors un lien personnel avec le Maître afin de pratiquer la discipline précise lui permettant d'atteindre la réalisation intérieure ou véritable Félicité.

La troisième partie, "Réflexions sur les commentaires par Babaji", correspond à Nididhhasan, ou destruction de l'ego. On apprend comment abandonner

.../...

A German Indologist

VERLAG W. HUCHZERMEYER

Lessingstr.64, 76135 Karlsruhe Tel. (0721) 85 62 01 Fax: 84 39 62

Deutsche Bank Karlsruhe 0529321 BLZ 660 700 04 USt-ID-Nr. DE 143660336

Fax: 0049 721 84 39 62 (8-20 hrs)

Swami Satyeswarananda
c/o Sanskrit Classics
P.O. Box 5368
San Diego, CA 92105
USA

28-9-96

Dear Swamiji,

I am a German Indologist, publisher and translator of Indian spiritual literature.

Recently, I read your title "Babaji" and very much enjoyed it. In fact, this subject has occupied my mind sincever I read the "Autobiography" a long time ago.

I would be interested in bringing out the book, in an abridged form, in my German translation. Actually, I have already done a first rough translation of the First Part, pp. 5-85 (second edition), which seems to contain the essence of your report.

You may know that the general interest in Yoga is somewhat less here than in the U.S. We have only a single specialized yoga yournal, which has a circulation of no more than 3,000. Therefore, there is less scope in Germany for bringing out such titles. I would suggest to attempt a simple edition, comprising the First Part, as mentioned above, without photos, except perhaps yours on the backcover.

As a small (living-room) publisher I pay, as a rule, no more than 5% royalties on the sales price. Please let me know whether that would be acceptable to you. I would require 5 years exclusive rights on this title, although they may be reissued earlier to any other party if I should stop publishing and distributing the book during this period.

I would start with a first edition of only a few hundred copies in order to limit my risk and test the demand. Naturally, it would be helpful if you could send me - in case of a positive response - addresses of persons in Germany, Austria, Switzerland who might have ordered English books from you so that I can reach their circles through my mailings.

However, please let me know at first how you basically feel about my proposal.

Yours sincerely,

W. Huchzermeyer

(Wilfried Huchzermeyer)

VERLAG W. HUCHZERMEYER
Lessingstr 64. 76135 Karisruhe Tel. (0721) 85 62 01 Fax 84 39 62

Deutche Bank Karisruhe 0529321 BLZ 660 700 04 USt-ID -Nr DE 143660336

Fax 0049 721 84 39 62 (8-20-hrs)

Swami Satyeswarananda
c/o Sanskrit Classics
P.O. Box 5368
San Diego, CA 92165
USA

Dear Swamji,

I am a German Indologist, publisher and translator of Indian spiritual literature.

Recently, I read your title "Babaji" and very much enjoyed it. In fact, this subject has occupied my mind sincever I read the "Autobiography" a long time ago.

I would be interested in bringing out the book, in an abridged form, in my German translation. Actually, I have already done a first rough translation of the First Part , pp 5-85 (second edition), which seems to contain the essence of your report.

You may know that the general interest in Yoga is somewhat less here than in the U.S. We have only a single specialized yoga journal, which has a circulation of no more than 3,000. Therefore, there is less scope in Germany for bringing out such titles. I would suggest to attempt a simple edition, comprising the First Part, as mentioned above, without photos, except perhaps yours on the back cover.

As a small (living-room) publisher I pay as a rule, no more than 5% royalties on the sales price. Please let me know whether that would be acceptable to you. I would require 5 years exclusive rights on this title, although they may be reissued earlier to any other party if I should stop publishing and distributing the book during this period.

I would start with a first edition of only a few hundred copies in order to limit my risk and test the demand. Naturally, it would be helpful if you could send me - in case of a positive response - addresses of persons in Germany.

Austria , Switzerland who might have ordered English books from you so that I can reach their circles through my mailings.

However, please let me know at first how you basically feel about my proposal.

Yours sincerely,

(Wilfried Huchzermeyer)

Marcel Jullien from Lyon, France, translated a few chapters of our *Kriya* book into French and sought permission later which was denied.

He was initiated in Ranchi to modified *Kriya*. He has a bookstore. He was a writer. He found our *Kriya* books so interesting *Kriya* literature; he could not resist translating into French as he was a serious seeker of truth. His subsequent letter is produced here.

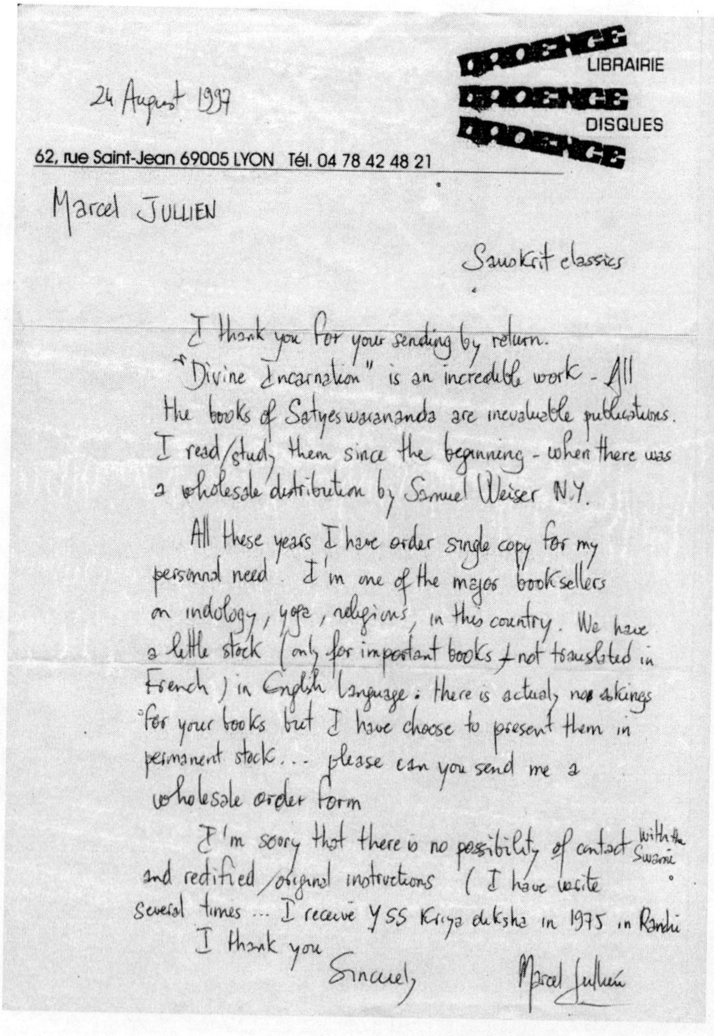

ORIENCE LIBRAIRIE
ORIENCE DISQUES
ORIENCE

24 August 1997

62, rue Saint-Jean 69005 LYON Tél. 04 78 42 48 21

Marcel JULLIEN

Sanskrit classics

I thank you for your sending by return.
"Divine Incarnation" is an incredible work - All the books of Satyeswarananda are inevaluable publications. I read/study them since the beginning - when there was a wholesale distribution by Samuel Weiser N.Y.

All these years I have order single copy for my personnal need. I'm one of the major booksellers on indology, yoga, religions, in this country. We have a little stock (only for important books & not translated in French) in English language: there is actualy no askings for your books but I have choose to present them in permanent stock... please can you send me a wholesale order form

I'm sorry that there is no possibility of contact with the Swami and rectified/original instructions (I have write several times... I receive YSS Kriya diksha in 1975 in Ranchi
I thank you

Sincerely

Marcel Jullien

24, August, 1997
62, rue Saint-Jean 69005 LYON, 04-78-42-48-21, France

Marcel Jullien

Sanskrit Classics

I thank you for your sending by return, "Divine Incarnation" is an incredible work. All the books of Satyeswarananda are invaluable publications. I read /study them since the beginning - when there was a wholesale distribution by Samuel Weiser, N. Y.

All these years I have order single copy for my personal need. I'm one of the major booksellers on Indology, Yoga, Religion, in this country. We have a little stock (only for important books not translated in French) in English language. There is actually no stoking of your books but I have choose [chosen] to present them in permanent stock. ... please can you send me a wholesale order form [?]

I'm sorry that there is no possibility of contact with the Swami and redified/ original instructions (I have write [written] several times ... I receive [received] YSS *Kriya diksha* [initiation] in 1975 in Ranchi.

I thank you.

Sincerely,

Marcel Jullien

People are so tempted for these books Swamiji wrote, of course at the instruction of Mahamuni Babaji, and Lahiri Manasay's using the right hand of Swamiji, to write; they simply do not understand the real purpose of these books is to benefit the spiritual seekers and not the intellectual fools who enjoyed them as reading like any other book.

Swamiji never answers to these type of letters except in some cases just to deny the permission officially in writing in a few lines. There was one such type of letter written from France. He also without permission already translated several pages.

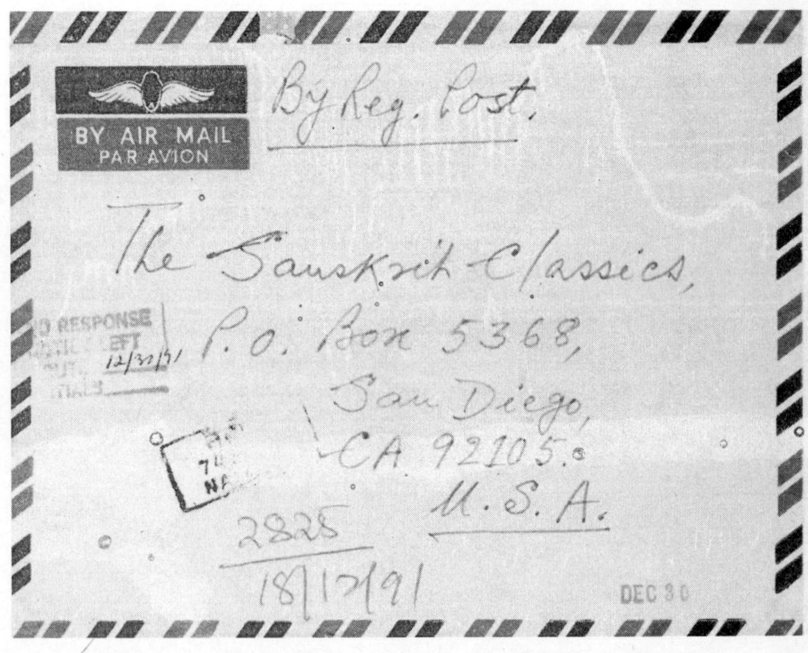

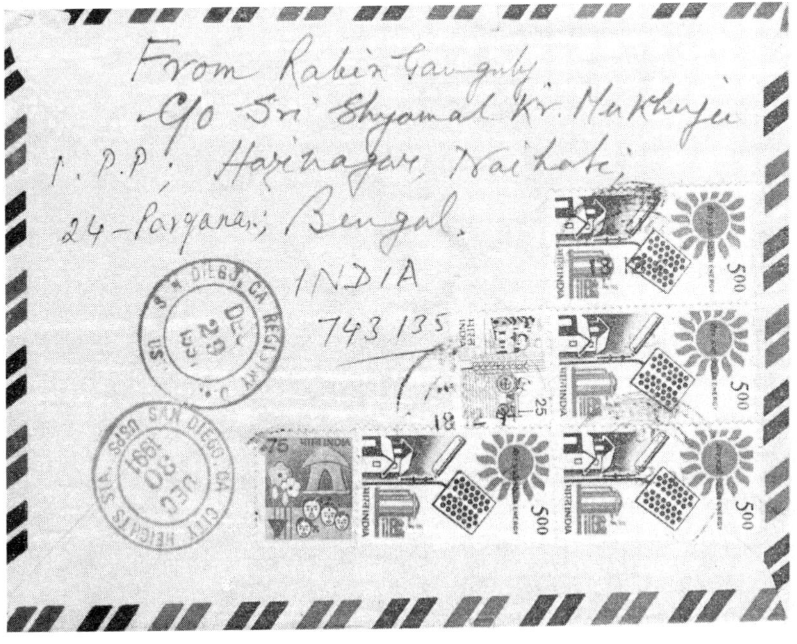
From Rabin Ganguly
C/o Sri Shyamal Kr. Mukherji
I.P.P.; Harinagar, Naihati;
24-Parganas; Bengal.
INDIA
743 135
SAN DIEGO, CA

পূজনীয় স্বামীজী মহারাজ,

12-12-91.

প্রথমে আমার আন্তরিক শ্রদ্ধা ও প্রণাম জানবেন। আপনার লেখা "বাবাজী" বইটি পড়ে মুগ্ধ হয়েছি। জানি না কি লিখব। আমার আপনার সাথে বাবাজী মহারাজের [illegible] হলো। আপনি ধন্য। আপনার সান্নিধ্য [illegible] পাবার আশা করি। আপনার চরণস্পর্শ করে নিজেকে ধন্য করতে চাই। আপনি কি India তে আসার কোন Plan করেছেন, যদি হয়ে থাকে তাহলে India তে দেখা করে আপনার আশীর্বাদ নেব, আর তা যদি না হয় তাহলে যদি San Diago তে যাই তাহলে কি সে সৌভাগ্য হবে? দয়া করে আপনার [illegible] জানাবেন। আশাকরি আমার [illegible] 2 নম্বর ইনল্যান্ড দিয়ে পাঠাবেন।

পার্থিব জগতে Misguided হয়ে দিন রাত কাজে করে চলেছি, তাই, যদি দয়া করে অনুমতি দেন তাহলে [illegible] করে [illegible] পারিবারিক [illegible] ভুলে। এখন নিজের কাছে আপনার অনুমতির উপর। পুনরায় আন্তরিক শ্রদ্ধা ও প্রণাম জানিয়ে শেষ করলাম।

"ইতি [illegible] গাঙ্গুলী"

C/O Sri Shyamal Kr. Mukherjee
India Paper Pulp Co. Ltd,
Hazinagar 743135, Naihati,
24 Pags, Bengal, INDIA.

Robin Ganguly 12/12/91
C/O Sri Shyamal Kr. Mukherjee
India paper Pulp Co. Ltd
Hazi Nagar 743135 Naihati'
24Pargs, Bengal, INDIA

Param Pujaniya Swamiji Maharaj:

Supremely Worshipable Swamiji Maharaj,

Kindly accept my heartfelt respect and *pranam* (bowing head traditionally). I am delighted reading your book Babaji; knowing how much near and dear relationship you have daily with Babaji. You are blessed. I expect your kindness and touching your feet I want to make myself blessed.

Do you make any plan to come to India? If you do come then I will meet you and have your blessings; and if you do not come then if I come to San Diego and please let me know if I come there would I have that opportunity and thereby I make my mind calm. Will be waiting to get a few line answer.

Many people are passing their days misguided in life. If you kindly permit me then I will arrange to publish the book in different languages and serve the people with affordable price. All are depending on your permission.

Again, I send my heartfelt respect and *pranam*.

Robin Ganguly.

The Conclusion:

At the end of the chapter, Swamiji did not find any consoling words for these enthusiastic people; professionally intellectual but spiritually naive.

For Personal Notes: